The Rehabilitation of Executive Disorders
A Guide to Theory and Practice

Edited by

Michael Oddy
Brain Injury Rehabilitation Trust, Horsham, UK

Andrew Worthington
Brain Injury Rehabilitation Trust, Birmingham, UK

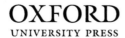

OXFORD
UNIVERSITY PRESS

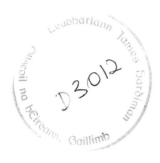

OXFORD

UNIVERSITY PRESS

Great Clarendon Street, Oxford OX2 6DP

Oxford University Press is a department of the University of Oxford.
It furthers the University's objective of excellence in research, scholarship,
and education by publishing worldwide in

Oxford New York

Auckland   Cape Town   Dar es Salaam   Hong Kong   Karachi
Kuala Lumpur   Madrid   Melbourne   Mexico City   Nairobi
New Delhi   Shanghai   Taipei   Toronto
With offices in
Argentina   Austria   Brazil   Chile   Czech Republic   France   Greece
Guatemala   Hungary   Italy   Japan   South Korea   Poland   Portugal
Singapore   Switzerland   Thailand   Turkey   Ukraine   Vietnam

Oxford is a registered trade mark of Oxford University Press
in the UK and in certain other countries

Published in the United States
by Oxford University Press Inc., New York

ISBN 978-0-19-856805-6

Printed in the United Kingdom by
Lightning Source UK Ltd., Milton Keynes

To Ann (M.O.)

To Lara for being there, to Stephie and
Amber for just being (A.W.)

Preface

The frontal lobes have long been the topic of vigorous debate in the realms of psychology, neurology, and psychiatry, providing the battleground for conflicts between so-called localizationists and their critics from the mid-nineteenth century. The ubiquitous Phineas Gage provides a clear description of the impact of lesions in this part of the brain, particularly bilateral lesions, but the significance of Gage's recovery and resulting personality change was not appreciated until many years after his accident in 1848. For decades the sequelae of frontal lobe damage were not easily encapsulated by the conventional investigative tools of the time. For example, Hebb (1939) found that a series of patients who had undergone surgical removal of frontal lobe tissue showed no loss in IQ scores. The apparent resilience of the frontal lobes helped popularize the removal of frontal lobe tissue as an effective treatment for psychiatric disorder. The paradox of retained IQ scores in the presence of clear cognitive impairment has now been resolved by a fuller understanding of the diverse nature of executive functions.

Executive disorders are common in a number of neurological conditions. In childhood, dysfunction within a complex series of fronto-striatal circuits is a popular paradigm for investigating many neurodevelopmental conditions (Bradshaw 2001). Many forms of acquired brain injury also have executive disorders as a common outcome. In traumatic brain injury and certain viral conditions, such as herpes simplex encephalitis, together with memory deficits, they represent the most common sequelae. Disruption of the vascular system involving the anterior cerebral arteries, for example due to haemorrhage or hypoxia, often causes executive deficits. Many forms of dementia begin with signs of executive disorder and they have been noted as occurring in association with a number of degenerative conditions including multiple sclerosis, Parkinson's disease, and motor neuron disease.

We use the term 'executive disorders' in preference to possible alternatives, although we have not insisted on the exclusive use of this term throughout the book. The concept of a dysexecutive syndrome (Baddeley and Wilson 1988) is still commonly used, but the notion of a discrete unitary syndrome is no longer tenable. Executive disorders is preferred because it implies a range of disorders rather than a single dysfunction or syndrome. The term is preferred to frontal lobe syndrome, not only for this reason, but also because executive disorders can occur following injury or illness that appears to spare the frontal lobes.

However, this does not mean that brain structure can be ignored. In Chapter 1, Stuss argues for an anatomical approach to the study of executive disorders on the grounds that this will facilitate the precise delineation of cognitive deficits following brain injury, which will provide a sound basis for designing and evaluating rehabilitation interventions.

Whatever neglect the frontal lobes suffered in the past, there is no doubt that in recent years they have provided some of the most intriguing and significant advances in our understanding of the brain. By their very nature executive disorders have a wide-ranging and often devastating effect. They have an impact on all areas of function, and consequently present a considerable challenge to individuals, their families and therapists.

This book is designed to provide an overview of current best practice in the rehabilitation of executive disorders. The book begins with three chapters indicating recent theoretical developments in our understanding of executive disorders. We share Kurt Lewin's view that 'there is nothing so practical as a good theory'. This is especially the case where the evidence for the efficacy of interventions is thin on the ground, as it undoubtedly is currently for the rehabilitation of executive disorders. The benefits in principle of a conceptually driven approach to cognitive rehabilitation have been recognized for some time (Riddoch and Humphreys 1994; Robertson 1999) but good evidence of effectiveness is harder to come by. In a review of executive rehabilitation techniques Worthington (2005) found that many successful interventions have a tenuous, often highly speculative, relationship to the theoretical rationale supposedly behind them. Cicerone et al. (2000) concluded from a systematic review of evidence-based practice that, given the small number of well-designed studies in the area, training in formal problem-solving strategies and their application could be offered as a 'practice guideline' (implying an intermediate level of evidence base) and that interventions which promote internalization of self-regulation strategies could be offered as a 'practice option'(the lowest level of evidence supported only by less well-designed studies)They found no evidence for rehabilitation approaches to executive disorders which merited the status of a 'practice standard' (i.e. based on the highest form of evidence—well-designed prospective randomized controlled trials). These conclusions were upheld by a further review of the evidence from studies conducted between 1998 and 2002 (Cicerone et al. 2005). In this situation, guidance from a good theory prevents intervention from being totally arbitrary.

The second section of the book consists of 11 chapters describing a variety of approaches to the rehabilitation of executive disorder. We adopt a broad definition of executive disorders and of the resulting behaviour changes and practical difficulties faced by those who suffer from them. Thus we include chapters on the management of anger and on the assessment and management of aggressive behaviour as these frequently coexist with executive disorders. We also include a chapter that explores the implications of executive disorder for physiotherapy following brain injury. Cognitive rehabilitation has arguably been slow to capitalize on the rapid development of technology over the last two decades, and hence we include a chapter on actual and potential uses of virtual reality and a chapter on how so-called 'smart' technology can be used to develop a prosthetic environment for those with severe executive disorders.

In the third section we consider some professional issues that arise in working with this client group. These include the use of medication for problems associated with executive dysfunction, assessments of capacity and risk, and ways of helping staff and families fulfil their respective roles in the rehabilitation of those with executive disorders.

References

Baddeley, A.D. and Wilson, B.A. (1988). Frontal amnesia and the dysexecutive syndrome. *Brain and Cognition*, 7, 212–30.

Bradshaw, J.L. (2001) *Developmental disorders of the fronto-striatal system*. Psychology Press, Hove.

Cicerone, K.D., Dahlberg, C., *et al.* (2000). Evidence-based cognitive rehabilitation: recommendations for clinical practice. *Archives of Physical Medicine and Rehabilitation* 81, 1596–1615.

Cicerone, K.D., Dahlberg, C., Malec, J.F., *et al.*, 2005. Evidence-based cognitive rehabilitation: updated review of the literature from 1998 through 2002. *Archives of Physical Medicine and Rehabilitation*, 86, 1681–92.

Hebb, D.O. (1939) Intelligence in man after large removal of cerebral tissue. Report of four left frontal lobe cases. *Journal of General Psychology*, 21, 73–87.

Riddoch, M.J. and Humphreys, G.W. (1994) Cognitive neuropsychology and cognitive rehabilitation: a marriage of equal partners? In: *Cognitive neuropsychology and cognitive rehabilitation* (ed. M.J. Riddock and G.W. Humphreys), pp. 1–15. Lawrence Erlbaum, Hove.

Robertson, I.H. (1999) Setting goals for cognitive rehabilitation. *Current Opinion in Neurology*, 12, 703–8.

Worthington, A. (2005) Rehabilitation of executive deficits: effective treatment of related disabilities. In: *Effectiveness of rehabilitation of cognitive deficits* (ed. P.W. Halligan and D.T. Wade), pp. 257–67. Oxford University Press, New York.

Horsham, UK   M.O.
Birmingham, UK   A.W.
February 2008

Acknowledgements

The editors would like to express their gratitude to the Brain Injury Rehabilitation Trust and to its parent organization the Disabilities Trust for support in the production of this volume.

Contents

Contributors

Nick Alderman
Kemsley National Centre for
Brain Injury Rehabilitation,
St Andrew's Hospital, Northampton
NN1 5DG, UK

Nicola Archer
Brain Injury Rehabilitation Trust,
1101 Bristol Road, Birmingham

Dawn Baker
Kemsley National Centre for Brain
Injury Rehabilitation, St Andrew's
Hospital, Northampton NN1 5DG

Chloe Cook
c/o Brain Injury Rehabilitation
Trust, Kerwin Court, Horsham
West Sussex

Sinead Corkery
Brain Injury Rehabilitation Trust,
York House, York

Jonathan J. Evans
Section of Psychological Medicine,
Faculty of Medicine, University of
Glasgow, Gartnavel Royal Hospital,
1055 Great Western Road, Glasgow
G12 0XH (e-mail:
jonathan.evans@clinmed.gla.ac.uk)

Mandy Fairweather
Brain Injury Rehabilitation Trust,
York House, York

Jessica Fish
MRC Cognition and Brain Sciences
Unit, Cambridge

Elizabeth Francis
Kent and Medway NHS and Social
Care Partnership Trust

John C. Freeland
Brain Injury Rehabilitation Trust,
York House, York

Camilla Herbert
Brain Injury Rehabilitation Trust,
Kerwin Court, Horsham, West
Sussex

David Johnson
Child Life and Health, University of
Edinburgh

Tom Manly
MRC Cognition and Brain Sciences
Unit, Cambridge

John D. McCrea
Disabilities Trust/Brain Injury
Rehabilitation Trust, Thomas
Edward Mitton House, Milton
Keynes

Michael Oddy
Brain Injury Rehabilitation Trust,
Kerwin Court, Horsham, West
Sussex, and University of Swansea

Helen O'Neill
Kemsley National Centre for Brain
Injury Rehabilitation, St Andrew's
Hospital, Northampton NN1 5DG

Roger Orpwood
Bath Institute of Medical
Engineering, University of Bath

Paul Penn
School of Psychology, University of East London, London E15 4LZ

Hugh Rickards
Birmingham and Solihull Mental Health Trust, and University of Birmingham

David Rose
School of Psychology, University of East London, London E15 4LZ

Rashmi Sharma
Brain Injury Rehabilitation Trust, Thomas Edward Mitton House, Milton Keynes

Karen L. Siedlecki
Taub Institute, Columbia University, 630 W 168th St, New York, NY 10032

Yaakov Stern
Taub Institute, Columbia University, 630 W 168th St, New York, NY 10032 (e-mail: ys11@columbia.edu)

Donald T. Stuss
Rotman Research Institute at Baycrest, 3560 Bathurst Street, Toronto, Ontario, Canada M6A 2E1. Departments of Psychology and Medicine (Neurology, Rehabilitation Sciences), University of Toronto, Canada (e-mail: dstuss@rotman-baycrest.on.ca)

Andy Tyerman
Community Head Injury Service, The Camborne Centre, Jansel Square, Aylesbury, Bucks HP21 7ET (e-mail: andy.tyerman@buckspct.nhs.uk)

Jackie Waller
Brain Injury Rehabilitation Trust, West Heath House, Birmingham

Barbara A Wilson
MRC Cognition and Brain Sciences Unit, Cambridge, and Oliver Zangwill Centre for Neuropsychological Rehabilitation, Ely

Andrew Worthington
Brain Injury Rehabilitation Trust, West Heath House, Birmingham

Peter Zeeman
Centre for Rehabilitation of Brain Injury, University of Copenhagen, Njalsgade 88 DK-2300, Copenhagen S, Denmark

Part 1

Theoretical developments

Michael Oddy and Andrew Worthington

An emphasis on separable functions has characterized much recent theorising about executive abilities at the expense of interest in structural divisions within the brain. The first chapter by Stuss argues that a return to a neuroanatomical approach to frontal lobe function offers the best chance of identifying functional relationships and fractionation of function. He concludes that the current evidence points to four major functions: deficient energization, executive deficits, impaired behavioural and emotional self-regulation and deficits in metacognition. He argues that careful delineation of precise impairments may be crucial to targetting pharmacological and cognitive rehabilitation interventions.

Siedlecki and Stern in Chapter 2 discuss the related concepts of brain reserve and cognitive reserve. These concepts have arisen in the light of growing evidence revealing a lack of correspondence between the extent of brain damage and the resulting functional impact. Clinicians have always known that recovery from brain injury is very variable and individual characteristics often seem to be more important than intensity of therapy in determining outcome. We considered a chapter on this topic essential to include as the research and theory promises new opportunities for understanding response to rehabilitation. For example, as Siedlecki and Stern describe, experience and education appears to have an influence on cognitive reserve. This suggests the possibility that these factors could influence rehabilitation and gives hope of a degree of plasticity that gives credence to the idea that some restoration of function can occur through educational and experiential means.

In Chapter 3, Oddy, Worthington, and Francis review the confusing area of motivational problems following brain injury. Motivation deficits are commonly encountered in rehabilitation and can challenge the most experienced of therapists. Such problems are frequently cited when clients fail to achieve their potential and clinicians often feel poorly equipped to deal with the difficulties they cause. Oddy *et al.* suggest a framework for identifying different ways in which goal directed behaviour can break down which in turn can be used as a basis for suggesting different interventions. They argue that motivational disorders are no different from other forms of cognitive disorder, and so-called motivational deficits can be understood in terms of selective breakdown of cognitive and emotional processes within their framework.

Rehabilitation of frontal lobe dysfunction: a working framework

Donald T. Stuss

Rotman Research Institute at Baycrest, and Departments of Psychology and Medicine (Neurology, Rehabilitation Sciences), University of Toronto

Introduction

Although 'dysexecutive syndrome' is difficult to define in a manner universally acceptable, most clinicians would claim that they recognize it when they see it. However, the difficulty in treating and managing such patients might be secondary to a lack of clarity in the operational definitions. The overall objective of this chapter is to present theoretical considerations and recent data that might be considered when developing or applying rehabilitation procedures for patients who suffer from what many call the 'dysexecutive syndrome'.

The chapter is composed of three sections. In this introductory section it is proposed that the terms 'executive' and 'frontal lobe' dysfunction need to be differentiated. Starting with a focus of functions related to anatomy (e.g. functions of the frontal lobes and frontal systems) minimizes the definitional confusion, and provides a more precise basis to study the efficacy of targeted rehabilitation efforts. The main body of the chapter presents a framework for understanding frontal lobe functions. Data are reviewed that indicate there are four different categories of function within the frontal lobes, of which 'executive' functions represent only one. These executive functions are comprised of different processes, with maximum representation in different frontal regions. The last section of the chapter addresses some potential applications of this framework to the rehabilitation of these disorders.

Executive or frontal lobe dysfunction?

In general terms, executive disorders impact the control of basic cognitive functions, and are usually characterized as impairments in such functions as initiation, planning, sequencing, inhibition, flexibility (shifting), and moni-toring. The clearest cause of disorders of this type is damage to the frontal lobes. As a consequence, 'executive dysfunction' and 'frontal lobe dysfunction' are often used interchangeably. Blurring the boundaries between anatomical and functional definitions can, however, result in confusion. For example, the impairments labeled executive have also been reported in patients without focal frontal pathology or in disorders where the pathology is not limited to the frontal lobes, and in some cases the amount of involvement of the frontal lobes may be questionable: e.g. toxic or metabolic encephalopathies, Alzheimer's disease, vascular injury to deep circulations, multiple sclerosis, or traumatic diffuse axonal injury. 'Executive dysfunction' has also been noted in psychiatric disorders such as schizophrenia, depression, and anxiety, and even secondary to chronic pain and sleep deprivation or fragmentation.

The suggested approach to establishing a theoretical framework for under-standing the complex impairments often described as 'dysexecutive' is multi-step. Focusing on deficits related to focal frontal lobe damage is the first step in establishing more precise operational definitions. Careful delineation of deficits as they occur after focal brain damage, and understanding the nature of such deficits, allows one to target rehabilitation and to test whether such targeted rehabilitation of deficits leads to improvement in functioning as well as real life. It is probably not wise at this stage to use degenerative disor-ders to study the functions of a particular neural unit (Aparicio *et al.* 2005). Although this first step might be criticized as 'localizationist' for a rehabilita-tion framework, it is set in the context of brain networks and systems. Before the system can be understood, the component parts need to be examined. This serves as a firm foundation when one treats patients with more complex dis-orders in whom the 'dysexecutive syndrome' appears to be prominent.

Understanding the nature of the deficits and their role in real-life disabilities may lead to well-constructed compensatory interventions. This approach provides the tools to determine whether certain rehabilitation approaches are effective, but only in specific populations. It is possible that targeted cognitive rehabilitation for a specific process or category of processes may never be effective, and that only a multi-component programme will suffice. What would be a clinical misfortune, however, is if the latent benefit of a targeted approach is never tested. The information in this chapter provides knowledge on which these hypotheses might be based.

Different categories of frontal lobe functioning

One important reason not to equate frontal lobe damage with executive disor-ders is that there are at least four separate categories of disorder related to damage in different frontal regions: deficient energization (initiation and sustaining of behaviour), executive deficits, behavioural and emotional self-regulation impairment, and disturbed meta-cognition (theory of mind) (Stuss 2007). Some authors use the term 'executive' for all four of these functional domains, but, based on evidence for operationally distinct categories of functions, the use of this term to encompass all these different categories appears to be inappropriate.

The existence of distinct functional domains within the frontal lobes is supported by developmental evidence, anatomical connectivity, and lesion effects. The human cortex develops from two discrete sources, hippocampal–archicortical and palaeocortical, providing the two major divisions within the frontal lobes (Sanides 1970; Pandya and Barnes 1987; Stuss and Levine 2002). The first (archicortical) resulted in the lateral prefrontal cortical cortex (LPFC), and the second (palaeocortical) in the ventral (medial) prefrontal cortex (VMPFC). Each determines a different category of functioning: LPFC determines spatial and conceptual reasoning, related to **executive** cognitive processes; VMPFC determines emotional processing, including the acquisition and reversal of stimulus–reward associations, which can be categorized as **behavioural/emotional self-regulatory**. These two categories map onto two of the three proposed frontal-subcortical circuits involved in cognitive and/or emotional processing (Alexander *et al.* 1986). A third functional category, the third of Alexander *et al.*'s frontal-subcortical networks related to more cognitive functioning, characterizes the medial frontal structures that regulate **energization** of all cognitive activities. The final category of frontal functions (**meta-cognitive**) is suggested by recent research on higher-order integrative functions of the frontal polar area 10 (Stuss *et al.* 2001a,b; Burgess *et al.*, in press). The behavioural data supporting these categories, with an emphasis on lesion research with some support from functional imaging, are summarized below. The categories and their general anatomical localization are illustrated in Figure 1.1.

Regulating energization and putative localization

Energization of cognitive functions is important for adequate performance of any function (this is commonly called activation, but that term has come to have multiple meanings and we prefer energization). Energization is the process of initiation and sustaining of any response mode. The obvious outcome of deficient energization would be slowing. Deficient energization is most consistently associated with lesions in more superior medial (anterior cingulate and superior) regions bilaterally, with some evidence for a more important role for the right SM area (Figure 1.2).

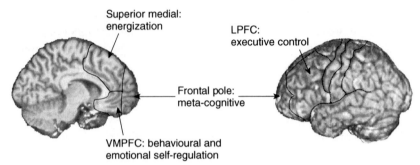

Fig. 1.1 Illustration of the gross localization within the frontal lobes of four separate functional categories: energization—superior medial; executive—lateral (these are divisible into right and left frontal lateral regions); behavioural/self-regulatory—inferior orbitofrontal/inferior medial; meta-cognitive/integrative—polar. Further specification may be possible. Note that this classification identifies categories of function and does not imply a totally localizationist approach.

Patients with superior medial (SM) damage are consistently slower than any other patient with focal frontal lobe damage on any demanding task (Stuss and Alexander 2007). This has been shown in Simple (button response to repeated single-feature stimuli) and Choice (respond to a defined target with the possibility of presentation of non-targets) reaction time (RT) tests, with potentially greater slowing the more demanding the task (Stuss *et al.* 2002, 2005). Although this energization impairment is most obvious in reaction time tests, the effect is evident in any speeded behaviour. For example, the impairment of patients with SM damage in producing words in the first 15 seconds of a verbal fluency task compared with control participants can be attributed to deficient energization (Stuss *et al.* 1998). Not only do patients with SM damage have difficulty initiating behaviours, they also have problems sustaining behaviour over time. Damage to the SM frontal area impairs the maintenance of consistent timing performance over prolonged periods of time in a self-sustaining tapping test (e.g. tap every 1.5 seconds (Picton *et al.* 2006)). For example, in a Choice RT task preceded by either a 1 second or a 3 second warning stimulus, all frontal patients benefited from the 1 second warning tone; when the warning interval was longer, the SM group alone among other frontal groups was deficient in benefiting from the warning stimulus (Stuss *et al.* 2005). This sustaining deficit was also evident in verbal fluency. Not only did the SM group have initial difficulty generating words, it was the only group in which the total number of words produced in the last 45 seconds was less than that produced in the first 15 seconds (Stuss and Alexander 2007).

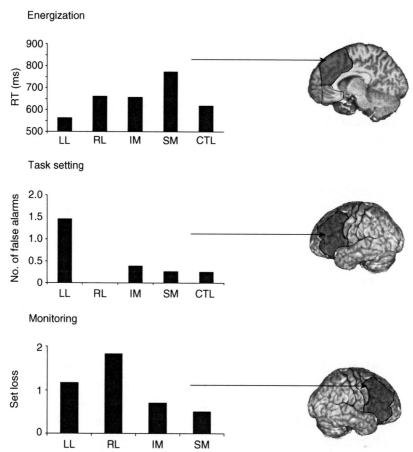

Fig. 1.2 Examples of data representing dissociation of energization and two processes within executive functions. (a) Energization—patients with superior medial frontal lobe damage are the slowest in a Choice RT task (respond with the dominant hand to a single-feature target presented with a 25 per cent probability (Stuss *et al.* 2005). (b) Task setting—damage to the left lateral region, in particular the left ventrolateral area, caused the greatest impairment in Concentrate (the number of errors occurring in the first 100 trials in a task requiring response to rapidly presented stimuli (Alexander *et al.* 2005). Monitoring, measured on the Wisconsin Card Sorting Test by difficulties in maintaining the selected criterion after being given all the detailed instructions for responding, was maximally impaired after right lateral damage (Stuss *et al.* 2000; Stuss and Alexander 2007). LL, left lateral; RL, right lateral; IM, inferior medial; SM, superior medial; CTL, control.

Perhaps the best measures to evaluate impaired energization are demanding but simple reaction time tests. This is illustrated in a test called **Concentrate**, which requires high levels of sustained attention (hence 'concentrate'). The subjects are required to press one of five response buttons situated directly under five LEDs, in response to the random illumination of one of the five LEDs (Alexander *et al.* 2005). Only patients with lesions in SM frontal regions had significant RT slowness, consistent across 500 trials.

These data and their interpretation are concordant with other lesion and imaging research and theories of the functions of this region (e.g. Luria 1973; Drewe 1975; Leimkuhler and Mesulam 1985; Richer *et al.* 1993; Passingham 1993; Godefroy *et al.* 1994; Picard and Strick 1996). The deficit has also been described clinically. Bilateral damage to the anterior cingulate gyrus and supplementary motor area produces abulia, or severe apathy, and at its worse akinetic mutism, a dramatic example of deficient energizing (Plum and Posner 1980; Devinsky *et al.* 1995; Alexander 2001). Changes in activity of the cingulate cortex occur as a function of sleep stages (Hofle *et al.* 1997), vigilance (Paus *et al.* 1997), and alertness (Luu *et al.* 2000a,b). Stuss and Benson (1984, 1986) called this phasic attention; Hockey (1993), in the information processing literature, called it effort system.

Executive cognitive functions and putative localization

Executive cognitive functions are defined as those high-level **cognitive** functions that provide control and direction of lower-level, more automatic functions. Neuropsychological studies suggest deficits in patients with primarily LPFC damage. In recent years, efforts have been made to investigate whether these executive functions can be fractionated functionally and anatomically. Using the paradigm of attention, our data suggest that at least two separate executive functions can be identified: task setting, and monitoring, the former associated with the left lateral frontal cortex, and the latter with the right (Stuss *et al.* 2002, 2005; Stuss and Alexander 2007).

Task setting is defined as the ability to set a stimulus–response relationship, either before a task starts (planning), or through trial and error during the initial learning of a new task. This stimulus–response connection requires formation of a criterion to respond to a defined target with specific attributes. The left lateral area is most associated with task setting, particularly ventrolateral. It is possible that other task-setting attributes (e.g. organization of the schemas necessary to complete a particular task, and adjustment of contention scheduling so that the automatic processes of moving through the steps of a task can work more smoothly) are related to other left lateral frontal regions, perhaps more caudal (dorsal).

The 'standard' measures of frontal lobe 'executive' functioning are complex and multifactorial, and individuals can fail for many reasons. However, if properly parsed, specific processes such as task setting can be isolated. For example, lesions in the right and left lateral regions caused the greatest impairment on the Wisconsin Card Sorting Test (WCST) (Stuss *et al*. 2000). However, depending on how the test is administered, the measurement can reflect different cognitive impairments. For example, using the dependent measure of 'set loss', defined as the number of times an error is made after at least three consecutively correct (one unambiguous) responses, impairment in the initial learning of the test was most associated with left ventrolateral frontal damage (see below on how the same measure in a different context relates to a different process). The difficulty in task setting can be shown to occur in different types of tests. For example, in the recognition measure of a word-list learning task, an individual has to set a criterion (bias; task set) for saying 'yes' that a word was one presented earlier. False-positive errors would index a task-setting problem. In two different studies in two different sets of patients with two different types of word lists, false-positive errors were related most to left lateral region pathology (Stuss *et al*. 1994; Alexander *et al*. 2003).

The same patterns are noted in RT tests. In the Concentrate test described above, analysis of speed of response indicated significant slowing after SM lesions. However, analysis of errors indicated that they occurred primarily in the first 100 of 500 trials, interpreted as poor task setting. Again, maximum impairment was related damage to left ventrolateral frontal areas (Alexander *et al*. 2005). In a variant of the Stroop test (Alexander *et al*. 2007), left ventrolateral region damage resulted in impairment in setting contingent response rules as indexed by the number of false alarms. Damage in this area also resulted in primarily false-positive errors in a complex Feature Integration RT test which required the detection and discrimination of complex target from non-target stimuli (Stuss *et al*. 2002).

Other lesion and imaging data support the association of the left lateral frontal region and setting specific stimulus–response contingencies (Perret 1974; Richer *et al*. 1993; Godefroy *et al*. 1994, 1999). Luria (1966) had postulated earlier that the left frontal lobe impairs a patient's ability to use task instructions to direct behaviour (verbal regulation of behaviour). Functional magnetic resonace imaging (fMRI) studies also support this hypothesis. In a meta-analysis of all neuroimaging studies between 2000 and 2004 of task switching and the Stroop test which assessed updating task representations(Derrfuss *et al*. 2005), the left inferior lateral region had the major localizations (see also Brass and von Cramon 2004).

Monitoring, on the other hand, is most associated with the right ventrolateral frontal area. Monitoring can be defined as the process of checking the task over time for 'quality control' and the adjustment of behaviour. Monitoring deficits can be demonstrated in many types of task. One simple index is the lack of a normal foreperiod effect in a RT test. As the inter-stimulus interval (ISI) increases between trials, there is normally a decrease in reaction time (Niemi and Naatanen 1981). We analysed the effect of damage to different frontal regions in both Simple and Choice RT tests in which the ISI varied from 3 to 7 seconds. All frontal patients demonstrate this normal foreperiod effect over time except the right lateral frontal group, interpreted as impaired monitoring of expectance (Stuss *et al.* 2005). This impaired foreperiod effect can also be seen after TMS stimulation in the right frontal region (Vallesi *et al.* 2007). Damage to the right frontal lateral region also impairs monitoring of time, either in time reproduction or time discrimination tests (e.g. Basso *et al.* 2003; Lewis and Miall 2003; Picton *et al.* 2006). In the complex Feature Integration task described above, damage to the right lateral frontal region resulted in errors of all kinds, interpreted as impaired monitoring, in contrast with the left lateral pathology which was associated primarily with false-positive errors (Stuss *et al.* 2002). In essence, damage to the right lateral frontal region impairs the ability to note that an error has occurred, and patients do not adjust their RT performance accordingly (Stuss *et al.* 2003). These data and interpretation are compatible with imaging and other lesion research in 'vigilance' and monitoring which also stress the importance of the right lateral regions (Wilkins *et al.* 1987; Pardo *et al.* 1991; Rueckert and Grafman 1996; Coull *et al.* 1998; Henson *et al.* 1999; Fletcher and Henson 2001; Shallice 2001, 2002).

The same deficit can be extracted from standard clinical tests. In such cases, the interpretation of the deficit is related to the context of administration. For example, if the WCST is re-administered with more explicit information about the task parameters (e.g. what the criteria were, and when to switch), set loss errors were now more associated with right ventrolateral frontal pathology (Stuss and Alexander 2007). The administration minimized the need for task setting, and set loss errors then became reflective of deficient monitoring and checking of performance over time. The right lateral frontal region also plays an important role in monitoring memory output and 'checking' performance as reported in lesion studies (Stuss *et al.* 1994; Alexander *et al.* 2003; Turner *et al.* 2007) and imaging research (Henson *et al.* 1999; Fletcher and Henson 2001).

Although the attempts to understand disturbed 'everyday functioning' were initiated under controlled conditions using the theory of disturbed executive functions, these 'real-life' measures appear to be more complex with necessary involvement of multiple functional systems. Moreover, these patients often had lesions that involved ventral medial frontal areas. For this reason, these measures are described with the group of behavioural/emotional self-regulatory measures (see below).

Behavioural/emotional self-regulatory functions and putative localization

The VMPFC region is involved in **emotional** processing, and damage here results in patients having difficulty in understanding the emotional consequences of their behaviour, even though their performance on commonly used neuropsychological tests of executive functioning is normal or even excellent. Because of the involvement of VMPFC in reward processing, it plays an important role in **behavioural self-regulation** as would be required in situations where cognitive analysis, habit, or environmental cues are not sufficient to determine the most adaptive response. Measurement of these abilities is more experimental in nature, and includes gambling tasks and naturalistic multiple subgoal tasks.

Different tests have been, or are being, developed to assess the role of the VMPFC in emotional processing (and the basic drives and rewards that provide input into high-level decision-making), such as tests assessing the acquisition and reversal of stimulus–reward associations. Such tests reinforce the distinction between 'executive' attentional and affective/emotional behavioural measures. For example, intra-dimensional shifts (reversal learning, interpreted as affective) are more sensitive to VMPFC lesions, while impairment in extra-dimensional (interpreted as attentional, or executive) set-shifting is observed after LPFC lesions (Dias *et al.* 1996, 1997).

One role that the VMPFC would obviously be involved in is higher-level decision-making tasks involving reward processing, particularly in unstructured situations. Gambling tasks have been developed for precisely that reason, and there was some initial suggestion that such tasks were both sensitive and specific to VMPFC lesions. However, as with many neuropsychological tests which are complex and multifactorial, it is likely that such tests depend on many processes, including executive, depending on how they are administered. The dissociation of the component processes within the gambling task may provide useful information.

Gambling tasks could be grouped under the umbrella label of 'self-regulatory disorder', defined as the inability to regulate behaviour according to internal goals and constraints, particularly in less structured situations. Excellent measures have been, and are being, developed, both as qualitative descriptions with naturalistic multiple subgoal tasks, and also more quantified paper-and-pencil laboratory versions.

Meta-cognitive processes and putative localization

The fourth category of frontal function appears to be maximally involved in the meta-cognitive and integrative aspects of human nature: integration of cognition and emotion, aspects of personality, social cognition, autonoetic consciousness, theory of mind, humour appreciation, and self-awareness. In general terms, meta-cognition implies a reflective representation of one's own mental states, beliefs, attitudes and experiences. Such self-reflection is essential for understanding the relationship of one's own thoughts to external events, as well as using this self-knowledge to understand the mental states of others. The obvious outcome of intact meta-cognitive processes is an ability to make inferences about the world, to empathize with and understand the actions of others, and to serve as a base for appropriate social judgements. Family reports often precisely describe the changes in behaviour that have occurred: lack of empathy, unconcern, and inability to appreciate humour that requires self-reflection (appreciation of slapstick humour may be intact).

The frontal region most often related to these meta-cognitive processes is Brodmann area 10, although relation to a more general area including the anterior medial regions is more reasonable at this stage of investigation. There is also some suggestion in this category of fractionation of component processes. There is an anatomical rationale for relating meta-cognitive processes to this general area. Area 10 is among the most recently evolved of human brain regions, and therefore may be uniquely positioned to integrate the higher-level executive cognitive functions with emotional or drive-related inputs, a bridging that would appear essential for meta-cognitive functions. Burgess *et al.* (2007, in press) have also interpreted the functions of area 10 as a 'gateway', facilitating stimulus-oriented or stimulus-independent attending.

There are no 'clinical' tests for this category of frontal lobe functions; the measures used are primarily experimental in nature (e.g. humour, visual perspective taking tasks, and comparison of performance on remember–know memory tasks). For some individuals, however, these tasks can be solved on the basis of factual knowledge, and may not be meta-cognitive.

Considerations for rehabilitation

An over-arching question one might ask is whether there is a 'dysexecutive' syndrome. This term has had historical usefulness. However, with the current ability to detect brain pathology earlier (e.g. in patients with tumours), with increased knowledge of the fractionation of frontal lobe functions, and if one accepts the operational definition of 'executive' as presented above, one might conclude that there is no dysexecutive syndrome—at least not in patients with focal frontal damage. Clearly, there are executive deficits, but these are disso-ciable and specific to different lateral frontal regions. In some types of patients with more diffuse pathology, it might be reasonable to characterize a patient's deficits as a 'dysexecutive' syndrome only if it is clearly understood that the label does not necessarily imply a definite frontal structural lesion. However, it is also reasonable to ask if some of the other categories of dysfunction as described above are present in such patients, since this could be potentially useful for rehabilitation purposes.

The brief summary of potential different categories of frontal functions, and the imprecision in operational definitions, illuminates some potential problems with construction of rehabilitation strategies. The data also suggest possible reasons for the minimal number of randomized controlled trials of executive rehabilitation (Turner and Levine 2004; Cicerone *et al.* 2005).

The objective of this chapter was to suggest for the rehabilitation specialist theoretical considerations in relation to 'executive dysfunction'. Operational definitions and clarity of terminology are important, at the very least for the purpose of common communication. The research data on frontal lobe function and dysfunction suggest that the term 'executive' may have been used in too global a manner. We have proposed that understanding the relationship of regional injuries to specific patterns of cognitive impairment is essential for accurate diagnosis and characterization of the patient. Specifying precise impairments may be critical to identification of patients who might benefit from specific medications or targeted cognitive rehabilitation.

We have also attempted elsewhere to describe in greater detail what impact this knowledge of different categories of frontal lobe function might have on establishing a rehabilitation framework in patients with traumatic brain injury (Cicerone *et al.* 2006) and focal frontal damage (Alexander and Stuss 2000; Levine *et al.*, in press). Whether the knowledge gained from such exper-imental research in patients has any value in the 'real world' of rehabilitation remains to be tested.

Acknowledgements

This chapter was prepared with the assistance of funding from CIHR GR14974, CIHR 108636, and J.S.F. McDonnell Foundation 21002032. Colleagues on the papers referenced are gratefully acknowledged. Figure and manuscript preparation were only possible with the assistance of Susan Gillingham. Personal funding for D. Stuss was provided partially by the Reva James Leeds Chair in Neuroscience and Research Leadership at the University of Toronto and Baycrest.

References

Alexander, M.P. (2001). Chronic akinetic mutism after mesencephalic-diencephalic infarction: remediated with dopaminergic medications. *Neurorehabilitation and Neural Repair*, **15**, 151–6.

Alexander, M.P. and Stuss, D.T. (2000). Disorders of frontal lobe functioning. *Seminars in Neurology*, **20**, 427–37.

Alexander, G.E., Delong, M.R., and Strick, P.L., (1986). Parallel organization of functionally segregated circuits linking basal ganglia and cortex. *Annual Review of Neuroscience*, **9**, 357–81.

Alexander, M.P., Stuss, D.T., and Fansabedian, N. (2003). California Verbal Learning test: performance by patients with focal frontal and non-frontal lesions. *Brain*, **126**, 1493–1503.

Alexander, M.P., Stuss, D.T., Shallice, T., Picton, T.W., and Gillingham, S., (2005). Impaired concentration due to frontal lobe damage from two distinct lesion sites. *Neurology*, **65**, 572–9.

Alexander, M.P., Stuss, D.T., Picton, T., Shallice, T., and Gillingham, S. (2007). Regional frontal injuries cause distinct impairments in cognitive control. *Neurology*, **68**, 1515–23.

Aparicio, P., Diedrichsen, J. and Ivry, R.B. (2005). Effects of focal basal ganglia lesions on timing and force control. *Brain and Cognition*, **58**, 62–74.

Basso, G., Nichelli, P., Wharton, C.M., Peterson, M., and Grafman, J., (2003). Distributed neural systems for temporal production: a functional MRI study. *Brain Research Bulletin*, **59**, 405–411.

Brass, M. and von Cramon, D.Y., (2004). Selection for cognitive control: a functional magnetic resonance imaging study on the selection of task-relevant information. *Journal of Neuroscience*, **24**, 8847–52.

Burgess, P.W., Gilbert, S.J., and Dumontheil, I. (2007). Function and localisation within rostral prefrontal cortex (area 10). *Philosophical Transactions of the Royal Society B: Biological Sciences*, **362**, 887–99.

Burgess, P.W., Simons, J.S., Dumontheil, I. and Gilbert, S.J. The gateway hypothesis of rostral prefrontal cortex (area 10) function. In: *Speed, control, and age: in honour of Patrick Rabbitt* (ed. J. Duncan, L. Phillips and P. McLeod). Oxford University Press, in press.

Cicerone, K.D., Dahlberg, C., Malec, J.F., *et al.*, (2005). Evidence-based cognitive rehabilitation: updated review of the literature from 1998 through 2002. *Archives of Physical Medicine and Rehabilitation*, **86**, 1681–92.

Cicerone, K., Levin, H., Malec, J., Stuss, D., and Whyte, J., (2006). Cognitive rehabilitation interventions for executive function: moving from bench to bedside in patients with traumatic brain injury. *Journal of Cognitive Neuroscience*, **18**, 1212–22.

Coull, J.T., Frackowiak, R.S., and Frith, C.D., (1998). Monitoring for target objects: Activation of right frontal and parietal cortices with increasing time on task. *Neuropsychologia*, **36**, 1325–34.

Derrfuss, J., Brass, M., Neumann, J., and von Cramon, D.Y., (2005). Involvement of the inferior frontal junction in cognitive control: meta-analyses of switching and Stroop studies. *Human Brain Mapping*, **25**, 22–34.

Devinsky, O., Morrell, M., and Vogt, B.A. (1995). Contributions of anterior cingulate cortex to behavior. *Brain*, **118**, 279–306.

Dias, R., Robbins, T.W., and Roberts, A.C. (1996). Dissociation in prefrontal cortex of affective attentional shifts. *Nature*, **380**, 69–72.

Dias, R., Robbins, T.W. and Roberts, A.C. (1997). Dissociable forms of inhibitory control within prefrontal cortex with an analog of the Wisconsin Card Sort Test: restriction to novel situations and independence from 'on-line' processing. *Journal of Neuroscience*, **17**, 9285–97.

Drewe, E.A. (1975). Go–no go learning after frontal lobe lesions in humans. *Cortex*, **11**, 8–16.

Fletcher, P.C. and Henson, R.N. (2001). Frontal lobes and human memory: insights from functional neuroimaging. *Brain*, **124**, 849–81.

Godefroy, O., Lhullier, C., and Rousseaux, M. (1994). Vigilance and effects of fatigability, practice and motivation on simple reaction tests in patients with lesions of the frontal lobe. *Neuropsychologia*, **32**, 983–990.

Godefroy, O., Cabaret, M., Petit-Chenal, V., Pruvo, J.-P., and Rousseaux, M. (1999). Control functions of the frontal lobes. Modularity of the central-supervisory system? *Cortex*, **35**, 1–20.

Henson, R.N.A., Shallice, T. and Dolan, R.J. (1999). Right prefrontal cortex and episodic memory retrieval: A functional MRI test of the monitoring hypothesis. *Brain*, **122**, 1367–81.

Hockey, G.R.J. (1993) Cognitive energetic control mechanisms in the management of work demands and psychological health. In: *Attention: selection, awareness and control: a tribute to Donald Broadbent* (ed A.D. Baddeley and L. Weiskrantz), pp. 328–45. Clarendon Press, Oxford.

Hofle, N., Paus, T., Reutens, D., *et al.* (1997). Regional cerebral blood flow changes as a function of delta and spindle activity during slow wave sleep in humans. *Journal of Neuroscience*, **17**, 4800–8.

Leimkuhler, M.E. and Mesulam, M.M. (1985). Reversible go–no go deficits in a case of frontal lobe tumor. *Annals of Neurology*, **18**, 617–19.

Levine, B., Turner, G.R. and Stuss, D.T. Rehabilitation of frontal lobe functions. In: *Cognitive rehabilitation: evidence and application* (2nd edn) (ed D. Stuss, G. Winocur, and I.H. Robertson). Cambridge University Press, in press.

Lewis, P.A. and Miall, R.C. (2003). Brain activation patterns during measurement of sub- and supra-second intervals. *Neuropsychologia*, **41**, 1583–1592.

Luria, A.R. (1966). *Higher cortical functions in man*. Basic Books, New York.

Luria, A.R. (1973). *The working brain: an introduction to neuropsychology*. Basic Books, New York.

Luu, P., Collins, P., and Tucker, D.M. (2000a). Mood, personality, and self-monitoring: negative affect and emotionality in relation to frontal lobe mechanisms of error monitoring. *Journal of Experimental Psychology: General*, **129**, 43–60.

Luu, P., Flaisch, T., and Tucker, D.M. (2000b). Medial frontal cortex in action monitoring. *Journal of Neuroscience*, **20**, 464–469.

Niemi, P. and Naatanen, R. (1981). Foreperiod and simple reaction time. *Psychological Bulletin*, **89**, 133–62.

Pandya, D.N. and Barnes, C.L. (1987). Architecture and connections of the frontal lobe. In: *The Frontal Lobes Revisited* (ed E. Perecman), pp. 41–72. IRBN Press, New York.

Pardo, J.V., Fox, P.T., and Raichle, M.E. (1991). Localization of a human system for sustained attention by positron emission tomography. *Nature*, **349**, 61–4.

Passingham, R. (1993). *The frontal lobes and voluntary action*. Oxford University Press.

Paus, T., Zatorre, R.J., Hofle, N., Caramanos, J.G., Petrides, M., and Evans, A.C., (1997). Time-related changes in neural systems underlying attention and arousal during the performance of an auditory vigilance task. *Journal of Cognitive Neuroscience*, **9**, 392–408.

Perret, E., (1974). Left frontal lobe of man and suppression of habitual responses in verbal categorical behavior. *Neuropsychologia*, **12**, 323–30.

Picard, N. and Strick, P.L. (1996). Motor areas of the medial wall: a review of their location and functional activation. *Cerebral Cortex*, **6**, 342–53.

Picton, T.W., Stuss, D.T., Shallice, T., Alexander, M.P., and Gillingham, S. (2006). Keeping time: effects of focal frontal lesions. *Neuropsychologia*, **44**, 1195–1209.

Plum, F. and Posner, J.B. (1980). *The diagnosis of stupor and coma*. Davis, Philadelphia, PA.

Richer, F., Decary, A., Lapierre, M.-P., Rouleau, I., Bouvier, G., and Saint-Hilaire, J.-M. (1993). Target detection deficits in frontal lobectomy. *Brain and Cognition*, **21**, 203–11.

Rueckert, L. and Grafman, J. (1996). Sustained attention deficits in patients with right frontal lesions. *Neuropsychologia*, **34**, 953–63.

Sanides, F. (1970) Functional architecture of motor and sensory cortices in primates in the light of a new concept of neocortex development. In: *Advances in primatology* (ed C.R. Noback and W. Montana), pp. 137–208. Appleton-Century-Crofts, New York.

Shallice, T. (2001). Fractionating the supervisory system. *Brain and Cognition*, **47**, 30.

Shallice, T. (2002) Fractionation of the supervisory system. In: *Principles of frontal lobe function* (ed. D.T. Stuss and R.T. Knight), pp. 261–277. Oxford University Press.

Stuss, D.T. (2007) New approaches to prefrontal lobe testing. In: *The Human frontal lobes: functions and disorders* (2nd edn) (ed B. Miller and J. Cummings), pp. 292–305. Guilford Press, New York.

Stuss, D.T. and Alexander, M.P. (2007). Is there a dysexecutive syndrome? *Philosophical Transactions of the Royal Society B: Biological Sciences*, **362**, 901–15.

Stuss, D.T. and Benson, D.F. (1984). Neuropsychological studies of the frontal lobes. *Psychological Bulletin*, **95**, 3–28.

Stuss, D.T. and Benson, D.F. (1986). *The frontal lobes*. Raven Press, New York.

Stuss, D.T. and Levine, B. (2002). Adult clinical neuropsychology: lessons from studies of the frontal lobes. *Annual Review of Psychology*, **53**, 401–33.

Stuss, D.T., Alexander, M.P., Palumbo, C.L., Buckle, L., Sayer, L., and Pogue, J. (1994). Organizational strategies of patients with unilateral or bilateral frontal lobe injury in word list learning tasks. *Neuropsychology*, **8**, 355–73.

Stuss, D.T., Alexander, M.P., Hamer, L., *et al.* (1998). The effects of focal anterior and posterior brain lesions on verbal fluency. *Journal of the International Neuropsychological Society*, **4**, 265–78.

Stuss, D.T., Levine, B., Alexander, M.P., *et al.* (2000). Wisconsin Card Sorting Test performance in patients with focal frontal and posterior brain damage: effects of lesion location and test structure on separable cognitive processes. *Neuropsychologia*, **38**, 388–402.

Stuss, D.T., Gallup, G.G. and Alexander, M.P. (2001a). The frontal lobes are necessary for 'theory of mind'. *Brain*, **124**, 279–86.

Stuss, D.T., Picton, T.W., and Alexander, M.P. (2001b). Consciousness, self-awareness and the frontal lobes. In: *The frontal lobes and neuropsychiatric illness* (ed S.P. Salloway, P.F. Malloy, and J.D. Duffy), pp. 101–9. American Psychiatric Publishing, Washington, DC.

Stuss, D.T., Binns, M.A., Murphy, K.J., and Alexander, M.P. (2002). Dissociations within the anterior attentional system: effects of task complexity and irrelevant information on reaction time speed and accuracy. *Neuropsychology*, **16**, 500–13.

Stuss, D.T., Murphy, K.J., Binns, M.A., and Alexander, M.P. (2003). Staying on the job: the frontal lobes control individual performance variability. *Brain*, **126**, 2363–80.

Stuss, D.T., Alexander, M.P., Shallice, T., *et al.* (2005). Multiple frontal systems controlling response speed. *Neuropsychologia*, **43**, 396–417.

Turner, G. and Levine, B. (2004). Disorders of executive function and self-awareness. In: *Rehabilitation of neurobehavioral disorders* (ed J. Ponsford), pp. 224–68. Guilford Press, New York.

Turner, M.S., Cipolotti, L., Yousry, T., and Shallice, T. (2007). Qualitatively different memory impairments across frontal lobe subgroups. *Neuropsychologia*, **45**, 1540–52.

Vallesi, A., Shallice, T., and Walsh, V. (2007). Role of the prefrontal cortex in the foreperiod effect: TMS evidence for dual mechanisms in temporal preparation. *Cerebral Cortex*, **17**, 466–74.

Wilkins, A.J., Shallice, T., and McCarthy, R. (1987). Frontal lesions and sustained attention. *Neuropsychologia*, **25**, 359–65.

2

Cognitive reserve

Karen L. Siedlecki and Yaakov Stern

Cognitive Neuroscience Division, Taub Institute, Columbia University College of Physicians and Surgeons, New York

The concept of reserve emerged as a mechanism to explain the discontinuity between the degree of pathology in a condition and the severity of its clinical features. For example, patients with the same amount of brain pathology post-mortem may display strikingly different clinical expressions of dementia and/or Alzheimer's disease (AD). For instance, patients with high educational attainment (Stern *et al.* 1992) or large brains (Katzman *et al.* 1988) may have few or no clinical symptoms of the disease while alive but definite evidence of AD pathology of the brain at autopsy. In fact, it is estimated that approximately 25 per cent (Ince 2001) of individuals who have neuropathological evidence of AD post-mortem are not demented during their lives. Increased reserve is hypothesized to be associated with increased protection against clinical expression of dementia in that those individuals with a higher amount of reserve may be able to cope better with the pathological changes occurring in the brain. Because cognitive reserve has been extensively studied with AD patients, most of the work discussed in this chapter focuses on the relation between cognitive reserve and dementia. Support for the cognitive reserve theory has also been found in patients with Parkinson's disease, schizophrenia, and HIV. Theoretically, these models of cognitive reserve can also be applied to patients with acquired brain injury, although to date there are few studies that have specifically examined cognitive reserve in patients with traumatic brain injury (TBI) (but see Kesler *et al.* 2003; Ropacki and Elias 2003).

In the case of TBI, cognitive reserve might influence both the ability of the brain to resist injury and its ability to recuperate from or compensate for brain injury. There is evidence that reserve may play an important role in both these abilities. In this chapter, the relevant research on cognitive reserve in dementia is summarized, and where appropriate, the findings are applied to TBI.

Two main classifications of reserve have emerged: brain reserve and cognitive reserve (see Figure 2.1 for a taxonomical representation of reserve).

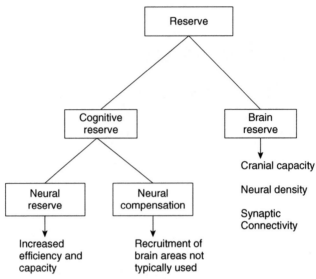

Fig. 2.1 Taxonomical representation of reserve.

Brain reserve

Brain reserve, as articulated by Satz (1993), is a threshold account of brain pathology. A threshold model predicts that once brain reserve is depleted past a certain threshold, clinical or functional deficits will become evident. Brain reserve typically refers to specific characteristics of the brain that may vary across individuals, including brain size, neural density, and synaptic connectivity. In each case more of that specific feature would impart greater reserve. There is evidence that brain size and head circumference are negatively correlated with both the severity and incidence of AD (Graves *et al.* 1996; Schofield *et al.* 1997) as well as with the degree of cognitive changes following TBI (Kesler *et al.* 2003). The hypothesized explanation of these findings is that larger brains have an increased number of neurons, and thus more neurons can be damaged or die before there is a manifestation of deficit (i.e. more damage is necessary to hit the critical threshold).

The concept of brain reserve plays an important role in TBI. Some early animal work on brain and behaviour indicated that the amount and type of functional neural networks evident prior to surgical removal of brain structures played a role in the subsequent outcomes (e.g. Schulkin 1989). Current work examining the relation between total intra-cranial volume (TICV) and change from pre-injury to post-injury intelligence quotient (IQ) has shown that TICV is predictive of outcome, i.e. larger TICV is associated with smaller changes in IQ (Kesler *et al.* 2003). This study gives evidence that absolute brain volume provides some protection against cognitive sequelae in instances of TBI. Because pre-injury TICV correlates with IQ, TICV might be considered a summation of brain reserve, IQ at birth, and the ongoing effects of lifetime cognitive stimulation on the brain.

Stern (2002) originally argued that brain reserve is a passive model of reserve because once a fixed threshold is reached, clinical changes emerge. Thus there is no active compensation for pathology. However, it is important to recognize that aspects of brain reserve can be altered by life experience. Katzman (1993) postulated that education may increase the growth of synapses in an infant or child, and Jacobs *et al.* (1993) reported that individuals with more education have more dendritic branching. Data from animal studies have indicated that exercise promotes brain vascularization, neurogenesis, and neuronal survival, and helps to resist brain insult (reviewed by Cotman and Berchtold 2002). There is also a positive relation between exercise and levels of brain-derived neurotrophic factor (BDNF), a protein which has neurotrophic and neuroprotective properties that may be linked to brain plasticity (Cotman and Berchtold 2002). Levels of neurotransmitters, suchas serotonin and dopamine, are also increased as a result of exercise (Blomstrand *et al.* 1989).

The research on humans is consistent with the results of the animal studies summarized above which provide evidence of the beneficial effects of exercise on cognitive functioning. In a meta-analysis of longitudinal intervention studies in adults over the age of 55, Colcombe and Kramer (2003) reported that fitness training in older adults increased performance on different cognitive tasks by an average of 0.5 SD compared with control groups. Specifically, executive control tasks appeared to benefit the most from exercise manipulations. Research has indicated that frontal regions of the brain may be most susceptible to the effects of ageing. These frontal regions are hypothesized to be largely involved in tasks that measure executive processing which may, in turn, be more likely to show improvements with exercise interventions. Deficits in executive functioning, along with decreased processing speed and a decline in short-term memory, are among the most common cognitive consequences of TBI (Bigler, 2006). Therefore it follows that exercise has the potential to promote brain repair in patients with brain injury and, in fact, evidence of cognitive improvements following motor enrichment after brain injury has been found in both animal and human studies (reviewed by Kleim *et al.* 2003).

Grealy *et al.* (1999) examined the effect of exercise with virtual reality on different tests of cognition in a group of 13 brain-injured patients with TBI.

Virtual reality environments (of a Caribbean island, a town and countryside, or mountains with snow and ski trials) were used while participants were exercising on stationary bicycles to enrich the environment and to enhance motivation of the participants. Grealy and colleagues reported improvements in measures of auditory learning, visual learning, and the digit symbol subtest of the participants compared with a population of 320 patients admitted to the same hospital who did not receive the virtual reality exercise paradigm. They did not find significant improvements in measures of long-term memory or task-switching. In a second study they reported significant improvements in reaction time and movement times after just one episode of the exercise virtual reality paradigm. However, because the exercise programme was performed in conjunction with the virtual reality environment, it is unclear if the same effects would be found with exercise alone. This is one of the few studies that examine the effect of exercise on cognition after brain injury and the results are consistent with findings from animal studies. Note, however, that some animal research suggests that forced exercise too soon after brain injury may have a detrimental effect (reviewed by Kleim *et al.* 2003).

The beneficial effects of exercise on cognition have also been demonstrated with young adults. After a 10-week intervention study, participants showed improvement on tests of processing speed, reasoning, and memory (Young 1979). However, the lack of a control group in this study limits the conclusions that can be made. In another study involving younger participants (between the ages of 18 and 48), Blomquist and Danner (1987) reported that those participants who showed an increase in fitness after an exercise intervention also showed an increased improvement on a retrieval task (although they did not show improvements on other cognitive tasks).

Collectively, these findings provide evidence that brain reserve may be malleable and suggest that exercise, in particular, may be beneficial.

Cognitive reserve

Stern (2002) suggested that cognitive reserve can be considered an active model of reserve, and has hypothesized that neural reserve and neural compensation are the two main components of cognitive reserve (see Figure 2.1). Cognitive reserve is considered an active model, as opposed to the threshold model which has been considered a more passive model (Stern 2002). Unlike the threshold model, where deficits set in after a certain level of depletion, cognitive reserve is an active model because the brain actively compensates for pathology.

Stern suggested that the neural implementation of cognitive reserve can be divided into neural reserve and neural compensation. Neural reserve refers to the differential efficiency or capacity of the brain prior to insult, and may be operationalized as more efficient circuits of synaptic connectivity. Neural compensation refers to the recruitment of brain areas not typically used by individuals without brain pathology in order to compensate for brain damage, and may reflect the use of alternative strategies. One way to conceptualize the difference between neural reserve and neural compensation is to consider that reserve may refer to the use of the same or additional networks in response to increased task demand, whereas neural compensation may refer to the use of additional networks that *are not typically used* in response to pathological changes in the brain. The cognitive reserve model is different from the brain reserve model in that it does not postulate a critical threshold at which time functional impairment occurs. Rather, the cognitive reserve model depends on the efficiency and compensation strategies employed at the neural level.

How is cognitive reserve measured? Education level (or literacy), occupational attainment, and participation in leisure activities have been proposed as surrogate measures of cognitive reserve since they are reflective of life experiences, and they may provide a set of skills that allow some individuals to manage pathological damage in AD better in the sense that the clinical manifestation of brain pathology is delayed or reduced. In TBI, increased cognitive reserve would theoretically help in resisting initial cognitive sequelae and may also help in recuperation and compensation for the injury through both neural reserve and neural compensation.

Education is correlated with IQ, and it has been suggested that IQ may be a more accurate marker of reserve than education (Alexander *et al.* 1997; Albert and Teresi 1999). However, Stern (2006) argues that reserve as measured by education, occupation, and other life experiences has value beyond that imparted from innate intelligence, and cites evidence that these life experience variables have separate and synergistic effects (e.g. Evans *et al.* 1993; Stern *et al.* 1995a). For example, Richards and Sacker (2003) used path analysis to examine the relations between cognitive reserve, as measured by the National Adult Reading Test (NART), and childhood cognition, educational attainment, and adult occupation. NART is a test of pronunciation of words that violate conventional grapheme–phoneme rules (e.g. superfluous, epitome). Using one's intellectual ability to guess the pronunciation would not necessarily help because the words violate conventional pronunciation rules. Therefore NART is an appropriate proxy for cognitive reserve because it reflects one's accumulated experience with reading. In their sample of the British 1946 birth cohort, Richards and Sacker found that childhood cognition (a measure of IQ) had the strongest independent relation with NART. Educational attainment had the next strongest independent relation with NART, and occupational attainment had the weakest unique relationship. These analyses support the argument that there are unique and independent relations of education and occupational attainment with cognitive reserve, even after accounting for childhood cognition.

Increased education has also been shown to be associated with a reduced relative risk of incident AD in a number of studies in the USA (Evans *et al.* 1993; Stern *et al.* 1994; White *et al.* 1994; Evans *et al.* 1997), as well as in China (Zhang *et al.* 1990), France (Letenneur *et al.* 1994), Finland (Anttila *et al.* 2002), and Sweden (Qiu *et al.* 2001). In one prevalence study, Rocca *et al.* (1990) investigated the prevalence of dementia in a small community in Italy in a door-to-door survey of individuals aged over 59 years. Twenty of the 798 participants were diagnosed with AD. Of those 20, 19 (95 per cent) had completed no more than 4 years of education. However, not all studies have reported an association between education and dementia (Paykel *et al.* 1994; Cobb *et al.* 1995; Graves *et al.* 1996; Hall *et al.* 2000). Discrepancies may exist because of differences between the studies, such as sample selection and measures used for diagnosis. For example, Paykel *et al.* (1994) used mainly the Mini Mental Status Examination (MMSE) (Folstein, Folstein, and McHugh 1975) to measure dementia as opposed to more sensitive neuropsychological measures, and less than 10 per cent of the sample used by Cobb *et al.* (1995) could be categorized as low education, thereby limiting the power to detect an education effect.

Kesler *et al.* (2003) specifically examined the reserve hypothesis in brain injury in a study with 25 participants who had sustained TBI. They used TICV as a measure of brain reserve, and pre-injury standardized test scores and education level as measures of cognitive reserve. Irrespective of injury severity, patients with lower TICV values had lower post-injury IQ and a larger decline in IQ from pre- to post-injury. Furthermore, both TICV and education predicted participants' post-injury IQ group (high, IQ > 90; low, IQ < 90). However, premorbid standardized test score (a measure of cognitive reserve) did not predict participants' post-injury IQ group. This study provides evidence that both brain reserve (as measured by TICV) and cognitive reserve (as measured by education, but not standardized test scores) may play a role in cognitive deficits after brain injury.

Other variables often used as indirect measures of cognitive reserve are occupational status and engagement in leisure activities. An association between incident dementia and occupational attainment has been found in a number of studies across multiple samples (Stern *et al.* 1994; White *et al.* 1994; Bickel and Cooper 1994; Schmand *et al.* 1997). For example, in a recent study from Sweden, Qiu *et al.* (2003) found that a specific subcategory of manual work (production of goods) was associated with an increased risk of AD after statistically controlling for education and other covariates.

However, other studies in France (Helmer *et al*. 2001), the UK (Paykel *et al*. 1994), and the USA have failed to find an independent relationship between occupation and dementia (Evans *et al*. 1997; Anttila *et al*. 2002), and Jorm *et al*. (1998) failed to find the same relation between occupation and prevalence of dementia in Australia longitudinally, as had been found in a cross-sectional analysis of the same sample.

The relation of leisure activity to incident dementia has been investigated longitudinally in prospective studies. In one study, Fabrigoule *et al*. (1995) followed a cohort of French participants over the age of 65 for 3 years after baseline screening which included an assessment of social and leisure activities. After controlling for age and cognitive performance, the activities of travelling, doing odd jobs or knitting, and gardening were significantly associated with a reduced risk of developing dementia. Alternately, Bickel and Cooper (1994) did not find a relationship between participation in leisure activities and a lower risk of subsequent dementia in a sample of older adults from Germany who were followed longitudinally.

In another prospective study, Scarmeas *et al*. (2001) obtained estimates from 1772 older adults on their engagement in 13 activities, including knitting, walking, visiting friends and family, watching television, volunteering, and playing cards. Participants were given one point for participating in each of the 13 activities in the previous month and subsequently received an activity score reflecting the total number of activities (ranging from 0 to 13). Individuals with high activity scores had a 38 per cent less risk of developing dementia as compared with those individuals with low activity scores, even after accounting for education, ethnicity, and occupation. Specific activities were more strongly related to a reduction in the risk of developing dementia— reading, visiting friends and family, going to movies and restaurants, and walking for pleasure or going for an excursion.

Ropacki and Elias (2003) operationalized cognitive reserve in a group of patients with closed head injury in a unique manner. They divided patients into two groups, one negative for premorbid history of alcoholism, drug abuse, psychiatric illness, or neurological disorders, and the other positive for any of the above. The positive group was considered to be the group with diminished cognitive reserve because of presumed previous assaults on neurocognitive functioning. Ropacki and Elias reported that patients with a positive history of premorbid disease suffered greater post-injury cognitive declines, specifically in measures of fluid ability, than did those with a negative history.

Correlates of reserve have also been found to have a relation to cerebral blood flow (CBF) in positron emission tomography (PET), which is often used as an indirect measure of brain damage since lower CBF indicates increased pathology. Studies have indicated that, after statistically controlling for clinical severity, those individuals with higher education (Stern *et al.* 1992), higher occupational status (Stern *et al.* 1995a), higher premorbid IQ (Alexander *et al.* 1997), and increased leisure activities (Scarmeas *et al.* 2003) have decreased CBF. This is consistent with the reserve hypothesis that at any given level of clinical severity demented individuals with more cognitive reserve have more brain pathology.

There is evidence that those individuals who have higher levels of cognitive reserve also have a more rapid cognitive decline once diagnosed with AD. This also supports the idea that, at any given level of clinical severity, those patients with higher cognitive reserve will have more extensive brain pathology (Stern *et al.* 1995b).

Normal age-related declines in cognitive abilities such as memory, processing speed, reasoning, and visuospatial ability are well documented (e.g. Salthouse 1996). There is additional evidence that individuals with higher education have slower cognitive and functional declines in *normal* ageing (Albert *et al.* 1995; Farmer *et al.* 1995; Butler *et al.* 1996), suggesting that reserve may also play a factor in resisting normal age-related changes.

However, the findings pertaining to normal ageing are mixed. Christensen *et al.* (1997) reported that in a community sample of older adults across 3.6 years, education slowed the rate of decline across crystallized ability measures such as language and knowledge but not across fluid ability measures such as memory, processing speed, and reaction time. Salthouse (2006) reported on the interactive effects of level of mentally stimulating activity (i.e. leisure activities) and age on cognitive functioning. After dividing the sample into high- and low-cognitive stimulation groups, the age-related trends for a spatial relations task, a memory task, and a processing speed task were nearly parallel across the two groups, even after controlling for education. However, consistent with Christensen *et al.* (1997), the trends across age were different for the two groups on a vocabulary test (a measure of crystallized intelligence), such that those who engaged in more stimulating activities showed less of a decline. Further, Lyekotsos *et al.* (1999) found that low level of education was associated with faster rates of decline in the MMSE, but only for those individuals who had less than 8 years of education. For those individuals with 9 or more years of education, there were no differences in the rates of decline over an 11-year period.

Neural reserve (efficiency and capacity)

Findings from studies using functional neuroimaging (fMRI) suggest that there is an increase in activation in the regions of the brain (or a recruitment of additional brain areas) when the difficulty of a task is increased in healthy young adults (Gur et al. 1988; Grady et al. 1996; Rypma et al. 1999). Most relevant to these findings is that there is evidence that individuals with more skill tend to recruit additional brain areas less, suggesting an increased efficiency.

Stern et al. (2003) examined whether cognitive reserve is related to aspects of neural processing using fMRI in a sample of young adults. A non-verbal recognition test was used which comprised a low-demand (one-item) test condition and a high-demand (titrated) test condition in which accuracy was equated across individuals to be approximately 75 per cent (thus list size varied across subjects in the high-demand condition). The authors used a voxel-wise analysis of the whole brain to examine the correlation between activation and NART scores (i.e. a measure of reserve) in order to evaluate how individual differences in cognitive reserve relate to changes in neural activity when moving from the low-demand to the high-demand condition. During both the study and test phase, Stern et al. reported that there was a systematic relationship between cognitive reserve as measured by NART and brain activation. There were significant positive and negative correlations between NART scores and the increase in activation from the low-demand to the high-demand condition, suggesting that neural processing differs as a function of cognitive reserve.

Neural compensation

There is evidence that AD patients may have greater and more extensive activation during the same task as controls (e.g. Deutsch et al. 1993; Grady et al. 1993). For example, Becker et al. (1996) presented seven AD patients and seven control participants with an auditory memory task consisting of one word, three words, or eight words while measuring regional cerebral blood flow with PET. During the eight-word task, the dorsolateral prefrontal cortex and the angular gyrus (BA39/40) became significantly active in the AD patients compared with activation in the three-word task, and these regions were not activated in the normal controls. Becker et al. argued that the recruitment of these additional brain regions provided evidence of the brain's attempt to compensate for the neuropathology.

The recruitment of additional networks has also been shown to be associated with increased performance in normal older people. Increased performance may be considered a separate issue, since changes in brain activation may be reflective of beneficial compensatory reorganization regardless of improvement in performance. However, once it has been established that an impaired group expressed some area to a greater degree than unimpaired individuals, it is useful to examine how this additional activation relates to performance. Cabeza *et al.* (2002) and Rosen *et al.* (2002) reported that in different memory tasks older adults showed increased activation or additional activated regions that were not activated by younger subjects. The older adults who showed the additional activation performed better than those older adults who did not. Recently, Cabeza *et al.* (2004) reported that task-independent age effects manifested in older adults as decreased activity in the occipital region and increased activity in the prefrontal cortex across tests of working memory, visual attention, and episodic memory. Specifically, older adults recruited contralateral prefrontal cortex (PFC) regions during the working memory task (by recruiting the right PFC) and visual attention task (by recruiting the left PFC). Their findings were consistent with an earlier study by Grady *et al.* (1994) in which occipital activity was lower, and PFC activity greater, in older adults than in younger adults in a face-matching task. Grady and colleagues suggested that the increased PFC activation compensated for the decreased occipital activation.

Cabeza (2002) proposed the Hemisphere Asymmetry Reduction in Older Adults (HAROLD) model to account for differences in brain activation across tasks in young and older adults. The HAROLD model has support from studies of episodic memory retrieval (e.g. Cabeza *et al.* 1997), episodic memory encoding/semantic retrieval (e.g. Stebbins *et al.* 2002), working memory (e.g. Reuter-Lorenz *et al.* 2000), source memory (e.g. Cabeza *et al.* 2002), perception (e.g. Grady *et al.* 1994), and inhibition (e.g. Nielson *et al.* 2002). However, some of the apparent bilaterality of activation could be a function of the analytical approaches used. Even if young and old express the same pattern (or areas) of activation, differences in the degree of expression could result in apparent differences in specific areas of activation.

Alternative explanations have been proposed to account for the finding of bilateral activation in older adults, typically based on the behavioural correlates of this additional activation. The compensation account, as described above, suggests that the recruitment of additional brain areas is a compensatory measure that allows older adults to perform better than when there is no additional activation. Alternately, the dedifferentiation account specifies that the decreased lateralization of brain regions reflects an age-related difficulty in selecting the appropriate specific neural mechanism. The compensation view generally implies that performance may be increased through the increased activation of brain regions (at least when compared with older adults who do not show a change in activation), whereas the dedifferentiation view is more ambiguous in its prediction, although it has been suggested that that performance may be hindered by the lack of neural specificity as a result of dedifferentiation (e.g. Zarahn *et al.* 2007).

There is support for each idea in different studies. The compensation view is supported by ageing studies, such as a study by Reuter-Lorenz *et al.* (2000) in which participants completed a verbal working memory task. The results indicated that those participants who had bilateral activation of their PFC had faster reaction times than those who did not. Additional support for the compensation view comes indirectly from studies showing recovery of function after brain injury. A number of studies have shown that homologous regions in the unaffected brain hemisphere are recruited after unilateral brain damage to aid in recovery (c.f. Cabeza 2002). Cabeza argues that since 'bihemispheric activity plays a compensatory role in people with brain damage, it is reasonable to assume it also plays a compensatory role in older adults' (Cabeza 2002, p. 90).

In addition to the patterns of increased bilateral activation of brain regions with increased age, evidence for the dedifferentiation view stems mainly from studies that have shown that correlations among cognitive abilities may increase with age (reviewed by Li and Lindenberger 1999). However, a number of other studies (reviewed by Zelinski and Lewis 2003) have failed to provide evidence in support the dedifferentiation hypothesis.

Stern *et al.* (2000) pointed out that differential activation of areas across groups could often be a function of differential task difficulty in the two groups. For example, in studies where AD patients show excess activation, one explanation is that the patients compensated for brain damage by recruiting different brain areas. However, an alternative explanation is that increased difficulty of the task for the AD patients elicits the additional brain networks compared with the controls. Thus, if the task was made more difficult, the controls might also recruit these additional areas. Further, there might be a level of difficulty at which controls would recruit more additional areas than patients. Stern *et al.* (2000) addressed this issue by controlling task difficulty in a verbal recognition task by adjusting the size of the list for each individual such that all participants were performing at 75 per cent accuracy. Brain activation was measured by cerebral blood flow using $H_2[^{15}O]$ PET. Healthy older adults (the controls) and three of the AD patients activated the left anterior cingulate, anterior insula, and left basal ganglia, and the list size increased as the activation increased. The remaining AD patients activated the left posterior temporal cortex, calcarine cortex, posterior cingulate, and vermis, and the activation of these areas increased with list size. Of note, the increased activation of the network used by the controls and three AD patients was associated with increased performance.

A more recent study (Scarmeas *et al.* 2004) examined differential brain activation (using PET) mediated by cognitive reserve in AD patients compared with healthy older adults in a paradigm similar to the one described above. In this study, the memory task comprised recognition tests for non-verbal stimuli (i.e. shapes) in two conditions. In the low demand condition, one stimulus presentation was followed by a yes–no recognition test, and in the titrated demand condition the task was again calibrated for each individual subject such that each subject was approximately 75 per cent accurate at recognizing the shape stimuli. A factor score was determined from three measures of cognitive reserve (i.e. NART, WAIS-R vocabulary subtest score, and years of education) and used as the independent variable in a voxel-wise multiple regression in which the activation difference between the low-demand and titrated-demand conditions was used as the dependent variable.

The results indicated that the slopes were significantly more positive in the left precentral gyrus and hippocampus, and significantly more negative in the right fusiform, right middle occipital, and left middle temporal gyri in the AD subjects. This suggests that there is a relation between cognitive reserve and brain activation during memory tasks and, specifically, that there are brain regions which may be reorganized in response to pathological changes associated with AD. Scarmeas *et al.* (2004) concluded that the brain regions in which the slopes between cognitive reserve factor score and brain activation are different across disease status may mediate 'the differential ability to cope with (i.e. delay or modify) clinical manifestations of AD'.

Stern *et al.* (2005) have also examined differential brain networks associated with cognitive reserve across healthy younger and older adults using PET. They found evidence of both neural reserve and neural compensation in a non-verbal recognition paradigm identical to the one described above. Specifically, young subjects with higher measures of cognitive reserve had an increased expression of a neural topography across the low-demand and titrated-demand conditions compared with those young subjects with lower cognitive reserve. Thus expression of the topography varied as a function of cognitive reserve level, suggesting that those with increased cognitive reserve were more responsive in their (or have a greater capacity for the) topographic expression. However, older subjects with higher cognitive reserve showed a decrease in expression of the network across conditions. Stern and colleagues argue that the decrease in expression probably represents a reorganization of the network, which therefore represents a compensatory mechanism (i.e. neural compensation).

Implications for neuroplasticity and neurorehabilitation

What are the implications of these findings in terms of neuroplasticity and neurorehabilitation? The reserve hypothesis provides a useful framework for examining the effects of TBI. As described above, Kesler *et al.* (2003) found that both brain reserve (as measured by TICV) and cognitive reserve (as measured by education, but not standardized test scores) may play a role in cognitive deficits after brain injury. Research has also indicated that there is an increased risk of developing dementia or neuropsychiatric disorders after TBI (Bigler, 2006). A possible explanation suggested by this finding is that reserve capacities are used during recovery from a brain injury and a result the brain is more vulnerable to later expression of potential disorders (Bigler, 2006).

The research regarding reserve also suggests that life experience imparted from education, occupation, and leisure activities protects individuals from clinical and functional expression of dementia or provides protection against cognitive deficits in other types of brain injury (such as TBI). A potential approach to reducing the risk of developing AD would be to systematically expose individuals to the life experiences associated with reserve. It is currently unclear whether interventions in the early stages of dementia consisting of, for example, leisure activities that are associated with a decreased risk of developing AD (like reading) would be an effective treatment. It may be the case that such cognitive interventions have to be applied at a younger age in order to be beneficial. Prospective studies examining the incidence of dementia in older cohorts have shown that leisure activity (as well physical and intellectual activity) is associated with a reduced risk of developing AD (e.g. Scarmeas and Stern 2003; Colcombe and Kramer 2003), although it is possible that this could be explained by the correlation between current and past activity level. One interesting question is whether engaging in these leisure activities post-TBI would have effects similar to engaging in physical activity after brain injury. Findings of brain changes that occur as a result of physical activity in animal studies are also promising, and collectively these results would suggest that the potential for plasticity still exists at older ages and after TBI or diagnosis of dementia.

Summary

The concept of reserve emerged from the observation that clinical manifestation of pathology was not directly related to the degree of brain pathology or damage. The cognitive reserve hypothesis provides a useful framework for examining what factors may contribute to the severity of cognitive consequences, and also what factors may help in recuperation from, and compensation for, brain injury.

Acknowledgements

The writing of this chapter was supported by federal grant AG26158 to Yaakov Stern. Karen L. Siedlecki was supported as a trainee by grant T32MH020004–09 from the National Institute of Mental Health.

References

Albert, M.S., Jones, K., Savage, C.R., *et al.* (1995). Predictors of cognitive change in older persons: MacArthur studies of successful aging. *Psychology and Aging*, **10**, 578–89.

Albert, S.M. and Teresi, J.A. (1999). Reading ability, education, and cognitive status assessment among older adults in Harlem, New York City. *American Journal of Public Health*, **89**, 95–97.

Alexander, G.E., Furey, M.L., Grady, C.L., Pietrini, P., Mentis, M.J., and Schapiro, M.B. (1997). Association of premorbid function with cerebral metabolism in Alzheimer's disease: implications for the reserve hypothesis. *American Journal of Psychiatry*, **154**, 165–72.

Anttila, B.M., Helkala, E.-L., Kivipelto, M., *et al.* (2002). Midlife income, occupation, *APOE* status, and dementia: a population-based study. *Neurology*, **59**, 887–93.

Becker, J.T., Mintun, M.= A., Aleva, K., Wiseman, M.B., Nichols, T., and DeKosky, S.T. (1996). Compensatory reallocation of brain resources supporting verbal episodic memory in Alzheimer's disease. *Neurology*, **46**, 692–700.

Bickel, H. and Cooper, B. (1994). Incidence and relative risk of dementia in an urban elderly population: findings of a prospective field study. *Psychological Medicine*, **24**, 179–92.

Bigler, E. (2006). Traumatic brain injury and cognitive reserve (85–116). In: *Cognitive reserve: theory and application* (ed Y. Stern). Taylor & Francis, New York.

Blomquist, K.B. and Danner, F. (1987). Effects of physical conditioning on information-processing efficiency. *Perceptual Motor Skills*, **65**, 175–86.

Blomstrand, E., Perrett, D., Parry-Billings, M., and Newsholme, E.A. (1989). Effect of sustained exercise on plasma amino acid concentrations and on 5-hydroxytryptamine metabolism in six different brain regions in the rat. *Acta Physiologica Scandinavica*, **136**, 473–81.

Butler, S.M., Ashford, J.W., and Snowdon, D.A. (1996). Age, education, and changes in the Mini-Mental State Exam scores of older women: findings from the Nun Study. *Journal of the American Geriatrics Society*, **44**, 675–81.

Cabeza, R. (2002). Hemispheric asymmetry reduction in older adults: the HAROLD model. *Psychology and Aging*, **17**, 85–100.

Cabeza, R., Grady, C.L., Nyberg, L., *et al.* (1997). Age-related differences in effective neural connectivity during encoding and retrieval: a positron emission tomography study. *Journal of Neuroscience*, **17**, 391–400.

Cabeza, R., Anderson, N.D., Locantore, J.K., and McIntosh, A.R. (2002). Aging gracefully: compensatory brain activity in high-performing older adults. *NeuroImage*, **17**, 1394–1402.

Cabeza, R., Daselaar, S.M., Dolcos, F., Prince, S.E., Budde, M., and Nyberg, L. (2004). Task-independent and task-specific age effects on brain activity during working memory, visual attention and episodic retrieval. *Cerebral Cortex*, **14**, 364–75.

Christensen, H., Korten, A.E., Jorm, A.F., *et al.* (1997). Education and decline in cognitive performance: compensatory but not protective. *International Journal of Geriatric Psychiatry*, **12**, 323–30.

Cobb, J.L., Wolf, P.A., Au, R., White, R., and D'Agostino, R.B. (1995). The effect of education on the incidence of dementia and Alzheimer's disease in the Framingham Study. *Neurology*, **45**, 1707–12.

Colcombe, S. and Kramer, A.F. (2003). Fitness effects on the cognitive function of older adults: a meta-analytic study. *Psychological Science*, **14**, 125–30.

Cotman, C.W. and Berchtold, N.C. (2002). Exercise: a behavioral intervention to enhance brain health and plasticity. *Trends in Neurosciences*, **25**, 295–301.

Deutsch, G., Halsey, J. H., and Harrell, L. E. (1993). Exaggerated cortical blood flow reactivity in early Alzheimer's disease during successful task performance. *Journal of Clinical and Experimental Neuropsychology*, **15**, 71.

Evans, D.A., Beckett, L.A., Albert, M.S., *et al.* (1993). Level of education and change in cognitive function in a community population of older persons. *Annals of Epidemiology*, **3**, 71–7.

Evans, D.A., Hebert, L.E., Beckett, L.A., *et al.* (1997). Education and other measures of socioeconomic status and risk of incident Alzheimer disease in a defined population of older person. *Archives of Neurology*, **54**, 1399–1405.

Fabrigoule, C., Letenneur, L., Dartigues, J.F., Zarrouk, M., Commenges, D., and Barberger-Gateau, P. (1995). Social and leisure activities and risk of dementia: a prospective longitudinal study. *Journal of the American Geriatrics Society*, **43**, 485–90.

Farmer, M.E., Kittner, S.J., Rae, D.S., Bartko, J.J., and Regier, D.A. (1995). Education and change in cognitive function: The epidemiologic catchment area study. *Annals of Epidemiology*, **5**, 1–7.

Folstein, M., Folstein, S., and McHugh, P. (1975). 'Mini-mental state': a practical method for grading the cognitive state of patients for the clinician. *Journal of Psychiatric Research*, **12**, 189–98.

Grady, C.L., Haxby, J.V., Horwitz, B., *et al.* (1993). Activation of cerebral blood flow during a visuoperceptual task in patients with Alzheimer-type dementia. *Neurobiology of Aging*, **14**, 35–44.

Grady, C.L., Maisog, J.M., Horwitz, B., *et al.* (1994). Age-related changes in cortical blood flow activation during visual processing of faces and location. *Journal of Neuroscience*, **14**, 1450–62.

Grady, C.L., Horwitz, B., Pietrini, P., *et al.* (1996). The effect of task difficulty on cerebral blood flow during perceptual matching of faces. *Human Brain Mapping*, **4**, 227–39.

Graves, A.B., Mortimer, J.A., Larson, E.B., Wenzlow, A., Bowen, J.D., and McCormick, W.C. (1996). Head circumference as a measure of cognitive reserve. Association with severity of impairment in Alzheimer's disease. *British Journal of Psychiatry*, **169**, 86–92.

Grealy, M.A., Johnson, D.J., and Rushton, S.K. (1999). Improving cognitive function after brain injury: the use of exercise and virtual reality. *Archives of Physical Medicine and Rehabilitation*, **80**, 661–7.

Gur, R.C., Gur, R.E., Skolnick, B.E., *et al*. (1988). Effects of task difficulty on regional cerebral blood flow: Relationships with anxiety and performance. *Psychophysiology*, **25**, 392–9.

Hall, K.S., Gao, S., Unverzagt, F.W., and Hendrie, H. (2000). Low education and childhood rural residence: risk for Alzheimer's disease in African Americans. *Neurology*, **54**, 95–9.

Helmer, C., Letenneur, L., Rouch, I., *et al*. (2001). Occupation during life and risk of dementia in French elderly community residents. *Journal of Neurology, Neurosurgery and Psychiatry*, **71**, 303–9.

Ince, P. (2001). Pathological correlates of late-onset dementia in a multicentre community-based population in England and Wales. *Lancet*, **357**, 169–75.

Jacobs, B., Schall, M., and Scheibel, A.B. (1993). A quantitative dendritic analysis of Wernicke's area in humans. II: Gender, hemispheric, and environmental factors. *Journal of Comparative Neurology*, **327**, 97–111.

Jorm, A.F., Rodgers, B., Henderson, A.S., *et al*. (1998). Occupation type as a predictor of cognitive decline and dementia in old age. *Age and Ageing*, **27**, 477–83.

Katzman, R. (1993). Education and the prevalence of dementia and Alzheimer's disease. *Neurology*, **43**, 13–20.

Katzman, R., Terry, R., DeTeresa, R., *et al*. (1988). Clinical, pathological, and neurochemical changes in dementia: a subgroup with preserved mental status and numerous neocortical plaques. *Annals of Neurology*, **23**, 138–44.

Kesler, S.R., Adams, H.F., Blasey, C.M., and Bigler, E.D. (2003). Premorbid intellectual functioning, education, and brain size in traumatic brain injury: an investigation of the cognitive reserve hypothesis. *Applied Neuropsychology*, **10**, 153–62.

Kleim, J.A., Jones, T.A., and Schallert, T. (2003). Motor enrichment and the induction of plasticity before or after brain injury. *Neurochemical Research*, **28**, 1757–69.

Letenneur, L., Commenges, D., Dartigues, J.F., and Barberger-Gateau, P. (1994). Incidence of dementia and Alzheimer's disease in elderly community residents of south-western France. *International Journal of Epidemiology*, **23**, 1256–61.

Li, S.-C., and Lindenberger, U. (1999). Cross-level unification: a computational exploration of the link between deterioration of neurotransmitter systems and dedifferentiation of cognitive abilities in old age. In: *Cognitive neuroscience of memory* (ed L.-G. Nilsson and H.J. Markowitsch), pp. 103–46. Hogrefe & Huber, Seattle, WA.

Lyekotsos, C.G., Chen, L.-S., and Anthony, J.C. (1999). Cognitive decline in adulthood: an 11.5-year follow-up of the Baltimore Epidemiologic Catchment Area study. *American Journal of Psychiatry*, **156**, 58–65.

Nielson, K.A., Langenecker, S.A., and Garavan, H.P. (2002). Differences in the functional neuronanatomy of inhibitory control across the adult life span. *Psychology and Aging*, **17**, 56–71.

Paykel, E.S., Brayne, C., Huppert, F.A., *et al*. (1994) Incidence of dementia in a population older than 75 years in the United Kingdom. *Archives of General Psychiatry*, **51**, 325–32.

Qiu, C.X., Backman, L., Winblad, B., Aguero-Torres, H., and Fratiglioni, L. (2001). The influence of education on clinical diagnosed dementia: incidence and mortality data from the Kungsholmen Project. *Archives of Neurology*, **58**, 2034–9.

Reuter-Lorenz, P.A., Jonides, J., Smith, E.S., *et al.* (2000). Age differences in frontal lateralization of verbal and spatial working memory revealed by PET. *Journal of Cognitive Neuroscience*, **12**, 174–87.

Richards, M. and Sacker, A. (2003). Lifetime antecedents of cognitive reserve. *Journal of Clinical and Experimental Neuropsychology*, **25**, 614–64.

Rocca, W.A., Bonaiuto, S., Lippi, A., *et al.* (1990). Prevalence of clinically diagnosed Alzheimer's disease and other dementing disorders: a door-to-door survey in Appignano, Macerata Province, Italy. *Neurology*, **40**, 626–31.

Ropacki, M.T. and Elias, J.W. (2003). Preliminary examination of cognitive reserve theory in closed head injury. *Archives of Clinical Neuropsychology*, **18**, 643–54.

Rosen, A.C., Prull, M.W., O'Hara, R., *et al.* (2002). Variable effects of aging on frontal lobe contributions to memory. *Neuroreport*, **13**, 2425–8.

Rypma, B., Prabhakaran, V., Desmond, J.E., Glover, G.H., and Gabrieli, J.D. (1999). Load-dependent roles of frontal brain regions in the maintenance of working memory. *NeuroImage*, **9**, 216–26.

Salthouse, T.A. (1996). The processing-speed theory of adult age differences in cognition. *Psychological Review*, **103**, 403–28.

Salthouse, T.A. (2006). Mental exercise and mental aging. *Perspectives on Psychological Science*, **1**, 68–87.

Satz, P. (1993). Brain reserve capacity on symptom onset after brain injury: a formulation and review of evidence for threshold theory. *Neuropsychology*, **7**, 273–95.

Scarmeas, N. and Stern, Y. (2003). Cognitive reserve and lifestyle. *Journal of Clinical and Experimental Neuropsychology*, **5**, 625–33.

Scarmeas, N., Levy, G., Tang, M.-X., Manly, J., and Stern, J. (2001). Influence of leisure activity on the incidence of Alzheimer's disease. *Neurology*, **57**, 2236–42.

Scarmeas, N., Zarahn, E., Anderson, K.E., *et al.* (2003). Association of life activities with cerebral blood flow in Alzheimer disease: implications for cognitive reserve hypothesis. *Archives of Neurology*, **60**, 359–65.

Scarmeas, N., Zarahn, E., Anderson, K.E., *et al.* (2004). Cognitive reserve-mediated modulation of positron emission tomographic activations during memory tasks in Alzheimer disease. *Archives of Neurology*, **61**, 73–8.

Schmand, B., Smit, J.H., Geerlings, M.I., and Lindeboom, J. (1997) The effects of intelligence and education on the development of dementia: a test of the brain reserve hypothesis. *Psychological Medicine*, **27**, 1337–44.

Schofield, P.W., Logroscino, G., Andrews, H., Albert, S., and Stern, Y. (1997). An association between head circumference and Alzheimer's disease in a population based study of aging. *Neurology*, **49**, 30–7.

Schulkin, J. (ed). (1989). *Preoperative events: their effects on behavior following brain damage.* Lawrence Erlbaum, Hillsdale, NJ.

Stebbins, G.T., Carrillo, M.C., Dorman, J., *et al.* (2002). Aging effects on memory encoding in the frontal lobes. *Psychology and Aging*, **17**, 44–55.

Stern, Y. (2002). What is cognitive reserve? Theory and research application of the reserve concept. *Journal of the International Neuropsychological Society*, **8**, 448–60.

Stern, Y. (2006). Cognitive reserve and Alzheimer disease. *Alzheimer Disease and Associated Disorders*, **2**, 112–17.

Stern, Y., Alexander, G.E., Prohovnik, I., and Mayeux, R. (1992). Inverse relationship between education and parietotemporal perfusion deficit in Alzheimer's disease. *Annals of Neurology*, **32**, 371–5.

Stern, Y., Gurland, B., Tatemichi, T.K., Tang, M.X., Wilder, D., and Mayeux, R. (1994). Influence of education and occupation on the incidence of Alzheimer's disease. *Journal of the American Medical Association*, **271**, 1004–10.

Stern, Y., Alexander, G.E., Prohovnik, I., *et al.* (1995a). Relationship between lifetime occupation and parietal flow: implications for a reserve against Alzheimer's disease pathology. *Neurology*, **45**, 55–60.

Stern, Y., Tang, M. X., Denaro, J., and Mayeux, R. (1995b). Increased risk of mortality in Alzheimer's disease patients with more advanced educational and occupational attainment. *Annals of Neurology*, **37**, 590–5.

Stern, Y., Moeller, J.R., Anderson, K.E., *et al.* (2000). Different brain networks mediate task performance in normal aging and AD: defining compensation. *Neurology*, **55**, 1291–7.

Stern, Y., Zarahn, E., Hilton, H.J., Flynn, J., De La Paz, R., and Rakitin, B. (2003). Exploring the neural basis of cognitive reserve. *Journal of Clinical and Experimental Neuropsychology*, **25**, 691–701.

Stern, Y., Habeck, C., Moeller, J., *et al.* (2005). Brain networks associated with cognitive reserve in healthy young and old adults. *Cerebral Cortex*, **15**, 394–402.

White, L., Katzman, R., Losonczy, K., *et al.* (1994). Association of education with incidence of cognitive impairment in three established populations for epidemiological studies of the elderly. *Journal of Clinical Epidemiology*, **47**, 363–74.

Young, R.J. (1979). The effect of regular exercise on cognitive functioning and personality. *British Journal of Sports Medicine*, **13**, 110–17.

Zarahn, E., Rakitin, B., Abela, D., Flynn, J., and Stern, Y. (2007). Age-related changes in brain activation during a delayed item recognition task. *Neurobiology of Aging*, **28**, 784–98.

Zelinski, E.M. and Lewis, K.L. (2003). Adult age differences in multiple cognitive functions: Differentiation, dedifferentiation, or process-specific change? *Psychology and Aging*, **18**, 727–45.

Zhang, M., Katzman, R., Salmon, D., *et al.* (1990). The prevalence of dementia and Alzheimer's disease in Shanghai, China: impact of age, gender and education. *Annals of Neurology*, **27**, 428–37.

3

Motivational disorders following brain injury

Michael Oddy*, Andrew Worthington†, and Elizabeth Francis‡

* Brain Injury Rehabilitation Trust, Horsham, West Sussex, and University of Swansea

† Brain Injury Rehabilitation Trust, Birmingham

‡ Kent and Medway NHS and Social Care Partnership Trust

Introduction

Impaired motivation is a frequently described consequence of acquired brain injury and is often attributed to disorders of the frontal lobes. However, the common use of the term motivation in everyday language and the myriad of related terms in the scientific and clinical literature mean that complex and contradictory concepts are often used without definition or clarity. For example, terms such as drive, need, want, and will are used in different and overlapping ways by various writers.

The aim of this chapter is to provide a unifying framework to classify motivational deficits following brain injury. It will be argued that the term 'motivation' is commonly used to describe goal-directed behaviour and that it is unnecessary to invoke a metaphysical élan or motivational force separate from the processes of emotion and cognition. The framework is based on theories of executive function, and it is argued that deficits ascribed to motivation can be explained as deficits in the function of executive control systems. It encompasses multiple stages in goal-directed activity from an initial idea or goal through to the accomplishment of that goal with a review process providing feedback to enable a learning mechanism that influences further goal oriented activity. This conceptualization of goal-directed behaviour will be used to classify different ways in which goal-directed behaviour or motivation breaks down and to suggest effective interventions. Although it is primarily a cognitive framework, it is acknowledged that affective or emotional processes as well as cognitive processes are involved. Following their brain injury, some patients show little or no interest in activities they previously valued highly. However, these patients also show an absence of emotional responsiveness in other respects, such as in response to potentially upsetting situations (Habib 2000). This suggests that the fundamental deficit is one of emotional responsiveness rather than a separate motivational responsiveness. Similarly, emotional or affective factors play a part in the maintenance and reinforcement of goal-directed behaviour in terms of reward systems and emotional reactions to the achievement of goals.

It is hoped that the framework will bring clarity to the different and overlapping terms and concepts used to describe what are apparently 'motivational' deficits following brain injury.

Review of current concepts in disorders of motivation

In this section the terms and concepts that have been used to describe deficits in motivation following brain injury will be reviewed. This will be followed by an attempt to classify them in terms of the unifying framework

Low levels of arousal

Changes in arousal level during the acute stage are extremely common in brain injury, particularly diffuse injury. However, they can also occur as chronic deficits. Arousal deficits are characterized by lethargy and drowsiness (Lishman 1987), and are frequently associated with severe brainstem injuries. Whyte (1992) defines arousal as the general receptivity to sensory stimuli and preparedness to respond. Thus arousal is seen as a general state without a specific target and stimulus. Deficits in arousal concern the energizing (quantitative) aspects of motivation rather than the directional (qualitative) aspects.

Following severe brain injury individuals often pass through stages of unconsciousness. These include a stage of unconsciousness which may be followed by a stage of persistent vegetative state and then the minimally conscious states where responsiveness is erratic or inconsistent. These differ from the locked-in syndrome, commonly associated with damage to the ventral pons (Smith and Delargy 2005) in which a person is conscious and aware of their environment and circumstances but unable (or minimally able) to respond physically or verbally to this.

Lack of energy when fully alert

The term anergia is used as a descriptive term to characterize the lack of energy that is observed in some patients who appear fully alert (Jorge et al. 1993).

Similarly, the term adynamia is often used as a general term to describe a lack of energy or goal-directed activity following brain injury (e.g. Simpson *et al.* 2001). The term adynamia is sometimes used more specifically to refer to a condition of flaccid paralysis resulting from muscle weakness (Beaumont *et al.* 1996), first described by Gamstorp (1956), in which an imbalance of potassium precipitates the onset of weakness.

Lack of initiation of activity

Several terms (abulia, aspontaneity, and akinesia) are used to denote problems with initiating behaviour. Aspontaneity appears to be used primarily in a purely descriptive fashion. Akinesia (and hypokinesia) is used to denote any poverty or slowness of movement (Beaumont *et al.* 1996) not attributable to sensory or motor neuron pathway damage. It takes many forms and may be manifested, for example, in a blank expression, an absence of blinking, reduced swinging of the arms when walking, or poverty of spontaneous speech. Lack of spontaneous initiation is commonly seen in Parkinson's disease (PD), whereas near-normal movement patterns may be provoked by external stimuli (akinesia paradoxica). Loss of movement due to akinesia has to be differentiated from physical deficits such as hemiplegia or psychiatric states such as catatonia. Therefore akinesia is a distinct motor disorder usually attributed to basal ganglia dysfunction or to lesions of the corpus callosum by involvement of the diencephalic structures (Heilman and Watson 1991). In comparison, psychic akinesia refers to a loss of spontaneous mental processing, also called auto-activation disorder (Laplane and Dubois 2001), in the context of normal externally triggered mental function. This concept is subtly different from, but overlaps, the notion of abulia.

Abulia is derived from the Greek word *boul* (will) (Marin 1990). Individuals suffering from abulia are said to lack spontaneity in actions and speech and to show psychomotor retardation. The individual is alert but shows little or no initiative, and is slow to initiate movements in response to commands, either internal or external. Fisher (1983) suggested that abulia is a specific neurological syndrome associated with psychomotor retardation, presenting in its extreme form as akinetic mutism. The features of this syndrome include decreased responsiveness, absence of enthusiasm, lack of interest, apathy, and lack of spontaneity. Motor responses are slow and hesitant, but paradoxically perseveration may be present, particularly with repetition of verbal responses. The person may show reduced emotional expression and feeling. The individual is characteristically alert and depression is not prominent, although it may appear to be. The patient may be temporarily roused by external stimulation but lapses back after this ceases. Fisher uses a 'butter sculpture' analogy to denote the inert appearance of the patient who may nevertheless be triggered into action by a well-learned automatic response such as answering a telephone when it rings. Brown and Marsden (1998) describe abulia as a kind of psychic akinesia similar to, and associated with, motor akinesia. These authors add that this condition is characterized by apathy but not low mood. It needs careful differentiation from catatonia on initial presentation (Muquit *et al.* 2001) but has a very different pathophysiology (Al-Adawi *et al.* 2000). Abulia is considered to represent a disconnection of input from output so 'neither thought nor sensory information are linked to mental or physical action'. Eames (2001) notes that this is invariably accompanied by extrapyramidal disorders (cogwheel rigidity; impassive facial expression) and is particularly common following anterior cerebral artery lesions resulting from axonal damage or destruction of cells of the dopaminergic meso-cingulate system (Fisher 1983). As a result abulia often responds to dopamine agonists, such as bromocriptine or carbidopa/levodopa (Drubach *et al.* 1995; Al-Adawi *et al.* 2000; see also Chapter 15, this volume). Abulia has been reported following damage to fronto-subcortical circuits, involving the anterior cingulate (Grunsfeld and Login 2006), the putamen (Nagaratnam *et al.* 2001), and the internal capsule (Pantoni *et al.* 2001). Abulia secondary to an intra-cranial mass lesion has recently been proposed as an explanation for the philosopher Nietzsche spending the last 7 years of his life in a state of docile mutism (Owen *et al.* 2007).

In summary, abulia appears to be most commonly described as a cluster of symptoms characterized by a lack of spontaneity and slowness and rigidity of movement, but there is less consensus on whether it should be understood as a primary disorder of motivation or a disconnection between the desire to act and the ability to act on that intention (Vijayaraghavan *et al.* 2002).

Deficits in reward-based systems

Other descriptions of motivation disorders focus on the inability to take pleasure in the achievement of goals. Emotional indifference describes an inability to experience any emotions with the normal intensity. It is variously described as a lack of emotional responsivity to events, emotional blunting, and flat affect. Andersson *et al.* (1999a) suggested that a lack of emotional responsivity is associated with reduced psychophysiological reactivity. Emotional indifference is reported to be associated with right hemisphere lesions (e.g. Gianotti 1989).

Athymia is another term that refers to loss of affect-driven behaviour (Habib and Galaburda 1998). Subsequently Habib (2000) reintroduced the hybrid term athymhormia (reflecting its Greek roots of impulse or drive, and affect), first proposed in 1922, to describe the combination of drive and affect that underlies motivation. Habib proposed a model incorporating cortico-subcortical circuits (or loops) integrating cognitive processes (associative loop), emotion (limbic loop), and behaviour (motor loop), all critically implicating the striatum.

The term anhedonia is used to refer to a lack of the ability to experience pleasure as opposed to a more general emotional indifference, and is associated with a dopaminergic meso-limbic reward system implicating prefrontal cortex and ventral striatum (Robbins and Evritt 1996). Wood and Eames (1981) viewed hedonic responsiveness as an essential prerequisite for motivation. Eames (2001) describes this as a disorder of the reward-based drive system— the loss of the ability to experience pleasure. However, this use of the term drive is confusing, since the concept of drive in experimental psychology has been used to refer to the specific motivation to obtain one type of reward (e.g. hunger drive, sex drive, etc.) rather than a general 'pleasure centre' such as that first proposed by Olds and Milner (1954) following work with rats. Wood (2001) equated drive with effort, suggesting that this is determined by the strength of a need state (such as thirst), which establishes a motivational incentive to action. However, effort is also often seen as a reflection of motivation, and the relationships between the three terms drive, effort, and motivation are rarely made clear.

Apathy

Apathy is normally defined as a lack of interest or motivation. As such, it embraces the whole range of motivational deficits. Marin (1991) proposed a relatively elaborate theory of motivation which includes the concept of apathy as a syndrome separable from apathy as a symptom. In this model, apathy as a syndrome refers to the simultaneous decrease in the behavioural, emotional, and cognitive concomitants of goal-directed behaviour. Marin (1991) suggests that lack of concern, indifference, and reduced initiative share a common motivational deficit, with lack of effort and initiative being the major behavioural characteristics. Lack of interest, curiosity, concern, and insight are the cognitive characteristics, while emotional flatness, lack of responsivity towards positive, and negative events are the emotional characteristics, similar to the Habib model described above, of three interconnected motivation circuits for affect, cognition, and behaviour. Marin suggests that abulia and apathy are part of a continuum of motivational impairments with abulia at the extreme end of the spectrum. The central feature of apathy as a syndrome in this model is the reduction in goal-directed activity due to lack of motivation. In other words, the diagnosing clinician has to distinguish between a lack of goal-directed activity due to loss of motivation and as a result of other factors, such as depression. If lack of motivation is not the dominant feature, then apathy is a symptom of some other syndrome. Marin argues that by specifying that the emotional, cognitive, and behavioural aspects of apathy must all be present, diagnostic distinctions can be made and this avoids the circularity that at first sight appears present in this formulation. Nevertheless it is an idiosyncratic way of defining motivation. For example, he states that for individuals with depression, the lack of interest reflects despair, hopelessness, and pessimism about the likelihood of achieving their goals. The distinction appears to be that people suffering from depression are dissuaded from pursuing their goals as they are pessimistic about their chances of success whereas those suffering from apathy no longer value the attainment of goals.

There is certainly support for the notion that apathy can occur in the presence or absence of depression after brain injury (e.g. Kant *et al.* 1998; Andersson *et al.* 1999b). However, it is unclear whether it is helpful to consider apathy as a single syndrome across conditions (Rao *et al.* 2007). Moreover, the hypothesis is underspecified in key respects, for example whether the cognitive and emotional components of apathy always occur together or impaired motivation can result from all (or some) of the cognitive or emotional components alone.

In the present chapter it is proposed that motivation can break down in a number of different ways, which can be elaborated using established notions of executive function. Executive functions are typically considered to involve a cluster of behaviours, which includes the initiation, planning, and monitoring of goal-directed behaviour (Lezak *et al.* 2004). Much of the literature implicates frontal lobe damage in disorders of executive function. However, executive functions are also sensitive to damage in other parts of the brain, such as subcortical damage following anoxic conditions involving the limbic structures. Al-Adawi *et al.* (1998) suggest that apathy and motivational deficits are a manifestation of disrupted executive function and reflect disturbance within a frontal-subcortical circuit (the meso-limbic and meso-cortical circuitry). Thus motivational deficits arising from executive disorders may reflect impairment of the cognitive component of goal-directed activity (e.g. planning, organizational skills, and self-monitoring). Motivational deficits also arise from impairment of the *affective* aspects of goal-directed behaviour, which can also be ascribed to an executive/frontal lobe deficit, as evidenced by the growing literature on the relevance of the ventro-medial prefrontal cortex in mediating the affective component of motivation (Robbins and Evritt 1996).

Framework for understanding and managing motivation disorders

Energizing aspect: arousal levels and fatigue

Arousal refers to a generalized state of responsiveness to environmental stimuli and preparedness to act or respond (Whyte 1992; Wroblewski and Glenn 1994). It is seen as a general state without a specific target or stimulus, analogous to cortical tone, which fluctuates during wakefulness or sleep, but which is underpinned by the brainstem reticular activating system.

Therefore injury to the brainstem often gives rise to low arousal, and may be associated with compression or herniation at the time of injury. Dysfunction at this level means that the individual presents as drowsy, sluggish, sleepy, and slow to respond. This may or may not be accompanied by a subjective sense of fatigue. However, fatigue is a common complaint following acquired brain injury (Quellet and Morin 2006) and can be seen as an additional general influence on the energizing aspect of goal-directed behaviour. Disturbances of arousal have been shown to undermine alertness and participation in rehabilitation (Worthington and Melia 2006).

Impaired arousal and fatigue have the potential to affect all stages in the proposed model of goal-directed activity. For example, arousal deficits may impede the initial stages of goal-directed activity by reducing the ability to respond to internal and external triggers and subsequently generate ideas.

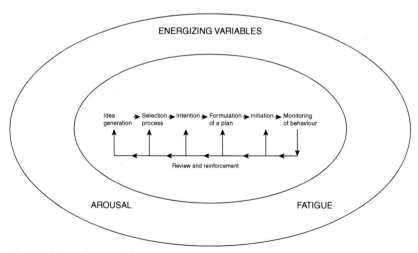

Fig. 3.1 Motivation model.

Stage 1. Idea generation

It is proposed that the first stage of goal-directed activity must involve the generation or production of goal-directed 'ideas'. These are seen as possible goals that the person may decide to pursue, either imminently or at a later date. The term 'ideas' does not imply subjective awareness or a conscious cognition at this stage, but is used to indicate that these potential goals have yet to be selected but constitute options from which a selection is made. 'Ideas' may arise from internal triggers which will include biological needs, akin to Wood's (2001) need states, as well as potential goals derived from cognitive processes, including goals such as curiosity, or altruistic goals. External triggers, such as unconditioned and conditioned stimuli, may also play a role here. Ideas may relate to short- or long-term goals. It is suggested that such goals only become conscious intentions if they are sufficiently complex to require high-level cognitive processes to be achieved. It is suggested that it is the invocation of the high-level cognitive processes that gives rise to consciousness or awareness of the goal.

A number of primary neurological factors can interrupt the ideas generation stage. If arousal level is impaired, there may be a paucity of ideas due to a reduced engagement with and hence reduced stimulation from the environment. Damage to specific centres, for example in the hypothalamus, may give rise to either a decrease or an increase in particular goal-directed ideas, such as hunger and thirst. Damage to frontal areas can lead to decreased emotional reactivity ('emotional indifference') and responsiveness, which may lead to a reduced production of ideas.

Attentional deficits affect the ability to select and attend to relevant aspects of the environment or context, and a reduction in the ability to produce cognitive ideas through reduced creative or divergent thinking (including bradyphrenia and psychic akinesia) will affect the production of ideas. Such deficits may manifest themselves as an apparent lack of concern, as the individual is unable to generate preferred activities or goals. The common problem of unawareness of deficit may inhibit the generation of certain goal-directed ideas.

Psychological influences on this process may include depression, although it is likely that depression influences later stages in this model (such as selection of ideas) rather than the generation of ideas. High levels of anxiety may produce distracting cognitions which prevent the emergence of ideas. It should be noted that the term ideas is not used here in the way that the terms motives or desires have been used. The suggestion is that 'ideas' themselves give rise to action without the need to infer a specific motivational force. The existence of an 'idea' gives rise to the following stages of goal-directed activity.

Stage 2. The selection process

This stage refers to the selection of goals. The first stage generates potential goals but not all of these can be pursued simultaneously and many will be completely discarded. Consequently there will be a need to prioritize and schedule goals. Hence concepts of goal hierarchy and biological imperative may be relevant, here incorporating notions of both reflexive and volitional or conscious selection. Different kind of goals will be sought under different kinds of prevailing conditions.

Potential goals need to be evaluated in terms of their desirability and their chances of attainment. 'Desirability' will depend upon a multitude of factors from biological survival to the way the goal fits into long-term life goals or strongly held values and beliefs. Some potential goals may need to be inhibited to make way for others or to conform to societal rules concerning acceptable behaviour.

Jahanshahi and Frith (1998) suggest that some patients have difficulty in suppressing externally triggered (pre-potent) goals to allow willed goals to be pursued. Frith (1992) suggests that such pre-potent goals are pursued because the individual lacks the ability to formulate a plan of action for more cognitively demanding goals. In other words, the deficit is not one of goal selection but one of plan formulation. In the framework proposed here, unlike Frith's proposal the distinction between routine action and 'willed' action is seen only as a matter of complexity. With more complex and novel goals higher cognitive processes need to be called into play. This has the effect of involving conscious awareness of the process. We take as evidence for this position the fact that 'willed' action can be impaired when routine action is spared, but we are not aware of patients for whom routine action is impaired whilst 'willed' action is spared. This suggests that the difference is that in 'willed' action more complex systems, but not entirely different systems, are involved.

In neurophysiological terms a lateral inhibition mechanism is proposed. Selection of a goal would automatically reduce activation thresholds in (anatomically and/or functionally) neighbouring networks on a gradient according to degree of incompatibility, such that the most strongly inhibited would be the goals which were most directly in competition with the selected goal. There is already evidence that such a mechanism operates, as selection of movement involves active suppression of unwanted movements in the prefrontal cortex (de Jong and Paans 2007).

Potential neurological influences on this process include slowed information processing. More specific influences will include:

(1) reasoning deficits which may result in difficulty in the prioritization of goals;

(2) selective attention deficits which may mean that the individual arbitrarily alights on certain goals at the expense of others;

(3) impulsivity which can be defined as the inability to inhibit competing goals or as the selection of goals without sufficient processing of their advantages and disadvantages;

(4) unawareness of deficit which may mean that certain goals are not selected (although it is more probable that goals related to deficits of which the individual is unaware may not arise in the first place);

(5) memory impairments which may interfere with the ability to retain and recall potential goals for selection.

Psychological factors such as personality and previous experience will intervene here. The Hullian concept of drive strength (Hull 1943) is relevant, whereby the strength of the drive to pursue a goal is related to need and the attractiveness of reward. This can be seen as a neurological influence, depending on the nature of the need (e.g. is it a biological or a social need?). The extent to which the goal is perceived as rewarding and valued may also be influenced by a number of psychological factors. The perceived effort-to-reward ratio will be of significance, as will the goal's congruence with over-arching goals and with the individual's values and beliefs. Learned helplessness can be seen as a decision not to pursue a goal, and perceived self-efficacy (Bandura 1977) in relation to the goal will also influence whether the goal is selected. Anxiety may prevent a goal being selected where there is anxious avoidance of a particular activity.

Stage 3. Formulation of a plan

Planning has been described by many writers as the central part of executive function. Norman and Shallice (1986) describe two systems. One, contention scheduling, enables frequently used existing behavioural routines or schemas to be played out in appropriate circumstances. However, when the situation demands a new untried plan, the supervisory (attentional) system is invoked. This system demands conscious attention and may involve adapting existing schemas or devising new schemas or plans.

Even for simple motor responses there will be a number of levels at which such planning takes place: providing an overall plan of the appropriate motor response, devising a programme of neuronal activity to effect this, and preparation for action. Functional neuroimaging implicates a complex motor planning circuit involving dorsolateral prefrontal, anterior cingulate, caudate, and lateral premotor areas (Dagher et al. 1999). At a higher level of sophistication, Lezak et al. (2004) suggest that in order to plan one must be able to conceptualize changes from present circumstances (look ahead), deal objectively with oneself in relation to the environment, and view the environment objectively (take the abstract attitude). Where these abilities are compromised by brain injury, the ability to formulate a suitable plan for the achievement of a goal may be reduced or lost. Failure to develop a plan of action has been found to be associated with damage to the prefrontal cortex (Frith 1992), and to the dorsolateral prefrontal circuit in particular (Cummings 1993).

Stage 4. Initiation

It is evident from the clinical presentations of patients with brain injury that some lack the ability to initiate plans although it is clear that such plans have been formulated. For example, some patients may be able to describe plans in great detail even though they seem quite unable to implement them. Others are able to implement such a plan when there are sufficient external triggers or prompts, such as Fisher's example of patients automatically responding to a telephone ringing (Fisher 1983). Brown and Marsden's (1998) description of motor and psychic akinesia can also be seen as descriptions of this kind of deficit. Cummings (1993) argued that injury to the anterior cingulate circuit gives rise to problems in initiation.

It is possible to view initiation as a problem occurring earlier in the sequence of goal-directed activity, such that 'ideas' or intentions are themselves not initiated. This is potentially confusing, and one should distinguish between generation of ideas and their initiation. The fact that some clients are able to describe clear intentions, and even action plans, but are unable to translate them into action suggests that there is an initiation function following the formulation of a plan. We suggest that the term 'initiation' should be reserved for this type of deficit, i.e. initiation of a formed and selected goal. We suggest the inability to *generate* ideas or goals adequately describes the other type of deficit.

The concept of willed intentions or volition has sometimes been invoked to explain disorders of initiation (Jahanshahi and Frith 1998, Vijayaraghavan *et al.* 2002). This has been used to explain the observation that actions consciously intended appear harder to initiate (e.g. in patients with Parkinson's syndrome) than automatic overlearned or reflexive actions. However, the fact that these actions are usually also impaired, at least to some extent, makes the current authors question whether there is a need to distinguish between conscious (subjectively aware) and unconscious goals. If there is no need to make this distinction, then the concept of willed action becomes redundant and the subjective experience of intentionality would appear to be an artefact of the increased complexity of the task and the greater attentional resources and cognitive processing required for its planning and execution.

There may be other reasons why initiation of goal-directed activity fails to occur. For example, those suffering from dyspraxia may not be able to initiate an activity because of motor programming difficulties, whilst those with attentional problems may be distractible and lose track of their planned goal.

Stage 5. Monitoring behaviour

If goals or intentions are to be followed through and successfully attained, the individual needs to monitor the primacy of the current goal (over competing goals), the success of the plan in moving towards the goal (and to modify the plan as necessary), and the time constraints to implement the plan. Damage to the prefrontal cortex is associated with maintenance and shifting of action (Norman and Shallice 1986; Jahanshahi and Frith 1998). Failure in any of these requirements results in going off at a tangent and hence failure to accomplish the goal, not completing the task because of time limitations, and being inflexible in terms of modifying the plan (an extreme form of which can be seen as being represented by perseveration). These are all well recognized and common symptoms of acquired brain injury.

Prospective memory deficits can be seen as an example of a failure to pursue a goal through failing to monitor or focus on the goal (see Chapter 5, this volume).

Stage 6. Review and reinforcement

The function of this stage is to review the achievement of a goal in order to learn from the experience so that this or similar goals can be attained more efficiently in future. The consequence of a failure in this process is that the person will fail to learn from experience and will repeat inefficient or even unsuccessful plans in the future. Once again, there is no implication that the person is necessarily aware of this process of review, but it will be reflected in their actions regardless of such awareness. It is suggested that awareness depends on the complexity of the goal-directed activity and hence the level and extent of cognitive processes involved.

Consequences which increase or decrease the probability that behaviour will be repeated (in response to the same conditions, triggers, or stimuli) play a role here. For example, classical and operant conditioning are examples of this process where the outcome or consequence of a behaviour alters the probability of that behaviour occurring in future. Damasio's somatic marker hypothesis (Damasio *et al.* 1991) explains deficits of this kind. This theory suggests that emotional connotations become attached to different forms of behaviour as positive or negative markers depending on their outcome. When this process fails due to brain injury negative (or positive) outcomes fail to influence future behaviour.

Anhedonia (loss of the ability to experience pleasure) will exert its influence at this stage because of its impact on the reinforcement of behaviour. Neuropsychological influences will include the ability to reflect on and evaluate success or achievement. Episodic memory appears to play a part here in that this is considered to free human beings from being 'slaves to their experience' and allows them to review recent experience in the light of previous experience (Baddeley 1990).

Additional influences will include the subjective value of reward, which may change from the anticipated value once attained, and repeated failure, which may lead to learned helplessness. The achievement of a goal may result in a variety of emotional experiences, and any change or reduction in the ability for affective experience is likely to have an impact on goal-directed activity.

Clinical utility of the proposed model

In working clinically with motivation deficits, it is important to assess and carefully tease out the contributing factors in order to guide the formulation and target appropriate interventions. This process of assessment and formulation is important, not only to aid in the selection of appropriate intervention strategies but also to enable clients and their families to understand the nature of their problems and to avoid the frustration and blame that can often occur in the context of (apparent) motivational deficits. As depression can give rise to an appearance of poor motivation, it is important to establish first whether the client is depressed and if so to treat this appropriately. In practice, however, depression is often misdiagnosed when the problem is one of a primary motivation disorder. Response to antidepressants should be closely monitored when the diagnosis is uncertain as this can help to distinguish the possibilities.

Energizing behaviour

There are a number of studies which describe the effectiveness of pharmacological interventions (many of which enhance dopaminergic function) on neurological influences on motivation (e.g. Van Reekum et al. 1995; Powell et al. 1996). However, choice of pharmacological intervention for energizing deficits depends on underlying pathophysiology. Eames (2001) argues that anergia (and similar sounding conditions like aspontaneity and apathy) may not respond to dopamine agonists (DAs) because the damage arises from DA target neurons in the meso-cingulate system. In such cases environmental modification or educational/behavioural management approaches may also have a role in helping to ameliorate primary influences, for example where problems with fatigue interfere with motivation (Burgess and Chalder 2005).

Generating ideas

To establish whether there is a problem at the level of idea generation will require determining whether the individual has ideas but is simply failing to act upon them. If the person does not have or is unable to report such ideas, it is important to determine whether this is general or restricted to certain aspects of behaviour such as eating. If it is a general paucity of ideas, simply providing the client with a list from which to select may help compensate for this problem. If this is not successful Levine *et al.* (2000, 2007) have described an intervention known as Goal Management Training. This is a multistage procedure which provides a structure for generating ideas or goals.

The role of unawareness of deficit on ideas generation and the goal-selection stage of motivation has been mentioned. In neurorehabilitation, unawareness of deficit needs to be carefully managed to optimize motivation through collaborative goal negotiation (van den Broek 2005), whilst continuing to sustain hope and optimism (Herbert and Powell 1989).

Selection process

Perhaps the most commonly arising problems here concern indecision over which goals to pursue and impulsivity of decision choice, sometimes resulting in disinhibited actions. If the problem arises from indecision, helping the client use a problem-solving strategy may reduce the impact of this problem. If the problem arises from impulsivity, a stop and think strategy may be implemented (see Chapter 4 for a discussion of these types of intervention). Techniques drawn from 'motivational interviewing' (Rollnick and Miller 1995, Bombardier and Rimmele 1999) may be useful here, helping the individual to draw upon their own beliefs, assumptions and overarching goals to select more specific goals.

Formulation of a plan

A number of studies have proposed ways to provide planning and problem solving training to people who have deficits in these areas (see Chapter 4, this volume). These approaches usually involve using one of two methods. The first is some form of framework with steps for the individual to work through in a prescribed and systematic fashion in order to arrive at a plan of action. An elaborate form of this approach, in which a medical practitioner was taught to use a checklist to systematically make a diagnosis, was described by von Cramon and Matthes-von Cramon (1994). For those for whom such an approach is too difficult, a predetermined routine can be used. This is common practice in brain injury rehabilitation in the context of both memory and exec-utive deficits. The routine may simply be taught to the client in a systematic and consistent fashion (e.g. Parish and Oddy 2007) or the client may be given a written or electronic series of instructions to follow (eg Clark-Wilson 1988).

Initiation

There is evidence for successful pharmacological intervention when the deficit concerns the translation of intentions into action. Both sinemet and bromocriptine may help alleviate symptoms (Eames 1989). Environmental manipulations that take advantage of the fact that automatic motor responses are often superior to intentional acts have also been tried. For example, the gait of patients with Parkinson's disease can be improved by drawing lines on the floor (Martin 1967). For more complex patterns of behaviour, a strict routine which, once triggered, will enable the individual to pass seamlessly from one phase to another (e.g. a personal hygiene and dressing routine) may enable greater independence. Self-instructional methods have also been applied to those with initiation difficulties. Evans (Chapter 4, this volume) describes the use of such an approach with a client who chose the phrase 'Just do it' to prompt himself in to action. Evans also describes the use of an external prompting system (the Neuropage) to help a woman with initiation problems.

Monitoring behaviour

If assessment reveals a problem at this stage of the process, compensatory means of helping the client monitor their behaviour may reduce the impact of the deficit. Alderman *et al.* (1995) described a method of teaching the client to use a form of self-monitoring. Evans *et al.* (1998) have described the use of electronic prompts to help a person to monitor time and to act at the appropriate time.

Review and reinforcement

Once again interventions need to be designed following a careful assessment of the exact nature of the deficit. At one level behavioural approaches address-ing the reinforcements available for behaviours may be relevant. Helping the client to monitor and reflect on their behaviour may be helpful.

Behavioural approaches may have a role to play in enhancing motivation by maximizing the experience of success and providing contingent feedback and reward. Interventions based on operant techniques, backward chaining, and errorless learning techniques may help to strengthen incentives and increase the reward value of goals and promote feelings of self-efficacy (see Worthington *et al.* (1997) for an example of cognitive-behavioural intervention being used to promote walking practice in two patients with reduced initiation). Behavioural interventions which facilitate intrinsic motivation for behaviour, and incorporate reinforcements that are meaningful and non-controlling, are likely to be most successful (Lepper *et al.* 1973; Langer and Rodin 1976) Where psychological factors such as attributions of success/failure and expectancies seem to be salient in understanding an individual's reduced motivation, cognitive interventions focusing upon attributions (e.g. to promote attribution of success to internal controllable stable factors (Weiner 1985)) and promotion of self-efficacy (e.g. working towards proximal subgoals that are relatively easily attainable) may be helpful.

Approaches to psychological influences on motivation in rehabilitation need to be multifaceted. There is a need to increase the expectation and possibility of success as well as to promote the individual's sense of control. It is important to secure positive supportive therapeutic relationships where emotional issues associated with adjustment and loss can be explored. Problems with depression need to be addressed, but sensitivity is required in order to deal with unawareness of deficit as the development of awareness may contribute to the emergence of depression thus having an adverse impact on motivation. The methods used in motivational interviewing may also be applied here.

Summary and conclusions

The framework of motivational deficits following brain injury proposed in this chapter is based on a model of goal-directed activity. The model suggests that loss of motivation can occur, not only to different degrees, but in a number of different ways and at different stages from the process of establishing the goal through to reviewing and refining the method of goal attainment. The advantages of this framework are that by identifying different forms of motivational breakdown different remedies may be suggested. Whilst many of the various forms of motivational breakdown will be familiar to clinicians, and are established in the literature, the framework suggests that double dissociations of types of motivational deficits may be observed. For example, there are patients who have no trouble generating ideas (which they can verbalize when asked to do so) but who cannot initiate goal-directed activity in relation to these. Frith (1992) has described these as patients who know what they want to do but cannot do it. There appear to be others who have difficulty in generating ideas but who, when provided with such ideas, can initiate relevant goal-directed activity. Further research to clarify the extent to which such deficits can occur independently or as a cluster in identifiable syndromes is required. Finally, given the terminological confusion in this area, a further advantage of the framework is the clear and unambiguous language with which to describe different motivational deficits.

The term motivation appears to have given rise to considerable confusion in relation to changes in goal-directed activity following brain injury. It is suggested that the above framework provides an alternative language with which to describe such changes. The stages, by indicating the processes that need to take place in the course of goal-directed activity, provide a means of identifying different ways in which the process can break down, leaving the term motivation for the study of why individuals select certain goals over others.

References

Al-Adawi, S., Powell, J.H., and Greenwood, R.J. (1998). Motivational deficits after brain injury: a neuropsychological approach using new assessment techniques. *Neuropsychology*, **12**, 115–24.

Al-Adawi, S., Dawe, G.S., and Al-Hussaini, A.A. (2000). Aboulia: neurobehavioural dysfunction of dopaminergic system. *Medical Hypotheses*, **54**, 523–30.

Alderman, N., Fry, R.K., and Youngson, H.A., 1995. Improvement of self-monitoring skills, reduction of behaviour disturbance and the dysexecutive syndrome: comparison of response cost and a new programme of self-monitoring training. *Neuropsychological Rehabilitation*, **5**, 193–221.

Andersson, S., Gundersen, P.M., and Finset, A. (1999a). Emotional activation during therapeutic interaction in traumatic brain injury: effect of apathy, self-awareness and implications for rehabilitation. *Brain Injury*, **13**, 393–404.

Andersson, S., Krogstad, J.M., and Finset, A. (1999b). Apathy and depressed mood in acquired brain damage: relationship to lesion localization and psychophysiological reactivity. *Psychological Medicine*, **29**, 447–56.

Baddeley, A.D. (1990). *Human memory: theory and practice*. Lawrence Erlbaum, Hove.

Bandura, A. (1977). Self-efficacy: toward a unifying theory of behavioural change. *Psychological Review*, **84**, 191–215.

Beaumont, G., Kenealy, P., and Rogers, M. (1996). *The Blackwell Dictionary of Neuropsychology*. Blackwells, Oxford.

Bombardier, C. and Rimmele, C. (1999). Motivational interviewing to prevent alcohol abuse after traumatic brain injury: a case series. *Rehabilitation Psychology*, **44**, 52–67.

Brown, P. and Marsden, C.D. (1998). What do the basal ganglia do? *Lancet*, **351**, 1801–4.

Burgess, M. and Chalder, T. (2005). *Overcoming chronic fatigue*. Robinson, London

Clark-Wilson, J. (1988). The use of a computer in aiding functional skill training: a single case study. *Clinical Rehabilitation*, **2**:199–206.

Cummings, J.L. (1993). Frontal-subcortical circuits and human behaviour. *Archives of Neurology*, **50**, 873–880.

Dagher, A., Owen, A.M., Boecker, H., and Brooks, D.J. (1999) Mapping the network for planning: a correlational PET activation study wiyth the Tower of London task. *Brain*, **122**, 1973–87.

Damasio, A.R., Tranel, D., and Damasio, H.C. (1991). Somatic markers and the guidance of behaviour: theory and preliminary testing. In: *Frontal lobe function and dysfunction* (ed H.S. Levin, H.M. Eisenberg, and A.L. Benton). pp. 217–229. Oxford University Press, New York.

De Jong, B.M. and Paans, A.M. (2007). Medial versus lateral prefrontal dissociation in movement selection and inhibitory control. *Brain Research*, **1132**, 139–42.

Drubach, D.A., Zeilig, G., Perez, J., Peralta, L., and Makley, M. (1995). Treatment of abulia with carbidopa. *Neurorehabilitation and Neural Repair*, **9**, 151–5.

Eames, P. (1989). The use of sinemet and bromocriptine. *Brain Injury*, **3**, 319–22.

Eames, P.G. (2001). Distinguishing the neuropsychiatric, psychiatric and psychological consequences of acquired brain injury. In: *Neurobehavioural disability and social handicap following traumatic brain injury* (ed R.L. Wood and T.M. McMillan), pp. 29–45. Psychology Press, Hove.

Evans, J.J., Emslie, H., and Wilson, B.A. (1998). External cueing systems in the rehabilitation of executive impairments of action. *Journal of the International Neuropsychological Society*, **4**, 399–408.

Fisher, C.M. (1983). Abulia minor vs. agitated behavior. *Clinical Neurosurgery*, **31**, 9–31.

Frith, C. (1992). *The cognitive neuropsychology of schizophrenia*. Lawrence Erlbaum, Hove.

Gamstorp, I. (1956). Adynamia episodica hereditaria. *Acta Paediatrica*, **45** (Suppl 108), 1–126.

Gianotti, G. (1989). Disorders of emotions and affect in patients after unilateral brain damage. In: *Handbook of Neuropsychology*, Vol 3 (ed F. Boller and J. Grafman), pp. 345–61. Elsevier, New York

Grunsfeld, A.A. and Login, I.S. (2006). Abulia following penetrating brain injury during endoscopic sinus surgery with disruption of the anterior congulate circuit: case report. *BMC Neurology* **6**. Available online at: http://www.biomedcentral.com/1471–2377/6/4

Habib, M. (2000). Disorders of motivation. In: *Behaviour and mood disorders in focal brain lesions* (ed J. Bogousslavsky and J.L. Cummings). Cambridge University Press.

Habib, M. and Galaburda, A.M. (1998). Disorders of action in limbic lesions. In: *Disorders of movement in psychiatry and neurology*. Blackwell, Cambridge, MA.

Heilman, K.M. and Watson, R.T. (1991) Intentional motor disorders. In: *Frontal lobe function and dysfunction* (ed H.S. Levin, H.M. Eisenberg, and A.L. Benton). pp. 199–213. Oxford University Press, New York.

Herbert, C.M. and Powell, G.E. (1989). Insight and progress in rehabilitation. *Clinical Rehabilitation*, **3**, 125–30.

Hull, C.L. (1943). *Principles of behaviour: an introduction to behaviour theory*. Appleton-Century, New York.

Jahanshahi, M. and Frith, C. (1998). Willed action and its impairments. *Cognitive Neuropsychology*, **15**, 483–533.

Jorge, R.E., Robinson, R.S., and Arndt, S. (1993) Are there symptoms that are specific for depressed mood with traumatic brain injury? *Journal of Nervous and Mental Disease*, **181**. 91–9.

Kant, R., Duffy, J.D., and Pivovarnik, A. (1998). Prevalence of apathy following head injury. *Brain Injury*, **12**, 87–92.

Langer, E.J. and Rodin, J. (1976). The effects of choice and enhanced personal responsibility for the aged: a field experiment in an institutional setting. *Journal of Personality and Social Psychology*, **34**, 191–8.

Laplane, D. and Dubois, B. (2001). Auto-activation disorder: a basal ganglia related syndrome. *Movement Disorders*, **16**, 810–14.

Lepper, M.R., Greene, D., and Nisbett, R.E. (1973). Undermining children's intrinsic interest with extrinsic reward: a test of the 'overjustification hypothesis'. *Journal of Personal and Social Psychology*, **31**, 479–86.

Levine, B., Robertson, I.H., Clare, L., *et al.* (2000). Rehabilitation of executive functioning: an experimental–clinical validation of Goal Management Training. *Journal of the International Neuropsychological Society*, **6**, 299–312.

Levine, B., Stuss, D.T., Winocur, G., *et al.* (2007). Cognitive rehabilitation in the elderly: effects on strategic behavior in relation to goal management. *Journal of the International Neuropsychological Society*, **13**, 143–52.

Lezak, M.D., Howieson, D.B., Loring, D.W., Hannay, H.J., and Fischer, J.S. (2004). *Neuropsychological assessment*. Oxford University Press.

Lishman, W.A. (1987). *Organic Psychiatry* (2nd edn). Blackwell Scientific, Oxford.

Marin, R.S. (1990). Differential diagnosis and classification of apathy. *American Journal of Psychiatry*, **147**, 22–30.

Marin, R.S. (1991). Apathy: a neuropsychiatric syndrome. *Journal of Neuropsychiatry and Clinical Neuroscience*, **3**, 243–54.

Martin, J.P. (1967). *The basal ganglia and posture*. Pitman, London.

Muquit, M.M.K., Ratshi, J.S., Shakir, R.A., and Larner, A.J. (2001). Catatonia or abulia? A difficult differential diagnosis. *Movement Disorders*, **16**, 360–2.

Nagaratnam, N., Fanella, S., Gopinath, S., and Goodwin, A. (2001) Prolonged abulia following putaminal haemorrhage. *Journal of Stroke and Cerebrovascular Diseases*, **10**, 92–3.

Norman, D.A. and Shallice, T. (1986). Attention to action: willed and automatic control of behaviour. In: *Consciousness and self-regulation*, Vol 4 (ed R.J. Davidson, G.E. Schwartz, and D. Shapiro), pp. 1–18. Plenum Press, New York.

Olds, J. and Milner, P. (1954). Positive reinforcement produced by electrical stimulation of the septal area and other regions of rat brain. *Journal of Comparative and Physiological Psychology*, **47**, 419–27.

Owen C.M., Schaller, C., and Binder, D.K. (2007). The madness of Dionysus: a neurosurgical perspective on Friedrich Nietzsche. *Neurosurgery*, **61**, 626–32.

Pantoni, L., Basile, A.M., Romanelli, M., *et al.* (2001) Abulia and cognitive impairment in two patients with capsular genu infarct. *Acta Neurologica Scandinavica*, **104**, 185–90.

Parish, L. and Oddy, M. (2007). Efficacy of rehabilitation for functional skills more than 10 years after extremely severe brain injury. *Neuropsychological Rehabilitation*, **17**, 230–43.

Powell, J.H., Al-Adawi, S., Morgan, J., and Greenwood, R.J. (1996). Motivational deficits after brain injury: effects of bromocriptine in 11 patients. *Journal of Neurology, Neurosurgery, and Psychiatry*, **60**, 416–21.

Quellet, M. and Morin, C.M. (2006). Fatigue following traumatic brain injury: frequency, characteristics and associated factors. *Rehabilitation Psychology*, **51**, 140–9.

Rao, V., Spiro, J.R., Schretlen, D.J., and Cascella, N.G. (2007) Apathy syndrome after traumatic brain injury compared with deficits in schizophrenia. *Psychosomatics*, **48**, 217–22.

Robbins, T. and Evritt, B. (1996). Neurobehavioural mechanisms of reward and motivation. *Current Opinion in Neurobiology*, **6**, 228–36.

Rollnick, S. and Miller, W.R. (1995). What is motivational interviewing? *Behavioural and Cognitive Psychotherapy*, **23**, 325–34.

Simpson, G. Tate, R., Ferry, K., Hodgkinson, A., and Blaszczynski, A. (2001). Social, neuroradiologic, medical, and neuropsychologic correlates of sexually aberrant behavior after traumatic brain injury: a controlled study. *Journal of Head Trauma Rehabilitation*, **16**, 556–72.

Smith, E. and Delargy, M. (2005). Locked-in syndrome. *British Medical Journal*, **330**, 406–9.

van den Broek, M.D. (2005). Why does rehabilitation fail? *Journal of Head Trauma Rehabilitation*, **20**, 464–73.

Van Reekum,R., Bayley, M., Garner, S., *et al.* (1995). *N* of 1 study: amantadine for the amotivational syndrome in traumatic brain injury. *Brain Injury*, **9**, 49–53.

Vijayaraghavan, L.V., Krishnamoorthy, E.S., Brown, R.G., and Trimble, M.R. (2002) Abulia: a Delphi survey of British neurologists and psychiatrists. *Movement Disorders*, **17**, 1052–7.

von Cramon, D. and Matthes-von Cramon, G. (1994). Back to work with a chronic dysexecutive syndrome. *Neuropsychological Rehabilitation*, **4**, 399–417.

Weiner, B. (1985). An attributional theory of achievement motivation and emotion. *Psychological Review*, **92**, 548–73.

Whyte, J. (1992). Attention and arousal: basic science aspects. *Archives of Physical Medicine and Rehabilitation*, **73**, 940–9.

Wood, R.L. (2001). Understanding neurobehavioural disability. In: *Neurobehavioural disability and social handicap following traumatic brain injury* (ed R.L. Wood and T.M. McMillan), pp. 3–27. Psychology Press, Hove.

Wood, R. and Eames, P. (1981). Application of behaviour modification in the rehabilitation of traumatically brain-injured patients. In: *Applications of conditioning theory* (ed G. Davey), pp. 81–101. Methuen, New York.

Wroblewski, B.A. and Glenn, M.B. (1994). Pharmacological treatment of arousal and cognitive deficits. *Journal of Head Trauma Rehabilitation*, **9**, 19–42.

Worthington, A.D.and Melia, Y. (2006). Rehabilitation is compromised by arousal and sleep disorders: results of a survey of rehabilitation centres. *Brain Injury*, **20**, 327–32.

Worthington, A., Williams, C., Young, K., and Pownall, J. (1997). Re-training gait components for walking in the context of abulia. *Physiotherapy Theory and Practice*, **13**, 247–56.

Part 2

Rehabilitation

Michael Oddy and Andrew Worthington

In the first chapter in Part 2, Evans provides a masterly overview of theory and practice in the rehabilitation of executive disorders providing a link between the section on theoretical developments and the section on rehabilitation. Fish and colleagues describe approaches to the remediation of prospective memory deficits, so often a major complaint of those suffering from executive disorders and those around them, but until recently a relatively neglected area of executive function. In Chapter 6, Alderman and Baker report their development of the original Multiple Errands Test first reported by Shallice and Burgess (1991). The authors argue that a multi-tasking exercise can be standardized for routine use as a tool for rehabilitation, but stress that this is an exceptional use of such a test, not something they would advocate for other tests.

The next two chapters tackle one of the most common but destructive aspects of acquired brain injury, so often closely associated with executive disorders. Aggression can be primarily organic in origin or secondary to psychological factors. Freeland focuses more on approaches to manage aggressive behaviour caused by brain damage whilst O'Neill suggests practical interventions to managing the experience of anger.

Moodiness and inappropriate social conduct are often associated with executive dysfunction and may be underpinned by poor communication skills. In Chapter 9, Corkery and Fairweather describe the ways in which executive disorder can affect communication and how high-level language deficits relate to executive dysfunction, again with a clear focus on how these difficulties can be managed. Zeeman in turn takes a broad view of the role of motor recovery and physical fitness in the management of executive disorder, demonstrating how executive disorders can affect the client's motivation and ability to benefit from physical activity in general and physiotherapy in particular.

The next two chapters focus on ability and participation rather than impairment. Worthington and Waller explore the wide-ranging impact of executive deficits on everyday function and suggest how this needs to inform our approach to functional rehabilitation. They provide an overview of methods of assessment and intervention that can be used to ameliorate executive disorders in everyday living skills. Executive disorders have far-reaching impact on all aspects of life and none is less important to the individual than the ability to work. It is seldom appreciated that whilst physical and sensory impairments restrict the types of work a person can do they rarely exclude employment altogether. Cognitive deficits, however, and executive deficits in particular, affect the ability to succeed in all forms of employment in one way or another. Tyerman reviews the evidence for the success of vocational rehabilitation with those with executive disorders and suggests a variety of ways in which sevices can be designed to help those with executive disorder return to work.

It is perhaps disappointing that computer technology which has had so much impact in areas such as banking, the media, and indeed some areas of medical practice has had so little effect on rehabilitation and brain injury rehabilitation in particular. Unlike the former industries brain injury rehabilitation is still obviously 'low-tech' as it tends to be very dependent on human interaction and these are difficult to replace with computers. However the chapters by Penn and colleagues and by Orpwood suggest ways in which such technology could replace or enhance the contribution of staff and become central to rehabilitation. Penn *et al.* describe the first steps taken to use virtual reality in assessment and rehabilitation of those with executive disorders. They emphasise the opportunity that virtual reality affords to put people in standardized but complex situations, to assess risk without taking risk. They also stress the fact that virtual reality may motivate clients, perhaps particularly young clients who are otherwise extremely difficult to motivate and engage.

Orpwood suggests how the use of sensors combined with devices which act in an 'intelligent' way may enable people with executive disorders to become much less dependent on other people for support. There are undoubtedly ethical issues to consider but there are surely advantages in technology that whilst monitoring people closely is far less intrusive than another person providing such monitoring. Orpwood makes the important point that now the difficulties in using so-called smart technology are not so much technological as psychological. It is the human interface with these devices that throws up the most challenging questions not the technology itself.

Reference

Shallice, T. & Burgess, P.W. (1991). Deficits in strategy application following frontal lobe damage in man. *Brain*, **114**, 727–741.

4

Rehabilitation of executive functioning: an overview

Jonathan J. Evans

Section of Psychological Medicine, Faculty of Medicine, University of Glasgow

Introduction

Executive functioning is the term used to encompass a range of cognitive skills including problem-solving, planning, initiation, self-monitoring, and error correction. Executive functions enable us to deal with problems that arise in everyday life and to cope with new situations. They are the cognitive skills necessary to identify, work towards, and achieve personal goals and to modify our actions when required (Burgess and Simons 2005). Much of everyday functioning is routine—patterns of action become automatic through many repetitions over the years. Complex tasks such as driving, preparing meals, and operating a computer, or at least components of them, can be carried out with little conscious attention. However, when a potentially dangerous situation arises or a novel problem is encountered, attention can be focused on the process of working out how to respond, formulating a plan of action, checking how effective the plan is when implemented, and modifying the plan if necessary. During familiar tasks that have multiple subtasks (e.g. shopping for several items requiring visits to a number of stores, preparing a more complex meal, completing work tasks), whilst individual component actions or sequences of actions may be carried out relatively automatically, some monitoring is required to ensure that overall goals are achieved. Thus everyday functioning is a highly complex and dynamic interaction of automatic routine behaviour and consciously controlled action (Norman and Shallice 1986). This system fails from time to time in the absence of any brain pathology. We all make errors that might be described as 'slips of action' (e.g. putting something away in the wrong cupboard, taking a turning when driving that is part of your usual routine route to work even though you are intending to travel somewhere else on that occasion)—in these circumstances it is as if the 'autopilot' is not being monitored effectively. However, brain injury or disease, particularly when it affects the frontal lobes, can also cause breakdown in the conscious control of action, greatly increasing the frequency of errors.

Executive functioning and the frontal lobes

Executive functions have long been associated with the frontal lobes and, like most cognitive functions, much has been learned about both the functions of the frontal lobes and the nature of executive functions from patients with brain injury. The most famous 'frontal lobe patient' is of course Phineas Gage, the American railway worker who became disinhibited and disorganized following an injury caused by an iron bar, a tamping iron, being accidentally blasted through his frontal lobes. Several other similar patients have been described since (Eslinger and Damasio 1985, Shallice and Burgess 1991; Cato *et al.* 2004). Based on his assessment of many patients with frontal lobe lesions, Luria (1966) conceptualized the frontal lobes as having a critical role in problem-solving, involving strategy selection, application of operations, and evaluation of outcomes. Stuss (2007 and Chapter 1 this volume) proposes that the prefrontal regions of the frontal lobes have four different (but related) functions. Executive cognitive functions are high-level cognitive skills (planning, monitoring, energizing, switching, inhibiting) that are involved in the control of more automatic functions and are mediated by the lateral prefrontal cortex. Behavioural–emotional self-regulatory functions are mediated by the ventral prefrontal cortex. Energization-regulating functions are dependent upon superior medial frontal regions and deficits here result in apathy or abulia. The frontal polar regions, particularly on the right, have a role in 'meta-cognitive aspects of human nature' (Stuss, 2007, p. 294).

Models of executive functioning

There are many theories of frontal lobe or executive functioning (see Burgess and Simons (2005) for a useful summary of some of them). As a clinician trying to understand the complexities of a patient after brain injury, it is not straightforward to decide which model is most helpful. However, several models or frameworks are rather similar, or at least overlap in some aspects, and although many are not strictly testable theories, they do provide a means of conceptualizing some of the problems with which patients present. As noted, Luria (1966) suggested that the behaviour of patients with frontal lobe lesions could be explained in terms of a failure of problem-solving, and more specifically a failure of verbal control of action. Norman and Shallice (1986) also made a distinction between automatic functioning and conscious control of action, attributing the frontal lobes with a supervisory attention system (SAS).

Shallice and Burgess (1996) later expanded on this concept and argued that the SAS can be fractionated into a set of basic subcomponents, or subprocesses, and presented evidence (based on neuropsychological dissociations and functional brain imaging) for this fractionation. They argued that responding appropriately to novelty requires three processes, each of which consists of a further set of subprocesses. Within their model (Shallice and Burgess 1996, p. 1407; Burgess and Simons 2005, p.222) they posit the need for (1) a set of psychological operations that lead to the generation of a plan or solution for solving a novel problem, (2) a special-purpose working memory that is required for the implementation of the plan, and (3) a system that monitors, evaluates, and accepts or rejects actions depending upon their success in solving the novel problem. This model is illustrated in Figure 4.1.

Clinical presentation of executive deficits

How do deficits in executive functioning present in everyday life? Executive deficits and their relationship with everyday difficulties are less tangible than many other cognitive problems. Memory impairment has obvious manifestations and consequences, as do language and perceptual deficits. Executive difficulties are a little more difficult to identify and distinguish from other problems. This is in part because the very concept of executive functions is a

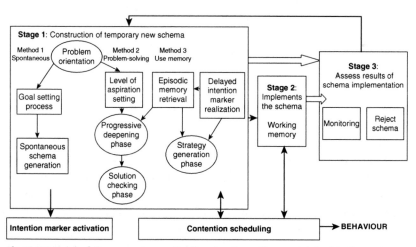

Fig. 4.1 Model of the supervisory attentional system. The model depicts three stages of supervisory system processing, each with a number of subprocesses: solid arrows, flow of control; unfilled arrows: information transfer. (Reproduced with permission from Burgess and Simons 2005, p.222 and Shallice and Burgess 1996, p.1407.)

rather broad concept which includes several different cognitive skills. Furthermore, by their very nature executive deficits are only evident in situations requiring planning, problem-solving, or novelty, and so patients with executive difficulties may function effectively in many basic aspects of everyday life. The patients described by Shallice and Burgess (1991) are good examples of this issue. For example, their patient FS, a 55-year-old woman who had suffered two head injuries and had an extensive lesion of the left frontal lobe, was described as working and living independently, but:

> she undertakes virtually no inessential or novel activities. She is very untidy, never putting things away. She seldom goes out in the evening, and virtually never travels away from her home town. Others always make arrangements when any joint activity is to be carried out. She is said by her sister never to organize anything. She shops every day buying only a few things on any occasion and never visits supermarkets. She had no activity planned for the following weekend and could give no example where anyone had relied on her to do anything. (Shallice and Burgess 1991, p.730)

One of the more obvious manifestations of executive deficits is impulsivity. Patients are reported by relatives to 'act without thinking'. The patient appears to fail to 'look ahead' and anticipate the consequences of his/her actions. For some this a relatively minor problem and, ironically, for some is even seen as a positive change in personality. However, for others impulsivity causes significant disability—tasks are not completed correctly, errors are made, and for this reason activities may take longer than usual despite being done at speed. In social contexts impulsivity may manifest itself in poor turn-taking which may contribute to breakdown of relationships and difficulties in establishing new ones.

For some patients the problem is not so much an inability to look ahead or anticipate consequences *per se*, but rather that apparent negative consequences of actions fail to influence decision-making. Damasio's somatic marker hypothesis (Bechara *et al.* 1994) refers to patients with ventro-medial prefrontal cortex whose behaviour seems governed by immediate reward, but is not affected by potential longer-term negative consequences of their actions. Emotion is central to the idea of somatic markers—emotions and feelings are associated by experience with predicted future outcomes. When a negative somatic marker is associated with a particular future outcome it acts as an alarm bell, and when a future outcome is associated with a positive somatic marker it becomes 'a beacon of incentive' (Damasio 1994, p. 174). Bechara *et al.* (2005) note that on the Iowa Gambling Test, which is designed to assess decision-making, some patients persisted with behaviour that would be disadvantageous over the longer term even when they were aware that the choices they were making were not going to be to their advantage in the long run, apparently being driven by more immediate short-term rewards. However, the concept of somatic markers remains controversial, with some (e.g. Maia and McClelland 2005) arguing that the behaviour of ventro-medial patients can be explained more parsimoniously in terms of an inability to respond to reversed contingencies (reversal learning).

Some people are disinhibited, saying things or behaving in a manner that is not within usual social norms, and appearing to fail to inhibit thoughts or actions. There is some overlap in the concept of impulsivity and disinhibition, although they are not identical and may be said to dissociate singly if not doubly. Some patients are impulsive but not disinhibited (e.g. patients who apparently act without thinking things through, but are not socially inappropriate, such as the case described by Evans (2008)), although whether it is possible to be disinhibited but not impulsive is perhaps less clear. Disinhibition takes many forms and may be caused by a number of different deficits in combination. For some there may be emotional lability combined with inhibition problems, and usually a more global cognitive impairment, (resulting in verbal or physical aggression). For others there may be impairment in the ability to appreciate the consequences of actions, so that hurtful or offensive things are said without awareness of the implications, although without the verbal or physical aggression shown by some. In practice it may be difficult to determine the cause of problem behaviours, but it is important to formulate carefully because the intervention that would be recommended may vary depending on the factors affecting the behaviour.

Other patients simply fail to engage in planning or problem-solving and so they have a limited behavioural repertoire. Routine tasks are carried out, but when faced with novelty or a lack of structure to prompt activity the patient is 'at a loss' as to what to do. Baddeley and Wilson (1988) described this as one of the core characteristics of the 'dysexecutive syndrome'.

For others, everyday problems relate to a failure to self-monitor or, as Duncan (1986) characterized it, 'goal neglect'. Duncan described the role of the frontal lobes in terms of 'goal maintenance'. He argued that the frontal lobes are involved in identifying 'goals' or behavioural objectives and managing actions that will lead to the achievement of those goals. Goal neglect is where the individual is able to identify what he/she needs to achieve and may be able to derive a plan, but during the course of the operation of the plan the main goals may become neglected and actions no longer lead to achieving the goal. Whilst not completely random, behaviour is no longer goal-directed. Thus patients may not have 'forgotten' what they were supposed to be doing (at least when asked directly), but have become distracted by irrelevant activity and so fail to stay on task and do not achieve their intended goal.

A common problem associated with frontal lobe damage is anosognosia (a deficit in insight or awareness). Awareness problems can arise for many different reasons and are not always the result of executive impairments—it is recognized that there are complex biological, psychological, and social influences on the development of awareness of deficits, particularly relatively subtle executive deficits after brain injury (Ownsworth *et al.* 2006; Yeates *et al.* 2007). Nevertheless, impairment in problem-solving combined with poor self-monitoring may contribute to the development of difficulties in being aware of everyday problems arising from executive dysfunction—patients may not notice their own mistakes or are unable to appreciate the implications of problems.

In practice, establishing whether a person is not functioning effectively because they are impulsive, are unable to plan, or are unable to maintain task goals is not always straightforward on the basis of self or other reports, observation, or neuropsychological test performance. In part this is because in each case the behavioural manifestations may be similar (tasks are not completed effectively or at all) and in part because patients (particularly those with larger frontal lobe lesions) will be likely to present with more than one executive deficit. There are no neuropsychological tests that have been specifically designed to map onto the component processes outlined in the model proposed by Shallice and Burgess (1996), or indeed any other model. However, as part of an assessment process it is possible, to some extent, to build a formulation of a person's difficulties based on their presenting problems and performance on a range of questionnaires and tests, or through more qualitative observation. Evans (2008) describes this process with reference to a range of tests of executive or frontal lobe function, as does Stuss (2007). Both note that careful interpretation of impaired performance is needed to properly formulate the person's difficulties. Many of the traditional frontal lobe tests (e.g. Wisconsin Card Sorting Test, Verbal Fluency, Trail Making, Tower of London), as well as the more recently developed tools (Behavioural Assessment of the Dysexecutive Syndrome (BADS); Hayling and Brixton), involve complex tasks, and so individuals can fail them for many reasons, some of which are not related to executive functioning. One approach to assessment of executive difficulties is to begin with multi-element tasks that make demands on a range of executive skills (e.g. Zoo Map or Modified Six Elements from the BADS) and if a patient is impaired to begin to try to tease out the explanation for his/her difficulties either using other tests that may make specific demands on key processes (e.g. the Tower test for planning, and WCST, Stroop, or Trails to look at monitoring and flexibility). Furthermore, hypotheses can be tested by observation of the person in everyday situations where predictions about the type of problems expected can be made. Some problems, such as initiation difficulties, are more difficult to assess with formal tests, as in almost all tests either the instructions or the context prompts action. With these problems, the most useful information usually comes from interviews with relatives or observation in the natural environment.

In summary, the assessment process should lead to a formulation of the person's problems that identifies the nature of any impairments in executive functioning with reference to a relevant theoretical model. As discussed, the Shallice and Burgess (1996) model (see also Burgess and Simons 2005) provides a helpful explanatory framework. The formulation must also aim to document the everyday problems experienced and try to account for these problems in terms of the cognitive impairments present. Having arrived at a formulation, rehabilitation interventions can be planned.

Approaches to the rehabilitation of executive functioning

Treatment interventions which may improve executive functioning or help manage executive dysfunction are discussed in this section. It should be noted that any intervention aimed at improving or managing executive functioning should be set in the broader context of the personal rehabilitation goals of the patient, and these goals must relate to the patient's participation in valued activities (Hart and Evans 2006). For example, a patient may have the goal of returning to work, and it may be clear that executive difficulties would prevent him from succeeding in the work environment. Any intervention for executive difficulties will almost always involve the need to identify how the strategies used could be applied in the work context. Because of the nature of executive impairment, generalization of strategies from one environment (e.g. the rehabilitation centre) to another (e.g. the workplace) may not be straightforward, and so this must be supported by the rehabilitation team. In the following sections approaches to the management of a number of forms of executive dysfunction are presented and discussed.

Managing awareness difficulties

Awareness difficulties can be very difficult to address, although it is perhaps too common for patients to be dismissed as having 'no insight' and for there to be something of a therapeutic nihilism in relation to the issue. Careful attention should be paid to the factors that are likely to be responsible in order to plan an intervention for addressing awareness deficits. Awareness difficulties may arise from poor attention which prevents self-monitoring, and hence the patient fails to notice problems as they occur. This is perhaps most evident in conversational situations. Similarly, impaired memory may mean that the patient cannot remember the nature or frequency of errors. Deficits in executive functioning may mean that the patient cannot anticipate the consequences of actions. For some there may be a lack of demand on cognitive skills, meaning that the patient simply lacks experience of errors, something that might be particularly relevant to returning to work. For others, denial of disability may represent a means of coping psychologically with the overwhelming consequences of injury. The intervention will vary depending on the cause of the insight problem. However, for most patients with insight difficulties, some combination of education about brain injury, supported exposure to functional difficulties, development of appropriate cognitive strategies in relation to deficits contributing to insight difficulties, and psychological support emphasizing positive coping will be appropriate. Fleming and Ownsworth (2006) reviewed the range of interventions that have been documented, noting that a number of sophisticated biopsychosocial models of awareness exist, and these can be used to formulate awareness deficits in patients and to guide treatment interventions. Champion (2006) provides a useful resource for conducting brain injury education groups, including sessions on executive functioning. Specific cognitive strategies aimed at improving self-monitoring (such as developing mental checking as used in Goal Management Training which is described below) may be used for those who have sufficient cognitive ability. Alderman *et al.* (1995) described a programme of self-monitoring training that they have successfully used with a person who had severe challenging behaviour in the context of poor awareness. Alderman and colleagues hypothesized that an underlying monitoring deficit was responsible for the development of the problem behaviour (repetitive verbal output), lack of awareness, and inability to respond to social feedback. Self-monitoring training was applied only in relation to the problem behaviour (it is not designed to improve insight in a more general sense), but was successful in first allowing the person to be more aware of their behaviour (reflected in more accurate counting of their own problem behaviour) and then to reduce the levels of problem behaviour via reinforcement schedules.

Work aimed at improving insight must be clearly set in the context of functional goals, although it is often the case that the patient's ultimate goal may not be achievable. For the more impaired patients it may not be possible to improve insight, and it will be necessary to focus on modifications to the environment that have the effect of reducing cognitive demands on the patient.

Managing impulsivity

Many of the interventions for executive dysfunction might be said to work by reducing impulsivity and as a result increasing the likelihood of more effective planning and decision-making. Some patients benefit from what might be referred to as 'Stop:Think' training. This is not a formalized training method, but a general approach of teaching patients first to be better at recognizing problems when they occur and using self-instructional self-statements to 'Stop' and 'Think' before acting. There are no formal evaluations of such training, but this approach is incorporated within Goal Management Training (Levine *et al.* 2000) and problem-solving therapy (von Cramon *et al.* 1991). Cicerone and Wood (1987) reported the case of a patient who was successfully taught using a training task (the Tower of London planning task) to improve his verbal control of his actions by first speaking aloud what he was going to do (e.g. say what move he was going to make) and then gradually internalizng his self-talk. Cicerone reported that with some generalization training the patient improved his everyday functioning. This approach of using some form of training and task and then moving to more 'real-life' contexts seems appropriate. Some patients may find the transition to applying a strategy in everyday life more challenging, and it may be helpful to use some form of prompt (cue cards in prominent places, alarms, SMS text or pager alerts) to support the patient in remembering to use the strategy on a day-to-day basis.

Sometimes what presents as impulsivity may be being caused by other factors. For example, in a case described by Evans (2008) a patient with memory problems found it very difficult to remember something he wanted to say in conversations. Therefore when he thought of something he wanted to say, his approach was to say it immediately before he forgot, often interrupting the other person speaking. To manage this he learned to make brief notes and also practised active listening skills to emphasize the importance of attending (listening) better during conversations.

Approaches to managing disinhibition will also vary according to the form of disinhibition and contributing factors. Alderman (2003) provides a comprehensive discussion of behaviour disorders and an overview of methods of managing challenging behaviour after brain injury. Behavioural management approaches have proved successful for those with more severe challenging behaviour, although such interventions are only likely to be effective in specialist services where high levels of consistency can be applied.

Training planning and problem-solving

Strategies for managing impulsivity are the first component of a broader problem-solving training approach. A number of studies have shown that training on exercises focused on cognitive flexibility, working memory, and planning improve some aspects of executive functioning in people with schizophrenia (Evans 2005). For brain injury, von Cramon *et al.* (1991) described and evaluated a problem-solving therapy (PST) group-based intervention. The aim of the therapy is to enhance patients' ability to perform each of the separate stages of problem-solving through practice on tasks that are designed to exercise the skills required for each of the separate stages. The stages are (a) identifying and analysing problems, (b) separating information relevant to a problem solution from unimportant and irrelevant data, (c) recognizing the relationship between different relevant items of information and if appropriate combining them, (d) producing ideas/solutions, (e) using different mental representations in order to solve a problem, and (f) monitoring solution implementation and evaluating solutions. Rath *et al.* (2003) described a similar group programme which was shown to improve performance on some measures of executive functioning, a role-played problem-solving task, and self-ratings of everyday problem-solving. In multicomponent interventions it is difficult to establish what the most important elements are but, as with the von Cramon programme, Rath and colleagues also note that a key component of the programme was to manage the tendency to respond impulsively by managing emotional responses to situations that arise. Learning to prevent impulsive responses may be vital for some patients because they do have the skills to generate and evaluate potential solutions to problems. For others, these latter skills need to be trained in addition to learning to manage impulsivity.

One particular component of the problem-solving process that has been shown to be impaired in people with head injury is the use of past experience in forming plans—solving a new problem by drawing on past experience of similar situations (Dritschel *et al.* 1998). Hewitt *et al.* (2007) showed that a brief training relating to the use of autobiographical memories improved performance of head-injured patients on a hypothetical practical problem-solving task. This technique has not been evaluated more extensively, but does suggest that building in specific reference to drawing on past experience as part of a problem-solving training programme may be beneficial.

Evans (2003) also describes a group approach, adapted from the von Cramon programme described above and from Goal Management Training of Robertson (see Levine *et al.* 2000) described in more detail below. The attention and problem-solving group is one component of a holistic rehabilitation programme. The first few sessions of the group programme address attentional difficulties and the later sessions are used to introduce a problem-solving framework. This framework is presented as a checklist of the stages of problem-solving. An accompanying template is also provided that can be used to proceed through the stages using a written format, but clients are encouraged, through practice at using the framework with the template, to internalize the framework so that in time its use becomes more automatic. Miotto and Evans (2005) have undertaken a formal evaluation of this group format and demonstrated improved outcome on some neuropsychological tests of executive functioning and everyday functioning as measured by the DEX questionnaire.

Managing initiation problems

The case examples of David (Evans 2003, p. 64) and RP (Evans *et al.* 1998) illustrate patients with initiation difficulties who benefited from rehabilitation interventions. At the age of 34, David suffered a stroke causing an internal capsule infarct. He had a number of attention and executive difficulties, including problems with initiation of actions. He was not depressed or lacking motivation, but found it difficult to start tasks he intended to do. He was trained to use a self-instructional approach involving a phrase which he selected ('Just do it') and successfully used to prompt himself to do things. RP had had a stroke affecting the medial frontal lobe bilaterally. She had severe initiation difficulties, which were compounded by attentional problems—she found it difficult to initiate actions, but when she did manage to do so, she was frequently distracted by irrelevant things in her environment. An external prompting system, the NeuroPage system, was used to provide an external alert and task information at the appropriate time. An evaluation showed that when using the system she completed activities without prompting from her husband, but without it she need very frequent prompts from him.

Goal Management Training

Levine *et al.* (2000) describe the use of a Goal Management Training (GMT) intervention derived from Duncan's (1986) concept of 'goal neglect'. The principle is that patients with frontal lobe damage fail to generate goal (or subgoal) lists of how to solve problems (and achieve goals) and/or may fail to monitor progress towards achieving subgoals or main goals. The training has five stages: (1) stop and think what I am doing; (2) define the main task; (3) list the steps required; (4) learn the steps; (5) whilst implementing the steps, check that I am on track, or doing what I intended to do. Several of these stages overlap with elements of problem-solving therapy, but GMT is less focused on making decisions about how to solve a problem and more focused on completing tasks for which the series of steps is relatively clear. Once again there is a strong focus on management of impulsivity (with stage 1 involving a stop and think training) as well as development of a mental checking routine (stage 5) to facilitate maintaining in mind the main task to be achieved. GMT has not been extensively evaluated as yet, although a recent study demonstrated that it was beneficial in healthy elderly (Levine *et al.* 2007).

In GMT the aim is for patients to use a self-instructional (mental-checking) routine to prompt goal maintenance. This may be difficult for some patients. An alternative approach is to use some form of external alert to prompt goal maintenance. The use of external alerting (via SMS text messaging) in combination with GMT has been shown to be beneficial in improving functional performance on an everyday prospective remembering task (Fish *et al.* 2007). The idea of this intervention is that rather than prompting specific actions at specific times (the way the NeuroPage system is most commonly used), a more general alert is delivered to prompt a 'goal review' by the patient. Fish and colleagues sent SMS text messages which said simply STOP; the patients had been trained to use this to prompt them to Stop, Think about what you are doing and what tasks you have to do, Organize (i.e plan for any tasks that need to be done later), and Proceed (i.e. carry on with current activity).

Using routine

If executive ability is concerned with dealing with novelty as opposed to routine, one approach to managing executive impairment is to compensate for the deficit by providing direct support to develop routines in new situations or on complex tasks. In other words, remove the responsibility for problem-solving or self-management and focus on development and maintenance of behavioural routines. We are all used to following recipe instructions very carefully until we have made a dish so often we remember all the quantities and steps involved. This principle of providing checklist support to remember what to do and to help monitor the stage we are at (i.e. to stay on task) can be applied to many tasks. Levine *et al.* (2000) illustrated the combined use of checklists and their GMT in teaching a woman who had suffered with encephalitis to be more effective in meal preparation. von Cramon and Matthes-von Cramon (1994) described the use of a checklist to support a man who had managed to train as a physician after a head injury. During his rehabilitation programme he was working in a pathology laboratory, but was described as impulsive in reaching diagnoses from autopsy information. With the provision of a set of rules/guidelines for the systematic process of diagnosis his performance improved. In this case he initially used a written checklist, but over time he was able to remember the steps which he applied as a routine. This is a good example of how a relatively complex skill can be trained to be routine. In perhaps more mundane contexts this means not leaving someone to work out independently which domestic tasks need to be done when, but using daily checklists of things to do or developing fixed routines of tasks.

Evidence-based practice

A number of systematic reviews of the effectiveness of cognitive rehabilitation have been undertaken in recent years and therefore it is important to consider their findings in relation to interventions for executive dysfunction. Some reviews have not included executive functioning (e.g. Cappa *et al.* 2005). However, Cicerone *et al.* (2005) concluded that there was sufficient evidence to recommend training of problem-solving strategies and their application in everyday life as a practice guideline for people with traumatic brain injury. Furthermore, cognitive interventions that promote internalization and self-regulation strategies through self-instruction and self-monitoring should be considered as practice options. Cicerone and colleagues noted that, as yet, there is insufficient evidence to make specific recommendations regarding interventions to improve self-awareness.

Summary

Executive functioning is a complex concept encompassing a large number of cognitive processes. Executive dysfunction takes many forms and presents a major challenge to rehabilitation services. Since the pioneering work of Luria, our knowledge of the executive functions of the frontal lobes and the impairments arising from damage to them has increased dramatically, but we still have a long way to go. There are a number of models of executive functioning that are helpful in explaining some of the problems we see in patients, but the relationship between models of frontal lobe executive functions and assessment tools is still somewhat tenuous. A range of approaches to interventions for executive dysfunction have been developed. The evidence base for their effectiveness remains limited, but is slowly growing. The task ahead is to develop and evaluate rehabilitation methods that are clearly set in a theoretical context and can be prescribed on the basis of assessment information.

References

Alderman, N. (2003). Rehabilitation of behaviour disorders. In: *Neuropsychological rehabilitation: theory and practice* (ed B.A. Wilson), pp. 173–96. Swets and Zeitlinger, Lisse.

Alderman, N., Fry, R.K., and Youngson, H.A. (1995). Improvement of self-monitoring skills, reduction of behaviour disturbance and the dysexecutive syndrome: comparison of response cost and a new programme of self-monitoring training. *Neuropsychological Rehabilitation*, **5**, 193–221.

Baddeley, A.D. and Wilson, B.A. (1988). Frontal amnesia and the dysexecutive syndrome. *Brain and Cognition*, **7**, 212–30.

Bechara, A., Damasio, A.R., Damasio, H., and Anderson, S.W. (1994). Insensitivity to future consequences following damage to human prefrontal cortex. *Cognition*, **50**, 7–15.

Bechara, A., Damasio, H., Tranel, D., and Damasio, A. (2005). The Iowa Gambling Task and the somatic marker hypothesis: some questions and answers. *Trends in Cognitive Sciences*, **9**, 159–62.

Burgess, P.W. and Simons, J.S. (2005). Theories of frontal lobe executive function: clinical applications. In: *The effectiveness of rehabilitation for cognitive deficits* (ed P. Halligan and D. Wade). Oxford University Press.

Cappa, S.F. *et al.* (2005) EFNS guidelines on cognitive rehabilitation: report of an EFNS task force. *European Journal of Neurology*, **12**, 665–80.

Cato, M.A., Delis, D.C., Abildskov, T.J., and Bigler, E. (2004) Assessing the elusive cognitive deficits associated with ventromedial prefrontal damage: a case of a modern-day Phineas Gage. *Journal of the International Neuropsychological Society*, **10**, 453–65.

Champion, A.J. (2006). *Neuropsychological rehabilitation: a resource for group-based education and intervention.* John Wiley, Chichester.

Cicerone, K.D. and Wood, J.C. (1987). Planning disorder after closed head injury: a case study. *Archives of Physical Medicine and Rehabilitation*, **68**, 111–15.

Cicerone, K.D., Dahlberg, C., Malec, J.F., *et al.*, 2005. Evidence-based cognitive rehabilitation: updated review of the literature from 1998 through 2002. *Archives of Physical Medicine and Rehabilitation*, **86**, 1681–92.

Dritschel, B., Kogan, L., Burton, A., Burton, E., and Goddard, L. (1998). Everyday planning difficulties following traumatic brain injury: a role for autobiographical memory. *Brain Injury*, **12**, 875–86.

Duncan, J. (1986). Disorganisation of behaviour after frontal lobe damage. *Cognitive Neuropsychology*, **3**, 271–90.

Eslinger, P.J. and Damasio, A.R. (1985). Severe disturbance of higher cognition after bilateral frontal lobe ablation: patient EVR. *Neurology*, **35**, 1731–41.

Evans, J.J. (2003). Rehabilitation of executive deficits. In: *Neuropsychological rehabilitation: theory and practice* (ed B.A. Wilson), pp. 53–70. Swets and Zeitlinger, Lisse.

Evans, J.J. (2005). Can executive impairments be effectively treated? In: *The effectiveness of rehabilitation for cognitive deficits* (ed P. Halligan and D. Wade). Oxford University Press.

Evans, J.J. (2008). Executive and attentional problems. In: *Psychological approaches to rehabilitation after traumatic brain injury* (ed A. Tyerman and N. King). Blackwell, Oxford.

Evans J.J., Emslie, H., and Wilson, B.A. (1998). External cueing systems in the rehabilitation of executive impairments of action. *Journal of the International Neuropsychological Society*, **4**, 399–408.

Fish, J., Evans, J.J., Nimmo, M., *et al.* (2007). Rehabilitation of executive dysfunction following brain injury: 'content-free cueing' improves everyday prospective memory performance. *Neuropsychologia*, **45**, 1318–30.

Fleming, J.M. and Ownsworth, T. (2006). A review of awareness interventions in brain injury rehabilitation. *Neuropsychological Rehabilitation*, **16**, 474–500.

Hart, T. and Evans, J.J. (2006). Self-regulation and goal theories in brain injury rehabilitation. *Journal of Head Trauma Rehabilitation*, **21**, 2, 142–55.

Hewitt, J., Evans, J.J. and Dritschel, B. (2006). Theory driven rehabilitation of executive functioning: improving planning skills in people with traumatic brain injury through the use of an autobiographical episodic memory cueing procedure. *Neuropsychologia*, **44**, 1468–74.

Levine, B., Robertson, I.H., Clare, L., *et al.* (2000). Rehabilitation of executive functioning: an experimental–clinical validation of Goal Management Training. *Journal of the International Neuropsychological Society*, **6**, 299–312.

Levine, B., Stuss, D.T., Winocur, G., *et al.* (2007). Cognitive rehabilitation in the elderly: effects on strategic behavior in relation to goal management. *Journal of the International Neuropsychological Society*, **13**, 143–52.

Luria, A.R. (1966). *Higher cortical functions in man*. Basic Books, New York.

Maia, T.V. and McClelland, J.M. (2005) The somatic marker hypothesis: still many questions, but no answers. *Trends in Cognitive Sciences*, **9**, 162–4.

Miotto, E. and Evans, J.J. Rehabilitation of executive functioning: a controlled cross-over study of an attention and problem-solving group intervention. Presented at Neuropsychological Rehabilitation, University of Galway, Ireland, 11–12 July 2005.

Norman, D.A. and Shallice, T. (1986). Attention to action: willed and automatic control of behaviour. In: *Consciousness and self-regulation*, Vol 4 (ed R.J. Davidson, G.E. Schwartz, and D. Shapiro), pp. 1–18. Plenum Press, New York.

Ownsworth, T., Clare, L., and Morris, R. (2006). An integrated biopsychosocial approach to understanding awareness deficits in Alzheimer's disease and brain injury. *Neuropsychological Rehabilitation*, **16**, 415–38.

Rath, J.F., Simon, D., Langenbahn, D.M., Sherr, L., and Diller L. (2003). Group treatment of problem solving deficits in outpatients with traumatic brain injury: a randomized outcome study. *Neuropsychological Rehabilitation*, **13**, 461–88.

Shallice, T. and Burgess, P. (1991) Deficits in strategy application following frontal lobe damage in man. *Brain*, **144**, 727–41.

Shallice, T. and Burgess, P. (1996). The domain of the supervisory process and temporal organisation of behaviour. *Philosophical Transactions of the Royal Society B: Biological Sciences*, **351**, 1405–12.

Stuss, D. (2007). New approaches to prefrontal lobe testing. In: *The human frontal lobes: functions and disorders* (2nd edn) (ed B.L. Miller and J.L. Cummings). Guilford Press, New York.

von Cramon, D. and Matthes-von Cramon, G. (1994). Back to work with a chronic dysexecutive syndrome. *Neuropsychological Rehabilitation*, **4**, 399–417.

von Cramon, D., Matthes-von Cramon, G., and Mai, N. (1991) Problem-solving deficits in brain injured patients: a therapeutic approach. *Neuropsychological Rehabilitation*, **1**, 45–64.

Yeates, G.N., Henwood, K., Gracey, F., and Evans, J.J. (2007) Awareness of disability after acquired brain injury (ABI) and the family context. *Neuropsychological Rehabilitation*, **17**, 151–73.

5

Rehabilitation for prospective memory problems resulting from acquired brain injury

Jessica Fish∗, Tom Manly∗, and
Barbara A. Wilson∗†

∗ MRC Cognition and Brain Sciences Unit, Cambridge

† The Oliver Zangwill Centre for Neuropsychological
Rehabilitation, Ely

Introduction

What is prospective memory, and why is it important in neuropsychological rehabilitation?

'Prospective memory' (PM) refers to the processes involved in remembering to do something in the future, requiring not just memory of an intention, but an ability to trigger the intention and carry out the necessary action at the appropriate time. This is one of the least understood aspects of executive function and yet even a cursory consideration of the everyday tasks that involve PM makes its functional significance obvious. Fundamental activities of daily life, such as remembering to post letters, pay bills, make phone calls, attend appointments, collect the children from school, and so on all have a PM component. The clinical neuropsychological interest in PM stems from this functional significance, along with the frequency with which PM is reported to be a problem in clinical practice. Everyday memory problems are frequent following brain injury (Kinsella et al. 1996), and it has been suggested that when people talk about having a poor memory, they often mean poor PM (Baddeley 1997).

PM impairments have been reported in an enormous range of disorders, including Parkinson's disease (Katai et al. 2003; Kliegel et al. 2005), depression (Rude et al. 1999), schizophrenia (Elvevag et al. 2003; Shum et al. 2004), and healthy ageing and dementia (Huppert et al. 2000), as well as following stroke (Brooks et al. 2004) and acquired brain injury (ABI) (Shum et al. 1999;

Groot *et al.* 2002). This disparate range of disorders is not particularly helpful in developing the theoretical understanding of PM—what do they share that would lead to a common impairment in PM? The lack of differentiation between types of PM problem may have also been hindered by inadequate assessment procedures. However, the practical significance of PM remains, and hence the importance of assessing it in clinical practice.

PM is by no means a unitary construct. Numerous separable cognitive operations contribute to completion of PM tasks, and disruption of any one component could compromise achievement. This can be demonstrated by thinking of the steps necessary for a typical PM task—remembering to post a letter. First, there must be a conscious intention to post the letter (without this you cannot have a PM failure). Unless a postbox is immediately to hand, you must either actively rehearse this intention until it can be executed at some time in the future, or intend to remember this intention when its execution is possible. Given that one may engage in many intervening tasks, this intention must be stored in such a way that it does not impinge upon current activity but, at the same time, it must have a special status in relation to all your other memories of things that you intended to do (cf. the intention superiority effect (Marsh *et al.* 1999; Freeman and Ellis 2003)). The intention must be accessed at the appropriate time or in response to the appropriate event, and actions associated with the intention must be initiated. In the letter-posting example, this would involve recalling the intention before leaving the house in order to take the letter with you, and again remembering the intention in order to post the letter upon passing the postbox. Additionally, it is desirable to remember the status of the PM task after completion—whether or not you posted the letter—to avoid unnecessary repetition. Ellis (1996) described these stages as encoding, retention, realization, and evaluation. Her descriptive model provides a useful basis for understanding the different areas of enquiry in PM research.

Theoretical insights towards the understanding of prospective memory

Many experimental studies (almost all concerning people without brain injury) have been useful in identifying relevant features in PM tasks, chiefly concerning how properties of the task influence performance. Many PM experiments have a dual-task design in which the act of remembering to do something at a future point must be maintained whilst completing a separate, attentionally demanding task (the 'ongoing' task). It is rather difficult to accept even the face validity of these laboratory tasks, particularly in terms of their usual time-scale compared with real-life intentions (minutes rather than hours or days). However, as Ellis (1996) points out, it is likely that intentions will be remembered intermittently between intention formation and enactment, so perhaps the seemingly diverse situations are not wholly irreconcilable. However, the relevance for the type of PM tasks that occur over periods of days, and of which patients complain, is as yet unclear.

A second strand of research concerning more general executive impairments has arguably been of greater influence in thinking about clinically significant PM problems than this form of purely PM-based research. Interestingly, both these research streams, while using different terms, focus on the formation and execution of intentions and arrive at a point where 'executive' function interacts with memory in goal-directed ways. We shall now briefly consider some relevant themes in both areas.

Theories of Prospective Memory Retrieval

Einstein and McDaniel (1996) differentiated between time- and event-based PM (in terms of the cue for action—'at 5.30 p.m.' versus 'on passing the post box'). Several studies from this group have investigated processes involved in PM retrieval—at the broadest level, these being strategic and automatic processes (McDaniel and Einstein 2000; McDaniel et al. 2004). Strategic processing refers to continuous monitoring of the environment for the prospective cue. This is analogous to the concepts of attentional and/or executive functioning which are more commonly used in clinical neuropsychology. Automatic processes are described as 'reflexive association', involving the environmental cue triggering activation of the stored memory trace of the intention and bringing it into conscious awareness. If this process fails, PM would fail. Automatic processes are supposedly involved to a greater extent in event-based tasks, and strategic processes more in time-based ones. This seems plausible as event-based tasks involve an inherent environmental cue, which time-based tasks often do not (other than time itself), and so continuous monitoring would not be adaptive under these circumstances.

Kliegel et al. (2001, 2004b) examined the effect of instructions emphasizing the importance of either the PM task or the ongoing task (simply 'the PM task is most important'). They found that these instructions affected PM performance only in the tasks that would require strategic monitoring. Specifically, the effect was initially found in time-based but not event-based tasks (Kliegel et al. 2001), and later in event-based tasks but only when the PM target was non-focal and not when it was focal (i.e. only when the target was not immediately obvious in the context of completing the ongoing task). Similar results hold true in experiments where factors such as (a) the PM cue distinctiveness is varied (perceptually or semantically), (b) the degree of association between target and action is manipulated, and (c) the nature of the ongoing task is varied (e.g. whether it is similar or different to the PM task and whether it is a novel or practised ongoing task). This indicates that different processes can be employed in the support of PM—referred to as 'multiprocess theory' (McDaniel and Einstein 2000; Einstein *et al.* 2005).

However, whether PM retrieval can really happen automatically is a matter of dispute. Smith (2003) argued that performance of even simple PM tasks involves cognitive resources that would otherwise be available for other tasks. Thus there should always be a cost of performing PM tasks on 'ongoing' tasks. Evidence supporting this view was provided by experiments in which a PM task was either embedded in the ongoing task or delayed until a later point in time. Slower responses were observed in the ongoing task when participants were expecting to perform the PM task than when they knew about the PM task but were not expecting to perform it until later on. This suggested deployment of attentional resources to the PM task even in the absence of a PM target stimulus. A further experiment compared the effects of embedded retrospective memory (RM) and PM tasks upon ongoing task performance, and found that although the level of performance was equivalent between PM and RM tasks, the detrimental effect upon ongoing task performance was specific to the PM task. This evidence was argued to support the position that although the mnemonic demands of PM and RM tasks are similar, there is an additional attentional demand of PM tasks. Interestingly, participants with good PM performance also exhibited longer response times to the ongoing task, suggesting that greater attentional resource allocation leads to better prospective remembering. This is inconsistent with reflexive–associative (automatic retrieval) models, and was argued to support a preparatory attentional and memory (PAM) process theory, which states that the involvement of capacity-consuming processes is *always* required for PM retrieval.

However, Einstein *et al.* (2005) report that spontaneous retrieval of intentions is at least possible, showing that costs to the ongoing task are evident only where the concurrent PM task requires monitoring. Further, Einstein and colleagues found that when PM targets were presented when they were not expected, and therefore when there would be no need for participants to engage monitoring processes, PM targets elicited longer response times than did new items, previously presented items, and items associated with a RM task. The authors infer from this that the items associated with a PM task were recognized spontaneously. They propose that task demands and individual differences will determine the extent to which monitoring or spontaneous retrieval is relied upon. They also predict that involvement of monitoring processes will reduce with increasing delay. Although it seems likely that strategic monitoring would not be continually engaged from the time of intention formation to action in the event of a long delay (indeed, it may be questionable whether such an intention would constitute a PM task), monitoring processes may well still be recruited, following intermittent recall of the intention, whether cued or spontaneous (cf. Ellis 1996).

The strategic monitoring processes in PM have a clear overlap with notions of executive function, and therefore problems with the prospective components of the PM tasks could well be viewed in some neurological patients as part of a wider part of the wider 'dysexecutive syndrome'. Indeed, several single-case studies have linked frontal lobe pathology with PM deficits (e.g. Shallice and Burgess 1991; Cockburn 1995; Evans et al. 1998). McDaniel et al. (1999) conducted the first group study that explicitly linked PM with frontal lobe function. They found poorer PM in older adults scoring poorly on tests of frontal lobe function—a composite score drawn from the Wisconsin Card Sorting Test, verbal fluency, and the mental arithmetic, mental control, and backward digit span subtests from the Wechsler Memory Scale–Revised (WMS–R) (Wechsler 1987)—compared with those scoring well on these tests. However, the effect observed was moderated by the differential ability on the ongoing task (general knowledge questions) between these two groups. After covarying for this factor, the difference in PM performance was only marginally significant. Supposed medial temporal lobe function (as measured by logical memory I, and verbal paired associates I and II from the WMS–R and the California Verbal Learning Test) was not related to PM performance. There is also evidence from cross-sectional studies that variance in PM performance at a group level may be better accounted for by measures of executive function than memory in TBI groups (Groot et al. 2002; Kopp and Thöne-Otto 2003; Martin et al. 2003). In a more direct test of this relationship, Burgess et al. (2000) conducted a neuropsychological investigation of multi-tasking, which identified left-hemisphere lesions to Brodman areas 8, 9, and 10 as affecting the delayed intention (PM) component of multi-tasking, whereas lesions to right dorsolateral prefrontal cortex impaired the planning component. There is now additional evidence from neuroimaging studies demonstrating involvement of specific regions of the frontal lobes in PM (Okuda et al. 1998; Burgess et al. 2001; Simons et al. 2006); however, as noted by Burgess et al. (2003), the network of regions involved is that typically associated with performance of any attentionally demanding task (areas in prefrontal and inferior parietal cortex). This pattern could have reflected the effortful nature of PM tasks compared with baseline tasks. Burgess et al. (2003), in a PET study of PM, reported that while activity in rostrolateral prefrontal cortex (rlPFC) increased under PM conditions compared with baseline, activity in rostromedial prefrontal cortex was (rmPFC) suppressed under PM conditions, arguing against a simple task difficulty hypothesis. The pattern has been replicated in subsequent studies (Simons *et al.* 2006), and suggests there are brain areas that are specifically involved in the realization of delayed intentions.

Executive function research relevant to prospective memory

Models of executive function, which may not explicitly deal with PM, still offer considerable insight, especially in consideration of contextual influences on PM performance. An example is the model of Norman and Shallice (1980), where emphasis is placed upon the nature of the situation in which an action is to be performed, the primary distinction being between routine and novel situations. In routine situations, actions and intentions can be carried out relatively automatically by a system referred to as 'contention scheduling'. Here, reinstatement of context results in activation of action schemas based upon prior experience, with little or no strategic involvement. However, in non-routine situations an appropriate schema may not exist. Therefore the construction and implementation of a new schema is required. The supervisory attention system (SAS) was proposed to oversee these processes. Shallice and Burgess (1996) described three stages within this system—strategy formation, implementation, and monitoring—with additional related sub-processes involving PM retrieval, episodic memory retrieval, and motivational components. This model can be seen in some ways as analogous to the multiprocess model of PM, although it is more comprehensive in nature.

Another line of research into executive or frontal lobe function that applies particularly well to PM deficits is that relating to 'goal neglect' (Duncan *et al.* 1996). This term describes a phenomenon whereby an intention that has been understood and well remembered (a goal) is not acted upon as intended. This can be seen as equivalent to an executive PM failure. Goal neglect was initially observed in patients with focal damage to the frontal lobes (Duncan *et al.* 1996), and subsequently in people with head injuries (Duncan *et al.* 1997). Duncan (2006), linking such work in neuropsychology with related research in human fMRI and primate physiology, proposed that a frontoparietal system, the 'multiple demand' network, adjudicates between various inputs simultaneously competing for attention. In the classic example of remembering to post a letter on the way to work, there will be many environmental stimuli other than postboxes to be aware of, and to which attention could be drawn. In the intact system, biasing processes are effective, resulting in the strongest competitive weight being assigned to the most behaviourally relevant input. In this case, the postbox would capture our attention and reactivate the intention to post the letter. If the system is damaged, it may be inefficient. Other competing inputs may have a stronger 'hold' on the focus of attention, resulting in goal neglect errors, in the context of more generalized disorganization of goal-directed behaviour. To continue the previous example, if one is navigating along a busy street, caught up in conversation, or thinking about what to have for dinner, one might be less likely to link the glimpse of a postbox with one's prior intention.

These models offer greater insight into the dynamics of PM processing than those that have emerged from the more constrained field of PM research, and have been much more influential in clinical neuropsychology and rehabilitation. For example, the goal neglect research was used as the theoretical standpoint in the development of Goal Management Training (GMT), a new rehabilitation programme for executive dysfunction (Levine *et al.* 2000; Levine *et al.* 2007).

Linking theory to practice

Many well-practised tasks can be triggered by the environment or context with little requirement for conscious mediation. However, although these circumstances describe some of our everyday tasks, such as switching off the lights when we are the last to leave the office, there are many everyday tasks that do not fit with this description, perhaps when the task is out of the ordinary, such as remembering to make a detour on the way to work to buy a birthday card. It seems likely, then, that in most everyday situations there will be at least some involvement of executive processes in PM task completion. Similarly, neuropsychological and neuroimaging findings suggest that there may be specific involvement of rlPFC and rmPFC in PM. However, it is unlikely that damage to rlPFC is the primary cause of PM difficulties because of the numerous potential routes to PM failure.

In terms of assessment it is clear that the sheer diversity of executive functions and number of factors affecting executive performance mean that impairment in one situation may not necessarily translate to impairment in another, depending perhaps on motivation, novelty, presence of competing stimuli, fatigue, and so on. Therefore an inclusive approach should be taken to patient assessment, formulation, and intervention.

Assessment for rehabilitation of prospective memory

In order to appropriately target rehabilitation for PM difficulties, it is obviously important to gain an understanding of which of the many components required for successful PM performance are the most problematic for a particular individual.

The theoretical studies discussed in the last section suggest a useful taxonomy of PM on which to base this approach. We suggest three different and potentially complementary approaches to the assessment of PM. The first is to use existing clinical tests which, to one extent or another, tax each of these components separately (e.g. planning, RM, and executive function). This may help to specify in which domain errors are most likely. However, it could be difficult to predict the extent of a PM deficit on the basis of such disparate test scores. The second approach involves the relatively few recent attempts to create analogues of PM tasks and incorporate them into standardized desktop tests. In essence, these involve asking clients to perform PM tasks such as 'pass me this message in 20 minutes time', along with distracter activities, such as completing puzzles (Raskin 2004; Wilson et al. 2005). Although there may be limitations inherent in this approach regarding the predictive validity of tests carried out over 20–30 minutes for everyday PM tasks (which remains to be established), it can be useful to observe patients combining mnemonic and executive processes in a single task, and to gauge this performance in relation to normative data. The third approach involves ecological measures of PM. The longer time-scale and everyday setting involved with this type of measurement means that there is a greater likelihood that nuisance variables will affect results. However, data collected in this way yield potentially more valuable results, particularly in terms of identifying reasons behind everyday PM failures.

Separate assessment of component processes

Considering the first approach, theoretical work has, as previously discussed, identified mnemonic and executive components of PM. Therefore assessment of memory and executive function should be informative in understanding the reasons behind everyday PM failure and the situations that are likely to be problematic. This should subsequently help in appropriately focusing rehabilitation strategies.

To illustrate, in the context of a standard neuropsychological assessment, if a client with reported everyday PM problems has impaired performance on tests of memory and learning, it would indicate that the PM problem is related to the retention of intention content. That is, as well as not remembering to carry out the task, he/she forgets the details of the task, or indeed that there was a task at all. Therefore it is clear that any significant RM impairment is likely to cause problems in *completing PM tasks*, although whether there is, strictly speaking, a *PM deficit*, is another matter entirely. However, this information remains useful as the memory rehabilitation literature (e.g. Wilson 1987) indicates that compensatory methods, such as using internal mnemonic strategies (e.g. mental imagery) or external memory aids such as memory notebooks or electronic organizers, will be the most appropriate form of intervention. Additional benefits could also be found in supporting learning of the retrospective aspects of PM tasks (see below), although the precise nature of the intervention should also depend upon other factors such as severity of the problem, preservation of other cognitive functions, experience with technology, and so forth.

Alternatively, if a client has difficulty in completing PM tasks, in the context of relatively preserved RM abilities, there could be a number of causes. Is it due to a problem with spontaneous retrieval, initiation, planning, strategy application, distractibility, or motivation? These may be more difficult issues to address, and although the models of executive function outlined above are more useful than the specific PM models, these issues are not readily incorporated into a single extant model. Consequently, they may not be easily assessed using existing tests. Reduced performance on tests tapping aspects of executive function suggest that the introduction of strategies focusing upon executive components of PM tasks may be fruitful. However, it is widely acknowledged that intact performance on tests of executive function does not necessarily rule out problems with executive dysfunction in daily life (Burgess *et al.* 2006).

Non-cognitive factors involved in PM failure should also be addressed. Conventional wisdom would suggest that tasks which are particularly emotionally salient, or carry a particular reward, may be forgotten to a lesser extent than neutral tasks with little or no inherent reward. For example, Meacham and Singer (1977) found superior PM performance under high-incentive conditions compared with low-incentive conditions (the high-incentive condition involved a chance to win $5,whereas the low-incentive condition involved no additional external incentive). The difference in PM performance may have been related to a greater use of external strategies in the high-incentive condition. Are the sorts of task that are forgotten those that the person wants and/or needs to remember?

Clinical tests of prospective memory

The second approach to assessment, using an analogue PM situation in a clinical setting, is certainly promising, but it at present is not very well developed. A well-established test of everyday memory function that includes PM items is the Rivermead Behavioural Memory Test (RBMT) (Wilson *et al.* 1985), which has very good ecological and predictive validity. These aspects of the RBMT were expanded into a clinical test of PM, the Cambridge Prospective Memory Test (CAMPROMPT) (Wilson *et al.* 2005), which involves three time-based and three event-based PM tasks for enactment after varying delays over a 30-minute period. Although the CAMPROMPT shares a modest correlation with the RBMT, so far it lacks convincing evidence that it predicts everyday PM performance. Another test of PM, the Memory for Intentions Screening

Test (MIST) (Raskin 2004), claims good validity and a large set of normative data. However, to our knowledge it is not currently available, and findings of the test have not been published beyond the form of conference abstracts.

Kliegel *et al.* (2000, 2004a) developed an experimental paradigm that aimed to differentiate components of prospective remembering, which has potential clinical application. In the test, participants are asked first to formulate a plan of action regarding a multi-tasking situation. This plan is specified for action at a later point in time, when a particular item in a questionnaire is reached. After a delay period they are asked to recall their plan. After a further delay period, upon reaching the specified question, the planned actions should be initiated. From this, separate scores for intention formation (planning), retention (memory), re-instantiation (remembering at the appropriate time), and execution (one score for following the earlier plan, another for switching between tasks effectively) are derived. This paradigm has great potential, and certainly has better face validity than the majority of tests used in the experimental psychology literature, but still requires further development before it can be used in formal clinical assessment. A further limitation of this type of test is its serial nature—even though separate scores are derived, the components themselves are highly related, and failure of the memory component precludes success on the executive components, regardless of executive ability. This is not necessarily a problem when used in research looking at the executive components of PM as participants with poor memory for their intentions can be excluded from subsequent analysis, but further testing will be required in clinical assessment.

There have also been studies employing virtual reality (Brooks *et al.* 2004) and video (Knight *et al.* 2006) paradigms to assess PM, but they are very preliminary at present. Although further tests are in development, which may improve the situation, at present the available clinical tests of PM have limited sensitivity. Questionnaires to measure the frequency of reported everyday PM problems are available (e.g. PRMQ (Crawford *et al.* 2003)), but these are also still in development and so it may transpire that the most important tool in clinical decision-making, and goal-planning, is self and relative perception of everyday difficulties. Apart from the lack of demonstrated validity, a further problem with these tests and questionnaires is that they do not adequately specify the locus of the problem. They do not tell us whether the failure results from loss of the content of the intention, or indicate whether the problem may be linked to distraction, problems with initiation, or other executive aspects of the task.

Naturalistic prospective memory tasks

The issues in the assessment of PM outlined above informed our choice of paradigm in a recent study on the rehabilitation of PM (Fish *et al.* 2007) and illustrate the third approach to assessment—using ecological PM tasks. Our task involved making a telephone call to a voicemail service at four set times over a 3-week period. Although this differs from some PM tasks in terms of the ease with which the task can be executed and its lack of consequences (other than those related to self-perception of performance), in terms of face validity it seems to mimic fairly well the type of task one might have to perform on a day-to-day basis, such as taking medication or remembering to phone the bank. It also allows for an estimation of variability in performance, which may in itself be important in predicting real-life PM performance. We attempted to minimize the retrospective demands of the task by using an errorless learning procedure in encoding task content, which involved slowly reducing the amount of to-be-learned information presented in order for the participant to recall it correctly, known as vanishing cues (Glisky *et al.* 1986), and discouraging guessing throughout. Reminder cards summarizing task demands were also provided. Another important aspect of the design was the inclusion of a daily telephone call from one of the experimenters, in which reasons for omissions or late calls were discussed. This provided much useful information in terms of why people forgot to make calls. The primary aim of this study was to examine the effect of a cueing strategy on PM performance (see below). However, this procedure also has potential application for relatively informal PM assessment (i.e. non-standardized, providing qualitative information). Using this type of task in a 'behavioural experiment' format may provide insight into reasons for making PM errors. In the study, errors resulted mostly from being caught up in other tasks, but sometimes other issues emerged, such as 'I received some bad news and forgot about making the calls', 'I left my mobile phone at home', or 'I thought about it a lot, but never at the right time'. Equally, it could be a way of understanding individuals' perceptions of PM errors; for example, someone saying that they have a terrible memory, but in fact making all calls quite accurately, perhaps has unrealistic expectations of how easily tasks should be accomplished or perfectionist tendencies, which may both serve to inflate perception of difficulties, in turn causing worry in relation to performance (which may well also impact upon performance). In this sense, this sort of task could be used as a method of collecting evidence in cognitive-behaviour therapy. The day-to-day changes in activity in the context of the constant PM task can also provide information on types of activity that are likely to cause forgetting (e.g. being on the Internet, chatting with a friend).

Another way of assessing real-life PM functioning is to ask the client to record day-to-day PM task performance in a diary, including, for example, successes, failures, strategies used, and reasons behind mistakes. Sohlberg and

Mateer (2001) advocate this method particularly for attention lapses (and successes) because it can add to clients' understanding and sense of control. A limitation associated with this method is the cognitive demand it places on the client; remembering to record PM lapses is in itself a PM task, whether this is done on an as-they-occur basis or at one time point for the whole day. Additionally, documenting the day's events taxes RM heavily. This leaves open the possibility that important information could be omitted, or inaccurately reconstructed.

As PM is still a relatively new area of research which is currently in a period of rapid development, there is no well-established method for its assessment. However, use of emergent methods as described above, in combination with interviews with the patient and relatives in the context of a comprehensive neuropsychological assessment, can shed light on why PM problems occur, and in which situations they are most likely to occur.

Rehabilitation of prospective memory

Neuropsychological rehabilitation is about the achievement of individual goals rather than improvement in specific cognitive functions. Within a holistic framework (e.g. Prigatano 1999; Wilson 2002) it is likely that work on PM would form only a component of any rehabilitation plan. However, given the ubiquity of PM complaints following brain injury, it is likely that change in this area would be an implicit feature within many clients' goals.

When taking a holistic approach to rehabilitation, it is difficult to pinpoint the effect of specific interventions on specific functions (e.g. improvements in mood could exert benefits across a number of cognitive domains). Nevertheless it is useful here to examine the evidence base of techniques that might specifically improve, or reduce the impact of, PM difficulties. We first consider pharmacological interventions, then the merits of repeated PM practice, and finally the use of compensatory strategies.

Pharmacological treatments

McDowell et al. (1998) conducted an exciting preliminary study on the effects of dopaminergic medication on executive and working memory tasks in a group of TBI patients, and found selective effects on tasks with suspected prefrontal involvement. This might imply beneficial effects for PM tasks, in view of the documented contribution of executive functions towards PM task execution (McDaniel et al. 1999; Burgess et al. 2000, 2003; Kopp and Thöne-Otto 2003). However, there are as yet no reports of replication or clinical application of these findings. More recently, Rusted et al. (2005) and Rusted and Trawley (2006) have

specifically examined the effects of nicotine (a cholinergic agonist) on PM function, and have found beneficial effects for tasks suspected to involve strategic
processing (monitoring processes; see earlier discussion of Kliegel *et al.* (2001,
2004b)) but not automatic processing. These differential effects indicate that
there is potential for improving the executive-monitoring component of PM
with pharmacological agents, but not for making spontaneous retrieval more
likely. These results are promising but, as with the wider evidence base for pharmacological treatment of cognitive and behavioural problems following brain
injury, the results are preliminary (Warden *et al.* 2006).

Re-training approaches

Sohlberg *et al.* (1992a) used repeated practice of simple PM tasks (e.g. 'Raise
your hand when I ring this bell') over increasing delay periods in the rehabilitation of two patients with ABI. Patient 1 received 58 hours training over
4.5 months, and progressed from being unable to complete a PM task (even
without distraction) at a 60-second delay, to being able to complete a PM task
at an 8-minute delay with a success rate of 40–80 per cent. Patient 2 received
32 hours of training over 3.5 months, and showed an increase in PM span,
including distracter activity, from 4 to 8 minutes. A third case, reported separately (Sohlberg *et al.* 1992b), used similar methods, with the addition of
generalization measures. Overall, the patient's PM span increased from 5 to
12 minutes. However, generalization to both to naturalistic PM tasks and RM
tasks was limited. Raskin and Sohlberg (1996) investigated PM training in two
case studies, this time contrasting PM training with an RM drill (performing
simple actions on instruction and then recalling the action over increasing
delay intervals). Improvements in PM accuracy were observed with onset of
PM training, but not with the onset of RM drilling, suggesting that the PM
training specifically benefited PM performance. There was also some evidence
of carry-over to subsequent RM drilling phases. Overall, the PM span of both
patients increased by 5 minutes (from spans of 1 and 2 minutes at baseline).
There was also evidence that performance on real-life PM tasks improved, as
recorded by significant others.

The advantage of this type of repeated-practice training is that it does seem
to offer benefits to PM, and this implies some improvement at the impairment
level. Additionally, although the improvements in PM span may seem insub-
stantial, considering Ellis's observation on the intermittent PM retrieval prior
to enactment, the gains could actually be quite important. However, the
evidence base for this technique is limited. There is mixed evidence of generalization, reports of maintenance are absent, and there are no large group
studies supporting its efficacy. An additional factor related to its clinical utility

is the nature of the training; it involves a large time commitment and appears passive. This may limit clients' enjoyment and, subsequently, tolerance of this type of training.

Compensatory approaches: supporting retrospective memory to improve PM performance

Camp *et al.* (1996) have used spaced retrieval, an established technique for learning information, in training people with Alzheimer's disease (AD) to remember to perform a daily PM task displayed on a wall calendar. The training involved weekly sessions in which participants were repeatedly asked how they would remember the task and, provided that a correct answer was given ('By checking the calendar'), the delay before the next repetition was progressively increased. Of the 23 participants, 20 were able to learn the strategy for verbal report in three to seven sessions. Of those 20, 15 were also successfully using the calendar (defined as at least four out of seven days per week). Kixmiller (2002) reported a pilot study of PM training in a small group of people with AD, which combined principles of spaced retrieval and errorless learning (EL), an established technique in memory rehabilitation (Baddeley and Wilson 1994). Training took place over 2 weeks (six sessions), and involved graded reduction of trainer involvement in carrying out PM tasks, such as making a telephone call reporting particular information, from initially observing the trainer, to carrying out the task with verbal prompts, then independently with feedback, and so on. Performance on these naturalistic PM tasks, with a post-training lag of up to 7 weeks, was superior in the five trained participants compared with the two untrained controls. Clearly, this work requires extension, but it is certainly a promising approach.

External memory aids: supporting retrospective and prospective components

External memory aids are now widely available, can be very inexpensive, and have the potential to be highly effective in the compensation for PM problems, with minimal further support in mild to moderately impaired patients (Kapur *et al.* 2004). There can be difficulty in both learning and remembering to use electronic reminders, but, even in densely amnesic patients, electronic devices can be used to aid PM. For example, Kime *et al.* (1996) described the use of a cueing device, an hourly watch alarm, to prompt a densely amnesic young woman to check a diary. Diary checking increased over the course of the programme, and was maintained at follow-up over a year later. The authors suggested that this system drew upon preserved implicit memory processes. Thinking about this in terms of theories of PM function, perhaps these types of compensatory approaches have benefits over and above their specific aims regarding task achievement—the repeated performance of a task with the support of an external device may alter a PM task from one requiring monitoring or strategic initiation to one that can be achieved with relative automaticity, and make its fulfilment over time more probable.

There is a substantial body of evidence supporting the use of electronic memory aids in PM rehabilitation. The largest such studies are those examining the NeuroPage system (Wilson *et al.* 1997, 2001), which involves sending text-based messages, according to a pre-specified schedule, from a central administration point to a simple-to-use pager worn by the patient. On average, the 143 patients in the 2001 study increased their goal attainment by 30 per cent when using the pager relative to baseline performance. There was also evidence that in some cases these benefits were maintained during the return to baseline phase, although this was not a universal finding—some participants were able to maintain pager-level performance, whereas a minority dropped back to baseline levels. These discrepant patterns are thought to depend upon the presence or absence of executive dysfunction—those with intact executive abilities may benefit from the provision of a routine and be able to consolidate this routine better than those with executive dysfunction, who may benefit from the provision of a cue in addition to the provision of the message content. Other studies (van den Broek *et al.* 2000, Yasuda *et al.* 2002) have shown that reminding devices with voice-based output can be effective in improving PM performance in patients with ABI, although it can be quite dificult to learn to use them.

Supporting the executive component

Fish *et al.* (2007), extending previous work by Manly *et al.* (2002, 2004), reported that using a 'content-free' cueing strategy improved performance of a group of 20 participants with ABI on an everyday PM task, which was to make telephone calls at four set times per day over a period of 2 weeks. The strategy involved sending the mnemonic STOP! to participants' mobile phones at random times on five randomly selected days. Importantly, the times were not linked to the optimal times to perform the PM task. The mnemonic STOP stood for Stop, Think, Organize, and Plan, and was intended to encourage participants to pause current activity and briefly review their wider current and future goals. The reliable increase in PM performance between days with and without cues, along with previous findings from short-scale measures of executive function, constitutes encouraging evidence that similar cueing strategies could be used with success in aiding performance towards personally relevant goals and PM tasks, rather than experimental ones.

Integrative approaches

Fleming *et al.* (2005) reported the results of a PM training programme in a series of three case studies. This programme had a focus on developing awareness and using compensatory strategies. Pre–post gains were found on questionnaire and performance measures of PM, although the lack of a control group renders these findings inconclusive. More importantly, all three cases showed an increase in the number of useful diary entries made following training. Unfortunately, several factors limit the conclusions that can be drawn from this study. Two of the three cases had sustained their injuries very recently (2 and 4 months previously), meaning that their improvement may have been a result of spontaneous recovery or, conversely, may have resulted in smaller benefits, as this was very early post-injury to undergo such a programme. Additionally, although the diary monitoring measure suggested more entries were being made post-training, it does not necessarily follow that these entries were acted upon successfully, and this, of course, is the most important measure. There is evidence that educational approaches in the area of executive function rehabilitation can be effective (Problem-Solving Training (von Cramon *et al.* 1991); Goal Management Training (Levine *et al.* 2000)), and these programmes may well hold benefits for PM.

Conclusion

Several cognitive processes contribute towards everyday PM performance, and therefore it can fail for a number of reasons. Comprehensive assessment procedures should shed light upon the source of a particular patient's PM problem, and consequently inform the appropriate intervention approach. At present there is good evidence for using compensatory strategies, in the form of diaries and/or electronic memory aids, in promoting achievement of PM tasks in terms of both their prospective and retrospective demands. There is preliminary evidence that techniques targeting the retrospective components of PM tasks, such as errorless learning and spaced retrieval, could be useful in facilitating task performance, although further work is required in this domain. There is also encouraging evidence that using strategies focusing on the executive component of PM tasks can be helpful. Combining such mnemonic and executive strategies may result in the greatest benefit, although the appropriate combinations have to be determined by the client's goals and neuropsychological profile.

References

Baddeley, A. (1997). *Human memory: theory and practice.* Psychology Press, Hove.

Baddeley, A. and Wilson, B.A. (1994). When implicit learning fails: amnesia and the problem of error elimination. *Neuropsychologia*, **32**, 53–68.

Brooks, B.M., Rose, F.D., Potter, J., Jayawardena, S., and Morling, A. (2004). Assessing stroke patients' prospective memory using virtual reality. *Brain Injury*, **18**, 391–401.

Burgess, P. W., Veitch, E., De Lacy Costello, A., and Shallice, T. (2000). The cognitive and neuroanatomical correlates of multitasking. *Neuropsychologia*, **38**, 848–63.

Burgess, P.W., Quayle, A., and Frith, C.D. (2001). Brain regions involved in prospective memory as determined by positron emission tomography. *Neuropsychologia*, **39**, 545–55.

Burgess, P.W., Scott, S.K., and Frith, C.D. (2003). The role of the rostral frontal cortex (area 10) in prospective memory: a lateral versus medial dissociation. *Neuropsychologia*, **41**, 906–18.

Burgess, P.W., Alderman, N., Forbes, C., *et al.* (2006). The case for the development and use of 'ecologically valid' measures of executive function in experimental and clinical neuropsychology. *Journal of the International Neuropsychological Society*, **12**, 194–209.

Camp, C.J., Foss, J.W., Stevens, A.B., and O'Hanlon, A.M. (1996). Improving prospective memory performance in persons with Alzheimer's disease. In: *Prospective memory: theory and applications* (ed M.A. Brandimonte, G.O. Einstein, and M.A. McDaniel). Lawrence Erlbaum, Mahwah, NJ.

Cockburn, J. (1995). Task interruption in prospective memory: a frontal lobe function? *Cortex*, **31**, 87–97.

Crawford, J.R., Smith, G.V., Maylor, E.A.M., Della Sala, S., and Logie, R.H. (2003). The Prospective and Retrospective Memory Questionnaire (PRMQ): normative data and latent structure in a large non-clinical sample. *Memory* **11**, 261–75.

Duncan, J. (2006). Brain mechanisms of attention. *Quarterly Journal of Experimental Psychology*, **59**, 2–27.

Duncan, J., Emslie, H., Williams, P., Johnson, R., and Freer, C. (1996). Intelligence and the frontal lobe: The organization of goal-directed behavior. *Cognitive Psychology*, **30**, 257–303.

Duncan, J., Johnson, R., Swales, M., and Freer, C. (1997). Frontal lobe deficits after head injury: unity and diversity of function. *Cognitive Neuropsychology*, **14**, 713–41.

Einstein, G.O. and McDaniel, M.A. (1996). Retrieval processes in prospective memory: theoretical approaches and some new empirical findings. In: *Prospective memory: theory and applications* (ed M.A. Brandimonte, G.O. Einstein, and M.A. McDaniel). Lawrence Erlbaum, Mahwah, NJ.

Einstein, G.O., Thomas, R., Mayfield, S., *et al.* (2005). Multiple processes in prospective memory retrieval: factors determining monitoring versus spontaneous retrieval. *Journal of Experimental Psychology: General*, **134**, 327–42.

Ellis, J.A. (1996). Prospective memory or the realization of delayed intentions: a conceptual framework for research. In: *Prospective memory: theory and applications* (ed M.A. Brandimonte, G.O. Einstein, and M.A. McDaniel). Lawrence Erlbaum, Mahwah, NJ.

Elvevag, B., Maylor, E.A., and Gilbert, A.L. (2003). Habitual prospective memory in schizophrenia. *BMC Psychiatry*, **3**, 9 [electronic resource].

Evans, J.J., Emslie, H., and Wilson, B.A. (1998). External cueing systems in the rehabilitation of executive impairments of action. *Journal of the International Neuropsychological Society*, **4**, 399–408.

Fish, J., Evans, J.J., Nimmo, M., *et al.* (2007). Rehabilitation of executive dysfunction following brain injury: 'content-free' cueing improves everyday prospective memory performance. *Neuropsychologia*, **45**, 1318–30.

Fleming, J.M., Shum, D., Strong, J., and Lightbody, S. (2005). Prospective memory rehabilitation for adults with traumatic brain injury: a compensatory training programme. *Brain Injury*, **19**, 1–10.

Freeman, J.E. and Ellis, J.A. (2003). The intention-superiority effect for naturally occurring activities: the role of intention accessibility in everyday prospective remembering in young and older adults. *International Journal of Psychology*, **38**, 215–28.

Glisky, E.L., Schacter, D.L., and Tulving, E. (1986). Learning and retention of computer-related vocabulary in memory-impaired patients: method of vanishing cues. *Journal of Clinical and Experimental Neuropsychology*, **8**, 292–312.

Groot, Y.C.T., Wilson, B.A., Evans, J., and Watson, P. (2002). Prospective memory functioning in people with and without brain injury. *Journal of the International Neuropsychological Society*, **8**, 645–54.

Huppert, F.A., Johnson, T., and Nickson, J. (2000). High prevalence of prospective memory impairment in the elderly and in early-stage dementia: findings from a population-based study. *Applied Cognitive Psychology*, **14**, S63–81.

Kapur, N., Glisky, E.L., and Wilson, B.A. (2004). Technological memory aids for people with memory deficits. *Neuropsychological Rehabilitation*, **14**, 41–60.

Katai, S., Maruyama, T., Hashimoto, T., and Ikeda, S. (2003). Event based and time based prospective memory in Parkinson's disease. *Journal of Neurology, Neurosurgery, and Psychiatry*, **74**, 704–9.

Kime, S.K., Lamb, D.G., and Wilson, B.A. (1996). Use of a comprehensive programme of external cueing to enhance procedural memory in a patient with dense amnesia. *Brain Injury*, **10**, 17–25.

Kinsella, G., Murtagh, D., Landry, A., *et al.* (1996). Everyday memory following traumatic brain injury. *Brain Injury*, **10**, 499–507.

Kixmiller, J.S. (2002). Evaluation of prospective memory training for individuals with mild Alzheimer's disease. *Brain and Cognition*, **49**, 237–41.

Kliegel, M., McDaniel, M.A., and Einstein, G.O. (2000). Plan formation, retention, and execution in prospective memory: a new approach and age-related effects. *Memory and Cognition*, **28**, 1041–9.

Kliegel, M., Martin, M., McDaniel, M.A., and Einstein, G.O. (2001). Varying the importance of a prospective memory task: differential effects across time- and event-based prospective memory. *Memory*, **9**, 1–11.

Kliegel, M., Eschen, A., and Thöne-Otto, A.I. (2004a). Planning and realisation of complex intentions in traumatic brain injury and normal aging. *Brain and Cognition*, **56**, 43–54.

Kliegel, M., Martin, M., McDaniel, M.A., and Einstein, G.O. (2004b). Importance effects on performance in event-based prospective memory tasks. *Memory*, **12**, 553–61.

Kliegel, M., Phillips, L.H., Lemke, U., and Kopp, U.A. (2005). Planning and realisation of complex intentions in patients with Parkinson's disease. *Journal of Neurology, Neurosurgery and Psychiatry*, **76**, 1501–5.

Knight, R.G., Titov, N., and Crawford, M. (2006). The effects of distraction on prospective remembering following traumatic brain injury assessed in a simulated naturalistic environment. *Journal of the International Neuropsychological Society*, **12**, 8–16.

Kopp, U.A. and Thöne-Otto, A.I. (2003). Disentangling executive functions and memory processes in event-based prospective remembering after brain damage: a neuropsychological study. *International Journal of Psychology*, **38**, 229–35.

Levine, B., Robertson, I.H., Clare, L., *et al.* (2000). Rehabilitation of executive functioning: an experimental–clinical validation of Goal Management Training. *Journal of the International Neuropsychological Society*, **6**, 299–312.

Levine, B., Stuss, D.T., Winocur, G., *et al.* (2007). Cognitive rehabilitation in the elderly: effects on strategic behavior in relation to goal management. *Journal of the International Neuropsychological Society*, **13**, 143–52.

McDaniel, M.A. and Einstein, G.O. (2000). Strategic and automatic processes in prospective memory retrieval: a multiprocess framework. *Applied Cognitive Psychology*, **14**, S127–44.

McDaniel, M.A., Guynn, M.J., Glisky, E.L., Rubin, S.R., and Routhieaux, B.C. (1999). Prospective memory: a neuropsychological study. *Neuropsychology*, **13**, 103–10.

McDaniel, M.A., Einstein, G.O., Guynn, M.J., and Breneiser, J. (2004). Cue-focused and reflexive-associative processes in prospective memory retrieval. *Journal of Experimental Psychology: Learning Memory and Cognition*, **30**, 605–14.

McDowell, S., Whyte, J., and D'Esposito, M. (1998). Differential effect of a dopaminergic agonist on prefrontal function in traumatic brain injury patients. *Brain*, **121**, 1155–64.

Manly, T., Hawkins, K., Evans, J., Woldt, K., and Robertson, I.H. (2002). Rehabilitation of executive function: facilitation of effective goal management on complex tasks using periodic auditory alerts. *Neuropsychologia*, **40**, 271–81.

Manly, T., Heutink, J., Davison, B., *et al.* (2004). An electronic knot in the handkerchief: 'content free cueing' and the maintenance of attentive control. *Neuropsychological Rehabilitation*, **1**, 89–116.

Marsh, R.L., Hicks, J.L., and Bryan, E.S. (1999). The activation of unrelated and canceled intentions. *Memory and Cognition*, **27**, 320–7.

Martin, M., Kliegel, M., and McDaniel, M.A. (2003). The involvement of executive functions in prospective memory performance of adults. *International Journal of Psychology*, **38**, 195–206.

Meacham, J.A., and Singer, J. (1977). Incentive effects in prospective remembering. *Journal of Psychology*, **97**, 191–7.

Norman, D.A. and Shallice, T. (1980). Attention to action: willed and automatic control of behaviour. CHIP Report 99, Center for Human Information Processing, University of California San Diego, CA.

Okuda, J., Fujii, T., Yamadori, A., *et al.* (1998). Participation of the prefrontal cortices in prospective memory: evidence from a PET study in humans. *Neuroscience Letters*, **253**, 127–30.

Prigatano, G. (1999). *Priniciples of neuropsychological rehabilitation*. Oxford University Press, New York.

Raskin, S. (2004). Memory for intentions screening test. *Journal of the International Neuropsychological Society*, **10**(S1), 110.

Raskin, S.A. and Sohlberg, M.M. (1996). The efficacy of prospective memory training in two adults with brain injury. *Journal of Head Trauma Rehabilitation*, **11**, 32–51.

Rude, S.S., Hertel, P.T., Jarrold, W., Covich, J., and Hedlund, S. (1999). Depression-related impairments in prospective memory. *Cognition and Emotion*, **13**, 267–76.

Rusted, J.M., and Trawley, S. (2006). Comparable effects of nicotine in smokers and nonsmokers on a prospective memory task. *Neuropsychopharmacology*, **31**, 1545–9.

Rusted, J.M., Trawley, S., Heath, J., Kettle, G., and Walker, H. (2005). Nicotine improves memory for delayed intentions. *Psychopharmacology*, **182**, 355–65.

Shallice, T. and Burgess, P.W. (1991). Deficits in strategy application following frontal lobe damage in man. *Brain*, **114**, 727–41.

Shallice, T. and Burgess, P. (1996). The domain of supervisory processes and temporal organization of behaviour. *Philosophical Transactions of the Royal Society of London. Series B: Biological Sciences*, **351**, 1405–12.

Shum, D., Valentine, M., and Cutmore, T. (1999). Performance of individuals with severe long-term traumatic brain injury on time-, event-, and activity-based prospective memory tasks. *Journal of Clinical and Experimental Neuropsychology*, **21**, 49–58.

Shum, D., Ungvari, G.S., Tang, W.-K., and Leung, J.P. (2004). Performance of schizophrenia patients on time-, event-, and activity-based prospective memory tasks. *Schizophrenia Bulletin*, **30**, 693–701.

Simons, J.S., Schölvinck, M.L., Gilbert, S.J., Frith, C.D., and Burgess, P.W. (2006). Differential components of prospective memory?. Evidence from fMRI. *Neuropsychologia*, **44**, 1388–97.

Smith, R.E. (2003). The cost of remembering to remember in event-based prospective memory: investigating the capacity demands of delayed intention performance. *Journal of Experimental Psychology: Learning Memory and Cognition*, **29**, 347–61.

Sohlberg, M.M., and Mateer, C.A (2001). *Cognitive rehabilitation: an integrative neuropsychological approach*. Guilford Press, New York.

Sohlberg, M.M., White, O., Evans, E., and Mateer, C. (1992a). Background and initial case studies into the effects of prospective memory training. *Brain Injury*, **6**, 129–38.

Sohlberg, M.M., White, O., Evans, E., and Mateer, C. (1992b). An investigation of the effects of prospective memory training. *Brain Injury*, **6**, 139–54.

van den Broek, M.D., Downes, J., Johnson, Z., Dayus, B., and Hilton, N. (2000). Evaluation of an electronic memory aid in the neuropsychological rehabilitation of prospective memory deficits. *Brain Injury*, **14**, 455–62.

von Cramon, D.Y., Matthes-von Cramon, G., and Mai, N. (1991). Problem-solving deficits in brain-injured patients: a therapeutic approach. *Neuropsychological Rehabilitation*, **1**, 45–64.

Warden, D.L., Gordon, B., McAllister, T.W., *et al.* (2006). Guidelines for the pharmacologic treatment of neurobehavioral sequelae of traumatic brain injury. *Journal of Neurotrauma*, **23**, 1468–1501.

Wechsler, D. (1987). *The Wechsler Memory Scale–Revised*. Psychological Corporation, San Antonio, TX.

Wilson, B.A. (1987). *Rehabilitation of memory*. Guilford Press, New York.

Wilson, B.A. (2002). Towards a comprehensive model of cognitive rehabilitation. *Neuropsychological Rehabilitation*, **12**, 97–110.

Wilson, B.A., Cockburn, J., and Baddeley, A. (1985). *Rivermead Behavioural Memory Test (RBMT)*. Thames Valley Test Company, Bury St Edmunds.

Wilson, B.A., Evans, J.J., Emslie, H., and Malinek, V. (1997). Evaluation of NeuroPage: a new memory aid. *Journal of Neurology, Neurosurgery and Psychiatry*, **63**, 113–15.

Wilson, B.A., Emslie, H., Foley, J., *et al.* (2005). *Cambridge Prospective Memory Test (CAMPROMPT)*. Harcourt Assessment, London.

Wilson, B.A., Emslie, H.C., Quirk, K., and Evans, J.J. (2001). Reducing everyday memory and planning problems by means of a paging system: a randomised control crossover study. *Journal of Neurology, Neurosurgery and Psychiatry*, **70**, 477–82.

Yasuda, K., Misu, T., Beckman, B., Watanabe, O., Ozawa, Y., and Nakamura, T. (2002). Use of an IC Recorder as a voice output memory aid for patients with prospective memory impairment. *Neuropsychological Rehabilitation*, **12**, 155–66.

6

Beyond the shopping centre: using the Multiple Errands Test in the assessment and rehabilitation of multi-tasking disorders

Nick Alderman and Dawn Baker

Kemsley National Centre for Brain Injury Rehabilitation,
St Andrew's Hospital, Northampton

Introduction

Miller (1992) outlined three goals for neuropsychological assessment. Two were concerned with diagnosis and measuring change. The third concerned ways in which assessment helps reach an understanding of how cognitive impairment affects function and the design of rehabilitation programmes to address these needs.

However, there is scant evidence in the literature regarding how performance on executive function (EF) tests directly contributes to the formulations clinicians make concerning the causes of patients' problems, or influences the rehabilitation they offer. Instead, specific packages that aim to improve generalized aspects of EF (e.g. Goal Management Training (Levine *et al.* 2000)), strategies to address everyday functional problems arising from executive impairment, such as washing and dressing (Worthington 2003), and strategies to adddress behavioural symptoms of the dysexecutive syndrome (Alderman and Ward 1991) have evolved in isolation from tests routinely used in clinical settings. When tests have been employed, it has invariably been to quantify any change following implementation of a (typically) group-based experimental intervention (e.g. Gordon *et al.* 2006).

Why do EF tests have a tenuous relationship with rehabilitation? It is not uncommon for patients to perform satisfactorily on EF tests yet have significant problems with organizing and executing normally undemanding everyday tasks (Eslinger and Damasio 1985; Shallice and Burgess 1991; Goldstein *et al.* 1993; Duncan *et al.* 1995). Shallice and Burgess (1991) argued that such tests did not reflect the type of demands met in everyday life and that the very structure of such tests made them unrepresentative of real-world demands (Table 6.1). Burgess *et al.* (2006) have highlighted other reasons for a lack of correspondence between the results of EF tests and performance in everyday life. These include the fact that executive ability fractionates into a number of separate abilities and tests are unlikely to reflect all of these. Other reasons include the fact that some tests that were not developed for clinical use in the first place and may be ill-suited to such use.

Functional assessment, in which patients are observed in the situations in which they experience difficulties, is more frequently used than EF tests to inform formulation and rehabilitation. Evans (2001) argued that this often reveals the stage at which, for example, problem-solving breaks down, which is not readily observable on tests (e.g. Alderman 2002; Worthington 2003). Direct observation of patients' difficulties, and inferences regarding causation

Table 6.1 Characteristics of EF tests regarding their 'representativeness' of real-world demands as an explanation as to why some measures are better than others

EF tests that show poor 'representativeness' of real-world models		Characteristics of EF tests that show good 'representativeness' of real-world models
Characteristics	**Example: card sorting**	
Typically only a single explicit goal to achieve	Find rule to sort (categorize) cards	Task incongruence, so demands of test are open-ended or 'ill-structured'
Tests, or trials within tests, are of very short duration	Each sorting attempt typically takes only a few seconds	Multiple goals, so patient has to plan and organize behaviour over a lengthy/indeterminate time period
Task initiation is clearly prompted by the examiner	Examiner gives patient a card and verbal command to take specific action (sort under key cards to find 'rule')	Multi-tasking element so that the patient has to make decisions regarding when to switch between (competing) tasks
Clear (and frequent) immediate feedback is given regarding success of performance	Examiner gives patient feedback regarding whether the correct rule has been identified or not immediately following each separate sorting attempt	Contingent feedback from examiner regarding success/ failure is unavailable. A prospective memory element so that the patient is required to activate an intention after a delay

From Shallice and Burgess 1991; Burgess *et al.* 2006

gained from so doing, can make a direct and seamless contribution to inter-vention. Given this, is there any point in arguing for a role regarding EF tests in rehabilitation?

We propose that the traditional strengths of psychometric assessment (reliability, validity, standardized approach) can be harnessed to contribute to understanding how executive impairment underpins patients' difficulties and the subsequent design of rehabilitation interventions. To do so we suggest that EF tests require the following properties.

1. They must have good psychometric properties.

2. They must comprise an analogue of real-world situations that make demands on the same cognitive resources used by patients in their every-day function.

3. Test performance must have a robust and predictable relationship with functional handicap attributable to EF impairment beyond the testing environment.

4. Agreement must be reached that the advantages of repeated use of the test for rehabilitation purposes outweigh what might be lost regarding the validity of reassessment in the future.

In this chapter we will demonstrate how one of the more ecologically valid EF measures, the Multiple Errands Test (MET), can be meaningfully employed to inform formulation and rehabilitation, and illustrate this with examples from clinical work.

The concept of 'ecological validity'

Before describing MET, it may be useful to remind readers about the concept of 'ecological validity' as this has played a central role in the creation of a new generation of EF tests developed specifically for clinical use. This concept, originally conceived by Brunswick (1956), has been applied more recently to neuropsychological assessment (Burgess *et al.* 2006). Tests 'rich' in ecological validity score highly on two dimensions. The first is 'representativeness'—the extent a test corresponds in form and context to situations encountered by patients beyond that of formal assessment. The second is the 'generalizability' of test results—is performance predictive of difficulties in the real world driven by EF impairment?

Burgess *et al.* (2006) argued that EF tests should comprise analogues of everyday situations which highlight executive difficulties; in other words, tests need to be high in 'representativeness'. They critically examined the character-istics of many routinely administered tests of frontal lobe function and concluded that these did not reliably capture the nature of patients difficulties experienced in everyday life (Table 6.1).

By considering these characteristics, Shallice and Burgess (1991) were able to define what qualities need to be embedded in EF tests if they are to tap the same cognitive operations demanded by novel tasks and unfamiliar situations encountered beyond the consulting room. When tests have these qualities they will score highly in terms of their ability to model real-world analogues.

Tests that are high in 'representativeness' are also likely to have high 'generalizability', i.e. they generate scores that are predictive of the presence of executive impairment in everyday life. An example of a measure that scores highly on both dimensions is Zoo Map from the BADS (Alderman *et al.* 1996). It directly mirrors a 'real-world model' in that patients are required to show how they would plan to visit a number of locations within a zoo, whilst at the same time adhering to a set of rules. Whilst the task loads heavily on planning, demands are made on other 'executive' cognitive operations, including error utilization and cognitive flexibility. Its obvious parallel to the sort of everyday activity in which planning impairment would be apparent ranks highly on 'representativeness'. Scores from Zoo Map also demonstrate the 'generalizability' of test results in that they are reliable predictors of behavioural symptoms of EF impairment. For example, Knight *et al.* (2002) demonstrated that Zoo Map was correlated with ratings of EF impairment on the DEX questionnaire (Burgess *et al.* 1996a).

Tests rich in ecological validity that have been developed to reflect function have much to offer clinicians. First, because they make demands on cognitive resources that enable (or not) a person to function well in the real world, they are valid and reliable assessors of EF from which meaningful inferences can be drawn. Because of this, the contribution of such tests to assessment and formulation becomes more attractive. Secondly, in addition to helping clinicians more ably understand the behaviour of their patients, there may be more potential to use these measures directly in rehabilitation itself.

The Multiple Errands Test

MET was originally described by Shallice and Burgess (1991) and was one of two new assessment procedures devised to address the shortcomings of some existing tests. MET was developed as a task that was as close as possible to a formalized version of 'real-world' situations in which patients experienced problems (Burgess *et al.* 2006). It scores very highly on the 'representativeness' dimension as it comprises a multi-tasking test carried out in a shopping centre. Patients are required to complete a number of tasks of varying complexity whilst conforming to a set of rules whose function is to increase the planning, monitoring, and prospective memory demands of the test. In addition, there are a number of covert problems that had to be identified and actioned as subgoals in order to achieve some of the designated tasks (e.g. writing information on a postcard and sending it, without being given a pen).

Shallice and Burgess (1991) described three neurological patients who performed at above-average levels on measures of general ability and whose performance on frontal lobe tests was satisfactory. Despite this, relatives reported that their ability to function in everyday situations was poor. It was argued that these tests did not comprise good models of the real world. Table 6.1 shows those elements that were embedded in the design of MET so that it was a good real-world model. Consequently, the number of errors made by all patients exceeded two standard deviations above that of controls; performance was also more representative of the difficulties described by relatives.

Simplified versions of MET

Alderman *et al.* (2003) designed a simplified version of MET (MET-SV) which is more appropriate for use with the range of patients more routinely seen in clinical practice. MET-SV is also conducted in a shopping centre. The patient is required to achieve a number of straightforward tasks (purchasing items, recording information, meeting the examiner at a defined place and time) without breaking a set of imposed rules (Box 6.1). Knight *et al.* (2002) made the point tha it is not always possible to assess patients in the community and successfully adapted MET-SV for use within a hospital setting (MET-HV). Most recently, Pennington (2006) used MET-SV as the basis for creating a version for use in hospital wards (e.g. to assess patients during the early stage of their recovery).

MET performance is determined by the number of errors made, of which there are four categories (see Table 6.2). A consistent finding for all MET variants was that the mean number of errors made by ABI groups was significantly greater than that of controls. Furthermore, the moderate sample sizes reported by Alderman *et al.* (2003) enabled valid comparison of the types of errors made, not just the error categories. Twenty-five errors were shared by both groups. However, whilst another four were evident only amongst controls, 33 were unique to the ABI group (see Table 6.2 for examples of routine and ABI-specific errors). This finding enabled construction of a weighted scoring system based on the 'normality' of errors which increased the ability of the test to correctly discriminate people with ABI from healthy controls from 44 to 82 per cent.

The psychometric properties of the different versions of MET are robust, even though the tests are not employed in the carefully controlled environment

Box 6.1 MET-SV instruction sheet given to participants

Instructions

In this exercise you should complete the following three tasks.

1. You should buy the following items:

    small brown loaf   bar of chocolate

    packet of plasters   single light bulb

    birthday card   key ring

2. You should obtain the following information and write it down in the spaces below.

    (1) What is the headline from today's *Daily Mail*, *Daily Mirror*, or *Sun* newspaper?

    (2) What is the closing time of the library on Saturday?

    (3) What is the price of 1 pound or kilogram of tomatoes?

    (4) How many shops sell televisions?

3. You must meet me under the clock 20 minutes after you have started this task and tell me the time.

TELL THE PERSON OBSERVING YOU WHEN YOU HAVE COMPLETED THE EXERCISE

Whilst carrying out this exercise you must obey the following rules:

- You must carry out all these tasks but may do so in any order.
- You should spend no more than £5.
- You should stay within the limits of the shopping centre.
- No shop should be entered other than to buy something.
- You should not go back into a shop you have already been in.
- You should not buy any item from the stalls.
- You should buy no more than two items in the supermarket.
- Take as little time to complete this exercise without rushing excessively.
- Do not speak to the person observing you *unless* this is part of the exercise.

From Alderman *et al.* 2003

nbers were correlated with fewer tasks and
nis is consistent with observation of such
rs' demonstrate gross impairment in the
and appear overwhelmed by the test from
ions may be formed, their behaviour and
t that other cognitive operations pertinent
red. They have difficulties with retaining,
sly formed intentions. The 'dysfunction' of
e: despite formulating a plan they end up
nopping centre or hospital ward at a loss as

arising from a

what cognitive operations and underlying
iour using a 'dysfunction-led' approach can
ideas. Difficulties with multi-tasking are a
ng memory that results in problems with
tive operations which maintain prospective
ability to form or activate intentions.
rns of dysfunction suggest different treat-
e direct way than would performance on
rtson 2002). Rehabilitation is directed at
ulty cognitive operations that underlie the
g styles. The question of restoration versus
n will not be debated here (see Evans 2001).
T may be further used as a rehabilitation
its own right.

measurement tool

ile to monitoring difficulties may benefit
ue saliency and feedback. Some categories
ved to be driven by monitoring problems,
is no longer appropriate are not perceived.
position of feedback systems that highlight
e patient because of difficulties they have
rces (Alderman 2001). Certain kinds of
ne can be effectively used to present feed-
ded, which typically lead to reduction in

Table 6.2 MET error categories and examples

Error types	Inefficiencies	Rule breaks	Interpretation failures	Task failures
Description	Where a more effective strategy could have been applied	Where a specific rule (either social or explicitly mentioned in the task) was broken	Where the requirements of a particular task were misunderstood	A task not completed satisfactorily
Examples of 'routine' errors	Purchasing a multipack of items rather than just one (e.g. two lightbulbs)	Speaking to the examiner when this is not a requirement of the test	Believed it was necessary to complete the whole test in 20 minutes	Failed to meet the examiner under the clock
Examples of ABI-specific errors	Purchased newspaper to obtain and write down headline	Left the designated boundaries of the shopping centre	Purchased item not on the list	Failed to purchase birthday card

From Shallice and Burgess 1991; Alderman et al. 2003

of the consulting-room. Furthermore, the variable relationship between test performance and impairment in the real world shown on some 'ecologically valid' measures (Wood and Liossi 2006) is not characteristic of MET. For example, a positive correlation between MET errors and ratings on DEX has been consistently reported (Knight *et al.* 2002; Alderman *et al.* 2003; Dawson *et al.* 2005a,b; Pennington 2006).

MET discriminates different error-making styles

A further attribute of MET which may benefit formulation and rehabilitation was the important finding made by Alderman *et al.* (2003) that people did not perform poorly on the test for a single reason. Instead, two distinct error styles were evident, characterized by breaking rules *or* failing to succeed on tasks. Patients grouped by error style were also found to differ on other EF tests, how carers rated them on DEX, and with regard to the awareness they had about their MET performance. Alderman and colleagues tentatively concluded that patients who had monitoring difficulties (a working memory deficit) charac-teristically broke the rules of the test. In contrast, task failures were attributed to problems with 'intentionality'—the ability to create and maintain goal-related behaviour (a prospective memory impairment).

The ability to characterize the behavioural manifestation of EF impairment on MET by classifying patients as either 'rule breakers' or 'task failers' may play a key role in formulation, and as a consequence what can be done to help. Burgess *et al.* (2006) recommended that to create better executive tests for clinical use, a function-led approach should be employed as it is more likely to capture adequately the dynamic interplay between the cognitive resources of the patient and their interaction with the environment. Using this, cognitive operations underpinning observable behaviour and the theoretical constructs from which they stem can subsequently be worked out. Similarly, MET performance enables the clinician to formulate hypotheses to account for 'dysfunction', and to use this as a vehicle to drive rehabilitation. Table 6.3 illustrates this 'dysfunction-driven' approach. It parallels functional assessment, but also contributes at a deeper level to formulation than can be gained from observation of behaviour alone.

Explanations for MET error styles

'Rule-breaking' behaviour

Alderman *et al.* (2003) suggested that MET rule-breaking behaviour was attributable to impairment of the central executive (CE) component of working memory (Baddeley 1986). This model has been used previously to account for ABI behaviour disorders and poor response to some neurobehavioural

Table 6.3 A dysfunction-led approach to understanding the two different error styles that characterize MET performance

	Dysfunction →	Operations →	Construct
Explanatory status	Directly observable	Experimentally detectable or inferable	Theoretical
Error style characterized by rule breaking	Problems with monitoring and error detection: cannot consistently maintain awareness of rules whilst pursuing tasks	Unsuccessful allocation of attentional resources to multiple internal/ external stimuli	Working memory impairment
Error style characterized by failure to achieve designated tasks	Problems with execution of delayed intentions	Difficulties with: intention formation intention retention reinstating intention execution of reinstated intention	Prospective memory ('intentionality') impairment

with SET performance: higher nu[m]
less task switching on the SET. T[
patients on MET. Some 'task fail[
ability to formulate any intention[s
the start. For others, whilst inten[
post-assessment debriefing sugges[
to prospective memory are impai[
re-installing, or activating previou[
these patients is clearly observabl[
wandering randomly around the s[
to what to do (Worthington 1999)[

Rehabilitation strategies [
MET performance

Making a formulation regarding [
constructs account for MET behav[
successfully generate rehabilitation[
function of impairment of worki[
monitoring; or disruption to cogni[
memory, resulting in reduced [
Furthermore, these separate patte[
ment applications in a much mo[
other EF tests (Burgess and Robe[
restoring or circumventing those f[
two dissociable MET error-makin[
compensation of cognitive functio[
Instead, we will illustrate how M[
and outcome measurement tool in[

Use of MET as an outcome[

Multi-tasking problems attributa[
from interventions that highlight [
of ABI behaviour disorder are beli[
as cues which signal that behaviou[
This can be negated through the in[
salient factors not perceived by th[
with allocating attentional resou[
behaviour modification programm[
back to patients, when this is nee[

behaviour disorder (Alderman and Ward 1991; Alderman and Burgess 1994). Alternatively, at least one cognitive retraining procedure has been developed specifically to improve monitoring skills in people with ABI whose behavioural problems were attributed to working memory impairment (Alderman *et al.* 1995; Dayus and van den Broek 2000).

Similar approaches may benefit multi-tasking abilities. We have not tested this hypothesis directly yet, but accounts in the literature regarding the benefits of intermittent auditory alerting on another consulting-room measure of multi-tasking give rise to optimism, once the challenge of how the technology can be successfully applied to the real world has been overcome (Manly *et al.* 2002).

Alderman *et al.* (2000) have used MET-SV to demonstrate improvement in multi-tasking abilities for three patients with severe dysexecutive syndrome. They completed MET-SV shortly after admission, and then again 12 months or more later. Figure 6.1 shows that the total number of rule breaks made by this small group fell from 83 on initial assessment to 22 when retested some months later. The authors argued that, although their patients had not received any specific EF treatment, their ability to self-monitor had improved through exposure to intensive behaviour-modification programmes and other systems that exaggerated feedback within the neurobehavioural unit, and that this was manifested through better MET scores. There is some evidence that the ability to utilize feedback more effectively may generalize following

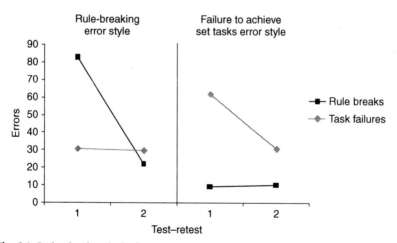

Fig. 6.1 Reduction in principal MET error style by 'rule breakers' following a period of intensive neurobehavioural rehabilitation (*n* = 3) and 'task failers' using a checklist (*n* = 3).

exposure to interventions in which patients are encouraged to monitor their behaviour accurately (Alderman *et al.* 1995). In addition, the number of task failures for these patients did not change significantly (test = 31; retest = 30), which Alderman and colleagues argued acted as a control condition for the behaviour-modification-monitoring hypothesis.

Use of MET as a tool to facilitate rehabilitation

Evans (2003) suggested that external aids are particularly helpful for patients with initiation and sequencing difficulties. Our 'dysfunction-led' approach to understanding which impairment of cognitive operations accounts for failure to achieve MET tasks highlighted how difficulties with prospective memory may explain this. Reduced ability to formulate intentions might be circumvented using a checklist which details for the person the action needed and the order in which to take it. Checklists can also contain embedded reminders of the need to take delayed action, thereby sidestepping problems in retaining and reactivating delayed intentions. An interesting finding by Alderman *et al.* (2003) was that some patients resorted to asking for help from the public. This was not beneficial to 'rule breakers': in fact, the opposite was found as there was a strong correlation (0.72) between the number of times help was requested and rule breaks. This is consistent with the working memory explanation as patients were observed to act on the information they obtained without consideration for the wider requirements of the task. However, the strategy was beneficial to people who had difficulty in attaining tasks: there was a negative correlation (−0.42) between asking for help and task failures. Again, this makes sense in the light of our 'dysfunction-led' approach to understanding MET error-making behaviour. Prospective memory difficulties underpin failure to achieve tasks, and so asking for help clarifies intention formation and initiation.

Given that some 'task failers' try to reduce the impact of their cognitive handicap by resorting to external guidance, using checklists to reduce the burden further also makes sense. Alderman *et al.* (2000) described another three patients categorized as 'task failers' on MET. This small group made 62 task failures. However, this was halved when the standard instructions were substituted by a numbered checklist that prompted specific action to take following completion of the previous step. There was no change in the number of rule breaks within this group on reassessment, which could be seen as a control condition for the intervention (Figure 6.1).

On the face of it, checklists may benefit people whose multi-tasking abilities are undermined by prospective memory impairment. However, further data presented by Alderman *et al.* (2000) suggest that it may not be that straightforward.

Table 6.2 MET error categories and examples

Error types	Inefficiencies	Rule breaks	Interpretation failures	Task failures
Description	Where a more effective strategy could have been applied	Where a specific rule (either social or explicitly mentioned in the task) was broken	Where the requirements of a particular task were misunderstood	A task not completed satisfactorily
Examples of 'routine' errors	Purchasing a multipack of items rather than just one (e.g. two lightbulbs)	Speaking to the examiner when this is not a requirement of the test	Believed it was necessary to complete the whole test in 20 minutes	Failed to meet the examiner under the clock
Examples of ABI-specific errors	Purchased newspaper to obtain and write down headline	Left the designated boundaries of the shopping centre	Purchased item not on the list	Failed to purchase birthday card

From Shallice and Burgess 1991; Alderman *et al.* 2003

of the consulting-room. Furthermore, the variable relationship between test performance and impairment in the real world shown on some 'ecologically valid' measures (Wood and Liossi 2006) is not characteristic of MET. For example, a positive correlation between MET errors and ratings on DEX has been consistently reported (Knight *et al.* 2002; Alderman *et al.* 2003; Dawson *et al.* 2005a,b; Pennington 2006).

MET discriminates different error-making styles

A further attribute of MET which may benefit formulation and rehabilitation was the important finding made by Alderman *et al.* (2003) that people did not perform poorly on the test for a single reason. Instead, two distinct error styles were evident, characterized by breaking rules *or* failing to succeed on tasks. Patients grouped by error style were also found to differ on other EF tests, how carers rated them on DEX, and with regard to the awareness they had about their MET performance. Alderman and colleagues tentatively concluded that patients who had monitoring difficulties (a working memory deficit) characteristically broke the rules of the test. In contrast, task failures were attributed to problems with 'intentionality'—the ability to create and maintain goal-related behaviour (a prospective memory impairment).

The ability to characterize the behavioural manifestation of EF impairment on MET by classifying patients as either 'rule breakers' or 'task failers' may play a key role in formulation, and as a consequence what can be done to help. Burgess *et al.* (2006) recommended that to create better executive tests for clinical use, a function-led approach should be employed as it is more likely to capture adequately the dynamic interplay between the cognitive resources of the patient and their interaction with the environment. Using this, cognitive operations underpinning observable behaviour and the theoretical constructs from which they stem can subsequently be worked out. Similarly, MET performance enables the clinician to formulate hypotheses to account for 'dysfunction', and to use this as a vehicle to drive rehabilitation. Table 6.3 illustrates this 'dysfunction-driven' approach. It parallels functional assessment, but also contributes at a deeper level to formulation than can be gained from observation of behaviour alone.

Explanations for MET error styles

'Rule-breaking' behaviour

Alderman *et al.* (2003) suggested that MET rule-breaking behaviour was attributable to impairment of the central executive (CE) component of working memory (Baddeley 1986). This model has been used previously to account for ABI behaviour disorders and poor response to some neurobehavioural

Table 6.3 A dysfunction-led approach to understanding the two different error styles that characterize MET performance

	Dysfunction	→	Operations	→	Construct
Explanatory status	Directly observable		Experimentally detectable or inferable		Theoretical
Error style characterized by rule breaking	Problems with monitoring and error detection: cannot consistently maintain awareness of rules whilst pursuing tasks		Unsuccessful allocation of attentional resources to multiple internal/external stimuli		Working memory impairment
Error style characterized by failure to achieve designated tasks	Problems with execution of delayed intentions		Difficulties with: intention formation intention retention reinstating intention execution of reinstated intention		Prospective memory ('intentionality') impairment

treatment interventions; there is some experimental evidence to support this (Alderman 1996). Disruption of the CE leads to monitoring difficulties because attentional resources cannot be effectively deployed to enable the patient to have concurrent awareness of several sources of information at the same time. Thus 'rule breakers' typically show good awareness of the rules after completing MET; however, observation of their behaviour during assessment, and their over-confidence afterwards regarding their performance, are clearly inconsistent with good recall of what the rules were. A CE account of this dissociation seemed to offer a reasonable explanation for behaviour as this would result in less capacity to maintain concurrent awareness of rules whist following a plan to achieve a task, resulting in rule neglect.

Although this is work in progress requiring more empirical support, some further support for this explanation comes from Hodgson (2006) who administered additional EF tests to ABI patients who had undertaken shopping centre and hospital-ward METs. These included Dual Task (DT), a specific measure sensitive to monitoring difficulties (Baddeley *et al.* 1997). Hodgson found a significant negative correlation between rule breaks and DT performance: high-frequency rule-breaking behaviour was associated with poorer ability to allocate attentional resources required to successfully undertake two tasks simultaneously. Rule breaks were not correlated with any of the other test scores, including the version of the Six Element Test (SET) from BADS (Burgess *et al.* 1996b). However, Hodgson further reported that rule-breaking was also associated with poor awareness of MET errors when patients were debriefed afterwards. These data further support the original explanation proffered by Alderman *et al.* (2003): these patients seem to be able to prioritize tasks and have good knowledge of the rules, but make errors because they lack the attentional resource required to follow their plan and concurrently maintain awareness of the wider requirements of the test.

'Task failing' behaviour

A prospective memory explanation for these errors is that when confronted with a demanding multi-tasking test, patients have difficulty with one or more of the following: the ability to formulate intentions to undertake particular courses of action, retain these, re-instate them when appropriate, and then act on them (Ellis 1996). Shallice and Burgess (1991) had previously highlighted the importance of prospective memory in multi-tasking by suggesting that an executive memory component created a temporal marker which subsequently triggered a delayed response. To test this, Hodgson used SET from BADS. On this, patients are required to independently undertake and switch between a number of different tasks. Hodgson found that MET task failures were associated with SET performance: higher numbers were correlated with fewer tasks and less task switching on the SET. This is consistent with observation of such patients on MET. Some 'task failers' demonstrate gross impairment in the ability to formulate any intentions and appear overwhelmed by the test from the start. For others, whilst intentions may be formed, their behaviour and post-assessment debriefing suggest that other cognitive operations pertinent to prospective memory are impaired. They have difficulties with retaining, re-installing, or activating previously formed intentions. The 'dysfunction' of these patients is clearly observable: despite formulating a plan they end up wandering randomly around the shopping centre or hospital ward at a loss as to what to do (Worthington 1999).

Rehabilitation strategies arising from a MET performance

Making a formulation regarding what cognitive operations and underlying constructs account for MET behaviour using a 'dysfunction-led' approach can successfully generate rehabilitation ideas. Difficulties with multi-tasking are a function of impairment of working memory that results in problems with monitoring; or disruption to cognitive operations which maintain prospective memory, resulting in reduced ability to form or activate intentions. Furthermore, these separate patterns of dysfunction suggest different treatment applications in a much more direct way than would performance on other EF tests (Burgess and Robertson 2002). Rehabilitation is directed at restoring or circumventing those faulty cognitive operations that underlie the two dissociable MET error-making styles. The question of restoration versus compensation of cognitive function will not be debated here (see Evans 2001). Instead, we will illustrate how MET may be further used as a rehabilitation and outcome measurement tool in its own right.

Use of MET as an outcome measurement tool

Multi-tasking problems attributable to monitoring difficulties may benefit from interventions that highlight cue saliency and feedback. Some categories of ABI behaviour disorder are believed to be driven by monitoring problems, as cues which signal that behaviour is no longer appropriate are not perceived. This can be negated through the imposition of feedback systems that highlight salient factors not perceived by the patient because of difficulties they have with allocating attentional resources (Alderman 2001). Certain kinds of behaviour modification programme can be effectively used to present feedback to patients, when this is needed, which typically lead to reduction in

Figure 6.2 shows the performance of the six patients again, but this time MET errors are shown for each person, rather than the group totals seen in Figure 6.1. Figure 6.2 is also different because each bar represents the magnitude of change between assessments ('number of errors on initial assessment' minus 'number of errors on reassessment'). For both error categories, Figure 6.2 also shows the 5 per cent cut-off derived from test–retest of neurologically healthy controls. In other words, any change in score above this is unlikely to be due to chance or practice. Figure 6.2 shows that each 'rule breaker' made significantly less rule-breaking errors when retested. However, when data are reconfigured in this way Figure 6.2 rather soberingly demonstrates that the checklist benefited only one of the three 'task failers'.

Case study of a 'task failer'

An individual case study will be described to illustrate how MET performance might account for this surprising and disappointing finding. In this example, MET-SV was used on many occasions: variations in how instructions were presented enabled the relative effectiveness of two different interventions to be evaluated.

LD, a 36-year-old skilled manual worker, sustained a TBI through assault. CT scan showed a large infarct in the right parieto-occipital and left fronto-parietal regions. He presented with severe dysexecutive syndrome and was

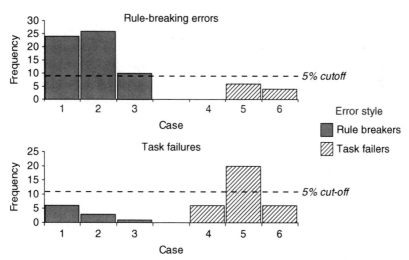

Fig. 6.2 Reduction in MET test–retest errors for individual 'rule breakers' and 'task failers'. (NB: Bars extending above the 5 per cent cut-off reflect reduction in errors that are statistically unlikely to be due to practice or chance based on performance of neurologically healthy controls.)

admitted to a neurobehavioural service. Before injury he was described as ambitious, hard-working, and a flexible problem-solver. At interview LD stated that he had no difficulties with planning and coped well with unfamiliar tasks and situations. However, ratings made about behavioural symptoms of executive impairment by staff using the DEX questionnaire were high. Mean sum of ratings was 36/80 which is uncharacteristic of neurologically healthy controls (falling at the 92nd percentile) but more typical of ABI (falling at the 62nd percentile). This was consistent with the view that LD presented with significant symptoms of executive impairment. Some items were rated very highly, reflecting particular impairments with planning, insight and awareness, perseverative behaviour, and restlessness. Functional difficulties symptomatic of executive dysfunction were also evident. For example, he was unable to clean and tidy his bedroom or prepare a simple microwave meal without explicit direction from staff. Problems were also evident prior to admission; for example, when preparing a meal for his daughter, LD was noted to cook all the sausages in a pack and then throw away those that were not needed.

High DEX ratings and functional difficulties were consistent with a dysexecutive syndrome. However, performance on EF tests was not. For example, DT performance fell within the 'average' range, whilst that on the BADS was consistent with his WTAR-predicted FSIQ ('low average') (Wechsler 2001). Furthermore, profile scores for both multi-tasking tests on BADS, Zoo Map (3, control mean = 2.44), and SET (3, control mean = 3.52) did not prompt specific concern.

In order to further investigate the discrepancy between LD's functional difficulties and his performance on EF tests, he completed MET-SV (Table 6.4).

LD's behaviour whilst undertaking MET-SV suggested that he lacked purpose as he wandered aimlessly about the shopping centre. There was no evidence of planning as he launched himself immediately into trying to achieve the goals of the exercise straight after the briefing from the examiner. He also attempted to seek external direction by questioning members of the public and asking the examiner for help.

Overall, LD's weighted error score (47) greatly exceeded the 5 per cent cut-off (12) for neurologically healthy controls, and falls more than two standard deviations above the mean achieved by the ABI sample reported by Alderman et al. (2003). Table 6.4 shows that LD's characteristic error style was failure to achieve tasks. Of the 12 tasks embedded in MET-SV, LD only achieved two. Some errors were also highly uncharacteristic of neurologically healthy controls. For example, he recorded the price of chilled tomato soup (not actual tomatoes as required) and entered the information on the wrong

Table 6.4 MET-SV weighted error scores for LD*

Trial	Task failures	Rule breaks	Interpretation failures	Inefficiencies	Total error score
MET-SV#1: standard administration	24	14	3	6	47
MET-SV checklist administration	11	4	0	3	18
MET-SV#2: standard administration	21	2	0	0	23
MET-SV booklet administration	9	1	1	4	15
MET-SV#3: standard administration	18	0	3	0	21

part of the recording sheet. His failure to purchase a light bulb and key ring, and record the closing time of the library and the number of shops selling televisions were all errors unobserved amongst controls. Other aspects of LD's performance were also out of the ordinary. For example, although he had no goods to purchase in the supermarket, he nevertheless joined a queue of customers waiting to pay, only leaving the store when it was 'his turn'.

The 'dysfunction-led' approach to understanding LD's poor MET performance began by considering his behaviour. His predominant type of error (requests for help) and random approach to the exercise reflected poor 'intentionality' in that his chief difficulty was creation and maintenance of goal-related behaviour.

Whilst LD's behaviour suggested that problems with intention formation, retention, and activation explained his difficulty with task attainment, this was not supported by performance on other EF tests. It will be recalled that his Zoo Map and SET profile scores fell in the normal range. However, Burgess has recently re-examined the BADS normative data and produced advanced scoring and norms for these two tests (P.W. Burgess, personal communication, 2007). These enable detailed analysis of performance that can be used to inform research and clinical practice. In the case of LD, these proved helpful in eliminating the discrepancy between the three multi-tasking measures. Specifically, with regard to task switching on the SET, LD achieved a 'below-average' performance that fell within the 6th–10th percentile. This is consistent with both the findings reported by Hodgson (2006) with respect to task failures, and the prospective memory hypothesis regarding such behaviour. With regard to Zoo Map, he spent no time planning on either trial; this falls at the first percentile for trial 1. The same behaviour was observed in trial 2, but as there is an overt strategy to follow through the written instructions, 'planning' is less relevant. LD was similarly observed to neglect planning on MET-SV. It was also interesting to note that LD's performance on the second trial of Zoo Map, in which success is more likely if the written instructions are followed, fell within the 90th–94th percentile. Following the instructions greatly reduces load on planning and provides support regarding the use of an external aid.

Consequently, LD undertook MET-SV for a second time to test the effectiveness of providing him with a structured plan to follow. As in the second trial of Zoo Map, instructions were modified so that they comprised a series of numbered steps to follow, each of which was to be ticked when completed prior to moving on to the next. It was anticipated that if LD followed the instructions, he would achieve all tasks. Table 6.4 confirms that improvement was evident; weighted task failures fell from 24 to 11, and the number of tasks achieved increased from 2/12 to 6/12. Whilst this was progress, the expectation that the numbered checklist would result in LD achieving all tasks was not met. However, some positive benefit was evident after he completed MET-SV for a third time using the standard administration: Table 6.4 shows that the weighted error score for task failures increased in the absence of the checklist to a level compatible with that achieved initially (21 vs 24).

Examination of the structured checklist used in the modified administration of MET-SV proved informative regarding possible reasons as to why he had not been completely successful. It was evident from LD's check marks on the instructions (showing that he had attempted a particular step) that he had failed to follow them in the order indicated. The problem was one of sequencing, which suggested that his difficulties with intention formation were more severe than originally suspected. Instead of systematically working through the numbered steps as instructed, he had randomly selected and attempted some, without completing them all. An additional measure was obtained whereby one point was awarded each time LD successfully moved on to the next consecutive step following completion of the one that preceded it (e.g. one point was given if he had moved on to step 3 after attempting step 2). The resulting 'sequencing score' amounted to just 3/13.

Again, the 'dysfunction-led' approach to account for MET performance suggested that further modification of the checklist was necessary to circumvent LD's sequencing difficulties. Thus he was given a small booklet. Each page

We are not advocating that neuropsychological tests designed for use in the consulting room be employed for rehabilitation purposes. The danger here is that people may be 'trained to pass tests'. However, we are arguing that MET is a special case, falling somewhere between being a functional assessment and a 'traditional' psychometric test. The principal advantage of MET is its ability to distinguish between two behavioural profiles that are functions of different forms of cognitive impairment, necessitating different interventions. This ability to differentiate between what underlies multi-tasking problems and to link these more seamlessly with rehabilitation is a great asset.

We are confident that other interventions for multi-tasking impairment will be generated as a consequence of being able to differentiate between, and explain, rule-breaking and task-failing errors on MET. Hopefully, this process of building bridges between the separate fortresses of assessment and rehabilitation for EF impairment will continue and better means of helping patients to overcome their difficulties will be identified.

References

Alderman, N. (1996). Central executive deficit and response to operant conditioning methods. *Neuropsychological Rehabilitation*, 6, 161–86.

Alderman, N. (2001). Management of challenging behaviour. In: *Neurobehavioural disability and social handicap following traumatic brain injury* (ed R.L.Wood and T.McMillan). Psychology Press, Hove.

Alderman, N. (2002). Individual case studies. In: *Evidence in mental health care* (ed S. Priebe and M. Slade). Brunner–Routledge, Hove.

Alderman, N. and Burgess, P. (1994). A comparison of treatment methods for behaviour disorders following herpes simplex encephalitis. *Neuropsychological Rehabilitation*, 4, 31–48.

Alderman, N. and Ward, A. (1991). Behavioural treatment of the dysexecutive syndrome: reduction of repetitive speech using response cost and cognitive overlearning. *Neuropsychological Rehabilitation*, 1, 65–80.

Alderman, N., Fry, R.K., and Youngson, H.A. (1995). Improvement of self-monitoring skills, reduction of behaviour disturbance and the dysexecutive syndrome: comparison of response cost and a new programme of self-monitoring training. *Neuropsychological Rehabilitation*, 5, 193–221.

Alderman, N., Evans, J.J., Emslie, H., Wilson, B.A., and Burgess, P.W. (1996). Zoo Map Test. In: *Behavioural assessment of the dysexecutive syndrome* (ed B.A.Wilson, N.Alderman, P.W.Burgess, H.Emslie, and J.J.Evans). Thames Valley Test Company, Bury St. Edmunds.

Alderman, N., Knight, C.K., Rutterford, N., and Swan, L. (2000). Ecological validity of a simplified version of the Multiple Errands Test: can it be used to drive treatment options and measure outcome in the rehabilitation of executive disorders? Presented at Impact 2000: an International Conference on Brain Injury, Nottingham, 13–15 September 2000.

Alderman, N., Burgess, P.W., Knight, C., and Henman, C. (2003). Ecological validity of a simplified version of the Multiple Errands Test. *Journal of the International Neuropsychological Society*, **9**, 31–44.

Baddeley, A., Della Sala, S., Gray, C., Papagno,C., and Spinnler, H. (1997). Review of studies using the pencil-and-paper version of the Dual Task. In: *Methodology of frontal and executive function* (ed P. Rabbitt). Psychology Press, Hove.

Baddeley, A.D. and Wilson, B. (1988). Frontal amnesia and the dysexecutive syndrome. *Brain and Cognition*, **7**, 212–230.

Brunswick, E. (1956). *Perception and the representative design of psychological experiments* (2nd edn). University of California Press, Berkeley, CA.

Burgess, P.W. and Robertson, I.H. (2002). Principles of the rehabilitation of frontal lobe function. In: *Principles of frontal lobe function* (ed D.T. Stuss and R.T. Knight), pp. 557–72. Oxford University Press, New York.

Burgess, P.W., Alderman, N., Emslie, H., Evans, J.J., and Wilson, B.A. (1996). The Dysexecutive Questionnaire. In: *Behavioural assessment of the dysexecutive syndrome* (ed B.A. Wilson, N. Alderman, P.W. Burgess, H. Emslie, and J.J. Evans). Thames Valley Test Company, Bury St. Edmunds.

Burgess, P.W., Alderman, N., Evans, J.J., Wilson, B.A., Emslie, H., and Shallice, T. (1996). Modified Six Element Test. In: *Behavioural assessment of the dysexecutive syndrome* (ed B.A. Wilson, N. Alderman, P.W. Burgess, H. Emslie and J.J. Evans). Thames Valley Test Company, Bury St. Edmunds.

Burgess, P.W., Alderman, N., Forbes, C., *et al.* (2006). The case for the development and use of 'ecologically valid' measures of executive function in experimental and clinical neuropsychology. *Journal of the International Neuropsychological Society*, **12**, 194–209.

Dawson, D.R., Anderson, N., Burgess, P.W., *et al.* (2005a). The ecological validity of the Multiple Errands Test—Hospital Version: preliminary findings. Presented at Meeting of the International Neuropsychological Society, St. Louis, MO, February 2005.

Dawson, D.R., Anderson, N., Burgess, P.W., *et al.* (2005b). Naturalistic assessment of executive function: the Multiple Errands Test. Presented at the American Congress of Rehabilitation Medicine, Chicago, IL, September 2005.

Dayus B. and van den Broek, M.D. (2000). Treatment of stable delusional confabulations using self-monitoring training. *Neuropsychological Rehabilitation*, **10**, 415–27.

Duncan, J., Burgess, P.W., and Emslie, H. (1995). Fluid intelligence after frontal lobe lesions. *Neuropsychologia*, **33**, 261–8.

Ellis, J. (1996). Prospective memory or the realization of delayed intentions: a conceptual framework for research. In: *Prospective memory: theory and applications* (ed M. Brandimonte, G.O. Einstein, and M.A. McDaniel), pp. 1–22. Lawrence Erlbaum, Hillsdale, NJ.

Eslinger, P.J. and Damasio, A.R. (1985). Severe disturbance of higher cognition after bilateral frontal lobe ablation: patient EVR. *Neurology*, **35**, 1731–41.

Evans, J.J. (2001). Rehabilitation of the dysexecutive syndrome. In: *Neurobehavioural disability and social handicap following traumatic brain injury* (ed R.L. Wood and T. McMillan). Psychology Press, Hove.

Evans, J.J. (2003). Rehabilitation of executive deficits. In: *Neuropsychological rehabilitation: theory and practice* (ed B.A. Wilson). Swets and Zeitlinger, Lisse.

Goldstein, L.H., Bernard, S., Fenwick, P.B.C., Burgess, P.W., and McNeil, J. (1993). Unilateral frontal lobectomy can produce strategy application disorder. *Journal of Neurology, Neurosurgery and Psychiatry*, **56**, 274–6.

Gordon, W.A., Cantor, J., Ashman, T., and Brown, M. (2006). Treatment of post-TBI executive dysfunction: application of theory to clinical practice. *Journal of Head Trauma Rehabilitation*, **21**, 156–67.

Hodgson, H. (2006). Multiple Errands Test errors—rule breaks and task failures. Separable and independent information processing impairments?. Unpublished MSc thesis, submitted to University College London.

Knight, C., Alderman, N., and Burgess, P.W. (2002). Development of a simplified version of the Multiple Errands Test for use in hospital settings. *Neuropsychological Rehabilitation*, **12**, 231–55.

Levine, B., Robertson, I., Clare, L., *et al.* (2000). Rehabilitation of executive functioning: an experimental-clinical validation of goal management training. *Journal of the International Neuropsychological Society*, **6**, 299–312.

Manly, T., Hawkins, K., Evans, J.J., Woldt, K., and Robertson, I.H. (2002). Rehabilitation of Executive Function: Facilitation of effective goal management on complex tasks using periodic auditory alerts. *Neuropsychologia*, **40**, 271–81.

Miller, E. (1992). Some basic principles of neuropsychological assessment. In: *Handbook of neuropsychological assessment* (ed J.R. Crawford, D.M. Parker, and W.M. McKinlay). Lawrence Erlbaum, Hove.

Pennington, E.A. (2006). Development of a simplified version of the Multiple Errands Test for use on a hospital ward. Unpublished doctoral thesis, submitted to University of Leicester.

Shallice, T. and Burgess, P.W. (1991). Deficits in strategy application following frontal lobe damage in man. *Brain*, **114**, 727–41.

Wechsler, D. (2001). *Wechsler Test of Adult Reading—adapted for UK use*. Psychological Corporation, San Antonio, TX.

Wood, R.L. and Liossi, C. (2006). The ecological validity of executive tests in a severely brain injured sample. *Archives of Clinical Neuropsychology*, **21**, 429–37.

Worthington, A. (1999) Dysexecutive paramnesia: strategic retrieval deficits in retrospective and prospective remembering. *Neurocase*, **5**, 47–57.

Worthington, A.D. (2003). The natural recovery and treatment of executive disorders. In: *Handbook of clinical neuropsychology* (ed P.W. Halligan, U. Kischka, and J.C. Marshall). Oxford University Press.

7

Assessing and rehabilitating aggressive behaviours in persons with dysexecutive symptoms

John C. Freeland

Brain Injury Rehabilitation Trust, York

Introduction

The prefrontal cortex is not only strongly associated with dysexecutive disorders but also modulates much of the activity of the limbic system and hypothalamus. This modulation is associated with the social judgement aspects of aggression (Zald and Kim 2001) In the field of acquired brain injury there is a broad acceptance of the connection between dysexecutive symptoms such as impulsivity, impaired problem-solving, perseveration, or compromised insight and the incidence of aggression. This connection is now receiving much attention in the study of adolescents (Santor et al. 2003), psychiatric populations (Bjorkly 2006), and alcohol-related violence and prisoners (Hoaken et al. 2003). In their review of frontal lobe dysfunction and violent/criminal behaviour, Brower and Price (2001) found cumulative evidence from imaging studies to support a strong association between increased aggression and prefrontal activity.

Aggression is common after traumatic brain injury. Recently, Baguley et al. (2006) followed a group of survivors of moderate to severe traumatic brain injury, and found that, even at 5 years, 58 per cent were reported to have exhibited some aggression over the previous month. Grafman et al. (1996) studied 520 head-injured Vietnam-era veterans and found that those with frontal lobe lesions were reported to display significantly more aggression than veterans with non-frontal lesions. Early attempts to formulate treatment methodologies for aggression after brain injury attempted to blend the use of behavioural techniques with neuropsychological concepts. One of the earliest neurobehavioural formulations was that by Wood (1987), and in the early nineties several authors followed with general guides to behavioural treatment (Braunling-McMorrow 1992a; Corrigan and Jakus 1994; Wesolowski and Burke 1994).

Neurobiological underpinnings

Research regarding the neurological underpinnings of aggression has primarily focused on the prefrontal cortex, hypothalamus, and amygdala. The hypothalamus has a key orchestrating role in aggressive behaviour because of its central role in modulating the sympathetic nervous system. Stimulation in laboratory animals produces transitory aggression, both predatory and affective, while lesions to the hypothalamus can produce permanently aggressive animals. The amygdala and associated temporal cortex are central to much affective behaviour. Animals with bilateral lesions to the amygdala have been reported as tame and quiet, whereas electrical stimulation produces rage (Hollander *et al.* 2002) This line of research has led to the theoretical linkage of temporal epilepsy with aggression and is often cited as the theoretical basis for the widespread use of anti-epilepsy medications for aggression, especially episodic dyscontrol. The frontal cortex has regulatory functions in appetitive responses and responses to aversive stimuli, and the orbital frontal cortex (OFC) has been associated with both emotive and aggressive behaviours. Damage to the OFC in humans can produce general patterns of social disinhibition, which are sometimes referred to as pseudopsychopathy (Zald and Kim 2001). Imaging studies of aggressive and violent populations have consistently reported frontal lobe abnormalities (Brower and Price 2001).

Cognitive and functional underpinnings

Many clients are tested for cognitive and executive abilities in the course of their rehabilitation for neurological injury or illness, but this knowledge then fails to inform the ongoing rehabilitation. Nowhere is this a greater misfortune than with aggression. Using knowledge of the client's cognitive, executive, and language skills can lead to asking important questions during the initial assessment of behaviour. Despite the wide acceptance among clinicians that cognitive and communication deficits have a strong impact on aggression, this connection has not been subjected to rigorous empirical research. In a study of school-aged children, one of whom was identified as 'brain damaged', Carr and Durand (1985) manipulated both staff attention and task difficulty for a language task. For several of the children, task difficulty rather than staff attention was the critical stimulus to elicit dyscontrolled behaviours. This was one of the few studies to focus specifically on language difficulty as a trigger for aggression.

Specific deficits in social skills, pragmatics (Hartley 1995), memory deficits (Manchester and Wood 2001), and perceptual disorders can all strongly influence aggression and require consideration in hypothesizing causal relationships and later intervention approaches. An archetypical example would be complex staff requests which overburden a client's verbal memory, resulting in confusion and subsequent distress with consequent verbal abuse. Deficits in problem-solving are among the most common of the dysexecutive symptoms, especially social problem-solving, which is often a core factor in understanding the functional basis for aggressive behaviour.

Developing effective cognitive and communication systems to compensate for impairments is critical, even though they are seldom tracked for their specific effect on challenging behaviours. Optimized compensatory systems for communication impairment, visuospatial impairments, memory impairments, and executive impairments can often dramatically reduce challenging behaviour. The importance of an experienced and creative interdisciplinary team in the treatment of aggression after neurological injury cannot be underestimated. Similarly, cognitive failures such as forgetting information or breakdowns in intentional memory may result in behaviours which are difficult to assess in functional analysis because they seldom appear as antecedents on staff recordings.

Executive disorder and aggression have been explored in numerous studies with an overall general consensus that impulsivity is commonly associated with aggression. Interestingly the association of other dysexecutive symptoms has been less well investigated. In a study by Greve *et al.* (2002) the selection and use of cognitive strategies were significantly less efficient for brain-injured persons with impulsive aggression than for controls. However, Greve *et al.* (2001) did not find similar group differences on a neuropsychological test of perseveration and concept formation.

Assessment of aggression

As many factors contribute to aggression, assessment can be complex and fraught with pitfalls. Few aspects of human behaviour result in stronger and more firmly held opinions than aggression, and conceptualizing staff or family opinions as hypotheses may aid in more effective assessment. Because of the emotive nature of aggression, great care needs to be taken not to merely accept the opinions of the most vociferous or influential members of a team. Developing a culture within the rehabilitation milieu which recognizes the value of reliable data is of paramount importance. At its most basic level, assessment can focus on frequency, intensity, or variability. In its more complex aspects, assessment can explore the impact of subtle social conflicts, psychosexual competition, coincidence of delusions, long-term personality factors, or underlying confusion to highlight only a few. An informed neurobehavioural approach will not only recognize the specific aggressive behaviours but will consider the neurological, cognitive, emotional, and social factors which influence the expression of aggression, many of which relate to dysexecutive symptoms, especially impulsivity, concreteness, limited problem-solving, and egocentricity.

From the biological and neurological perspective, one of the most fundamental early distinctions to consider is the differentiation of agitation and more instrumental forms of aggression. Agitation is often associated with delirium and acute confusion. Corrigan and Bogner (1995) developed a reliable measure for these type of symptoms. The management of agitation often focuses on environmental modifications. Whereas the nature and extent of aggression associated with agitation in the early stages of recovery will often follow a gradual pattern of improvement, conversely, marked increases in aggression combined with other symptoms of agitation may be the harbinger of a delirium which could require medical diagnosis and not merely behavioural or psychopharmacological intervention. Unfortunately, full consideration of comorbid issues such as anxiety, mood disorders, or psychosis are beyond the scope of this chapter. Those with secondary neuropsychiatric symptoms or pre-existing psychiatric conditions require a more complex method of assessment to understand the impact of neuropsychiatric symptoms upon aggressive behaviour.

Another important aspect of the neurobehavioural assessment of aggression is the functional implications of the aggressive behaviours. What does the aggression accomplish and how are the behaviours being reinforced or punished (Meyers and Evans 1989)? Interventions from verbal reprimands to supportive counselling often turn out to strengthen the very behaviours they were meant to decrease, and without a strong functional analysis of behaviours, such relationships are often obscured by intuition and supposed common sense (Treadwell and Page 1996). Factors that are frequently overlooked in assessing behaviours include antecedents, consequences, social attention, access to reinforcers, demand characteristics of tasks, environmental factors, self-regulatory aspects of behaviour, and the social-communicative function of the behaviour. Careful review of information can show that the presence of certain people or environments influences the expression of aggression and may suggest antecedent control approaches in treatment (Ducharme 1999). There is a general recognition that understanding the internal thoughts and beliefs which precede the emotive behaviours concomitant to overt aggression is important, and techniques are similar to those used in treating depression (Khan-Bourne and Brown 2003).

One scale that has been widely reported in the measurement of aggression is the Overt Behavior Scale (Yudofsky *et al.* 1986), which was later modified to add antecedents and consequences by Alderman *et al.* (2002). The present author has developed a scale, the BIRT Aggression Rating Scale, which has extensive training material to ensure staff reliability in its use for classifying aggressive behaviours in three levels for verbal aggression and three for physical aggression. Careful review of antecedents and consequences can often uncover relationships showing how, for instance, verbal aggression might result in the withdrawal of staff demands to participate in a difficult and frustrating task. Thus the targeted behaviour is negatively reinforced (i.e. reinforcement by removing noxious stimuli) by removing the demand situation.

Rehabilitation of aggression

One of the critical elements in approaching aggressive behaviour is its inherent urgency—being berated, threatened, struck, etc. tends to elevate behaviours from the object of cold analytical scrutiny to crisis. One of the most important distinctions in treatment plan development is clarifying whether you are drafting a plan for crisis management, an interim plan, or a developed treatment plan. The first two areas often fall under the broad heading of risk management. Several authors have laid out practical prescriptive recommendations for this purpose (Ponsford 1995; Karol 2003) A number of key elements might be considered in crisis management guidelines: take a non-judgemental verbal approach; when feasible allow time for de-escalation; consider the use of distraction; paraphrase and clarify; make simple straightforward requests; consider verbal or gestural redirection to less stimulating environments.

Ducharme (1999) developed a conceptual framework for categorizing interventions for externalizing behaviours, which is conceptually well developed but not widely used. For our purposes, decelerative approaches mean those techniques which reduce the frequency or intensity of behaviour. Consequential approaches generally focus on the reinforcers or punishments which follow a behaviour, while antecedent methods refer to programmes which focus primarily on managing the issue leading up to a behaviour. Psychotherapeutic approaches include behavioural rapport/therapeutic alliance and cognitive-behavioural approaches. The skills training approaches come out of a number of areas including social learning theory for social skills training, communications skills from the speech and language area, and cognitive-behaviour therapy for problem-solving.

Treatment is a catch-all term for a holistic process which includes defining the problem, developing an assessment, developing a working hypothesis, designing and implementing the intervention, evaluating the impact of the intervention, and then considering maintenance and generalization.

Hypotheses which lead to skill training interventions are often the consequence of cognitive, executive, and language assessments, but can also be driven from assessment of the specific antecedents. For instance, a general problem-solving approach might be taken after neuropsychological testing revealed dorsolateral associated deficits in perserveration. In another instance collecting behavioural data on swearing might reveal that the verbal abuse is often preceded (i.e. the antecedent) by a staff request, and hence teaching assertive refusal skills might be appropriate.

A skill intervention approach which is perhaps the most logical to use with aggression is anger management, most of which is based upon the original work of Novaco (1975) In more recent research based on a student population, Deffenbacher et al. (1996) conducted a reasonably large study comparing cognitive and relaxation approaches which failed to demonstrate significant advantage to either approach. A review and model for anger management with survivors of brain injury was published by Demark and Gemeinhardt (2002) (see also Chapter 8, this volume). Only one evaluation of an anger management programme with acquired brain injury has been published (Medd and Tate 2000) but unfortunately the 13 participants did not reliably complete their anger logs. In a treatment study of five participants in a residential programme O'Leary (2000) used a combination of coping skills and anger management to demonstrate reductions in recorded incidents of verbal and physical aggression. The severity of the pretreatment aggression in this study was noted to pose a serious barrier to community living.

The use of communication approaches to address behavioural challenges was first reported by Carr and Durand (1985). Their work has been expanded upon in the field of brain injury (Braunling-McMorrow 1992b). A discourse-based approach to general conversation and interaction skills is reviewed by Hartley (1995). In educational settings, Ylvisaker and Feeney (1998) emphasized social skills, communication-based interventions which focus on the client's everyday context and routines, practice with the client's usual communication partners, and a careful functional analysis of behaviour. The support requirements of 80 participants who came into their community-based programme from residential treatment centres or correctional programmes at least 2 years post-injury showed substantial cost reductions for care in relation to the programme cost (Feeney et al. 2001).

Other skills-based approaches involve addressing the emotive and physiological underpinnings of anger and aggression. In a 10-week intervention with five persons with traumatic brain injury, Aeschleman and Imes (1999) completed a stress inoculation programme and used interview information with participants and relatives to measure impulsivity, which was predominantly weighted with measures of verbal and physical aggression. Participants showed a particularly effective reduction in frequency, especially for the more common verbal behaviours. Another allied approach to reducing underlying conflict as a means of reducing aggression has been problem-solving training (Corrigan and Jakus 1994).

Figure 7.1 is from a single client with a severe hypoxic brain injury who has progressed from a locked unit for challenging behaviours to a supported community living scheme. The dependent variable, the irritability–aggression index, was derived from observed aggression, taking both frequency and severity into account. The graph demonstrates the powerful effect of individually tailored incentive programmes which are labelled on the graph (Behaviour Incentive Programme and Politeness Guideline). In the Behaviour Incentive Programme, a system of check marks was provided for non-aggressive behaviour which could be accumulated to earn extra reinforcing activities, such as extra trips to the local pub etc. The Politeness Guideline focused on verbal abuse using similar techniques. Both these programmes demonstrated good effects above the neurobehavioural milieu in which this client lived.

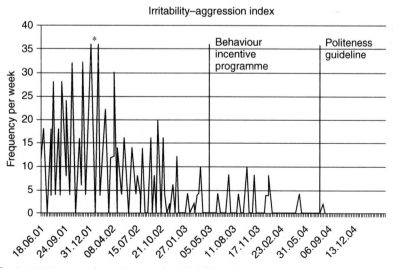

Fig. 7.1 BIRT aggression ratings scale: irritability index.

On examination of the initial period it is obvious that the aggressive behaviours peaked in late December 2001 (asterisk). What was not an obvious neurobehavioural intervention but probably had a very substantial impact on the reduction of behaviour was the reformulation of the client's visual impairment. In December 2001 he was seen by a senior neuropsychologist who recognized that his visual disorder was not cortical blindness but a severe, albeit slowly resolving, visual agnosia. The cognitive approach to his rehabilitation at that time changed markedly and concomitantly his challenging behaviours also began to decrease substantially. Developing effective cognitive and communication systems to compensate for impairments is critical even though they are seldom tracked for their specific effect upon challenging behaviours. Certainly one of the most critical areas for compensation in treating aggression is the communication area. Optimized compensatory systems for communication impairment, visual spatial impairments, memory impairments, and executive impairments can often dramatically reduce challenging behaviour. In this regard the importance of an experienced creative interdisciplinary team cannot be overestimated.

More direct behavioural interventions which encourage or promote behaviours can be divided into means of applying reinforcers, shaping behaviours, and cueing systems (Wesolowski and Burke 1994). Modelling or social learning might be added here, but is covered to some extent in skills-based approaches. Most interventions aimed at increasing prosocial behaviours rely upon the association of a target behaviour with its consequence by either the delivery of a desirable consequence (Andrewes 1989; Alderman and Knight 1997) or removal of an undesirable stimulus (i.e. negative reinforcement). Much of the ground-breaking work in this area goes back to earlier behavioural research with learning disabilities and school-aged children. General references (e.g. Kazdin 2001) remain very useful resources when considering treatment implementation. Often contingency reinforcement programmes are implemented making assumptions regarding the saliency or powerfulness of reinforcers. Behavioural observations will often provide cues as to more naturalistic and less staff-intensive reinforcers. In planning reinforcement strategies concern for satiation should be considered and a menu system explored. In many situations attention to behaviours other than the aggressive ones, a natural contingency of differentially reinforcing other behaviour or low rates of behaviour (DRL), are set up *de facto* (Alderman and Knight 1997). Schedules of reinforcement are an important consideration which are beyond the present survey. The reader is referred to Kazdin (2001) reference for a more detailed discussion.

Early behavioural literature used the term 'shaping' to describe means of guiding a client through successive approximations of a behaviour (Wood 1990a).

Generally these techniques used verbal instructions or directions, and less often physical guidance or gestures. In their discussion of addressing challenging behaviours, Ylvisaker and Feeney (1998) consider an array of communication dimensions aimed at supporting many aspects of executive function which often break down into aggression. Many of the issues of shaping, while not purely tied to antecedent control from a theoretical perspective, relate to very similar issues. Yuen and Benzing (1996) generated a list of 11 strategies which they term redirection. Wood (1990b) also used the term 'prosthetic' environment to encompass a social milieu providing important social cues.

Somewhat akin to shaping is the concept of antecedent control in which there is an intervention prior to situations leading to aggressive behaviour. Some aspects of antecedent control approximate shaping but tend to have a pre-emptive aspect more than a training aspect *per se*. A single case study of antecedent control techniques by Fluharty and Glassman (2001) gives a good example of treating aggression with numerous distraction techniques and of how specific issues such as bathing could be addressed. In a somewhat provocative but thought-provoking statement, Yody *et al.* (2000) estimated that 95 per cent of maladaptive behaviour was attributable to staff interactions, which speaks to the importance of antecedent issues and rapport. While it can be argued from a purely operant perspective that such strategies do not retrain or change behaviours, they do allow for the naturalistic reinforcement of other behaviours and may help to teach strategies related to executive function using a more modelling-based strategy. A recent clinical case illustrates the power of these techniques. A young male client with a very severe traumatic brain injury had demonstrated for some time a very lowered tolerance for noise and for other clients who were confrontational. For many months he had been exhibiting both verbal and physical aggression on a daily basis. Staff feedback such as 'Please don't yell' or 'That is not appropriate' merely served as triggers for further verbal and sometimes physical aggression A video-taped staff tutorial was prepared demonstrating his response to a distraction technique. All staff were required to view the tape, and a comparison of the 15 weeks prior to the tutorial with the 15 weeks after the tutorial showed a 62 per cent reduction in physical aggression and a 46 per cent reduction in verbal aggression. Graphs of his behaviour were circulated to staff an attempt to maintain the approach.

The use of cognitive-behaviour therapy (CBT) as a front-line treatment for aggression has been reported by a number of authors. The actual literature on the efficacy of this approach with brain injury is sparse. A decade ago a survey of members of the International Neuropsychological Society showed that over half reported a reliance upon CBT techniques (Mittenberg and Burton 1994).

Most work to date has been with very mild brain injury or post-concussional syndrome. Means of adapting CBT to a more cognitively impaired population was addressed by Manchester and Wood (2001). Alderman (2003) reported a case using CBT with the aim of improving self-awareness such as by enhancing self-monitoring. He made the point that some aspects of cognition guiding behaviour may be less effective in certain people with severe brain injury or with aphasia, but that CBT work with persons with learning disabilities is encouraging evidence that such obstacles can be overcome.

Decelerative techiques often focus upon extinction as a primary intervention. The theoretical problem with using extinction in these circumstances is the underlying assumption that attention is reinforcing the behaviours. In cases in which aggressive behaviours play a role in escape or avoidance, this may be a very misguided approach. A good functional analysis will generally clarify these issues. An important issue to convey to staff is the expectation of an extinction burst when such programmes are initiated. One specific risk with extinction procedures is that if they are inconsistently implemented, the behaviour may move from consistent reinforcement to a variable ratio (meaning that occasionally the behaviour is reinforced) and such schedules of reinforcement are even harder to extinguish.

Contingency management programmes are generally designed such that the absence of aggressive behaviours leads to the consequence of a reward, and a specific response cost procedure in which privileges or activities are restricted is the consequence of continued aggression. Such systems are criticized as ignoring memory deficits and the poor cause-and-effect reasoning found with dysexecutive disorders. However, a carefully articulated contingency management system will create more staff consistency, and operant learning is not wholly dependent on higher memory or executive abilities as evidenced by its effectiveness with animals without those cognitive systems. Taking this system somewhat further in terms of client engagement and specificity, a contingency management system can take the form of a contract (Braunling-McMorrow 1992a). These are best if behaviours, reinforcers, recording systems, and exceptions are all carefully delineated in plain language. They are also generally more effective if the client is an active participant in the design of the contract, and interestingly the client will often be stricter regarding contingencies than the staff. It is important that the concrete incentives are not overemphasized with staff at the expense of social praise and positive feedback.

Another form of contingency contracting is a token economy. There is a limited amount of literature on this topic after the early report by Eames and Wood (1985) although several reasonably well-known rehabilitation units have focused on challenging behaviours using these systems. Some units go as far as printing their own token money. Alderman (1996) reported a study which separated clients based upon their response to the token economy, but the nature of the token system was not discussed in depth. More commonly, privilege systems, also called level systems, organize the availability to such activities as unescorted community access based upon behaviour and these can provide a system which naturally reinforces prosocial behaviour.

Another strategy for addressing challenging aggressive behaviours is termed differential reinforcement of incompatible behaviour (DRI), in which a specific incompatible behaviour is targeted and reinforced. A variation of this technique is differentially reinforcing other behaviour (DRO) in which any other appropriate behaviour is reinforced. A final variation on this theme is differentially reinforcing low rates of behaviour (DRL). DRL and DRO have most frequently been used for behaviours which are not in themselves inappropriate, but at a very high rate can be distressing. For instance, question asking is very reasonable but when an amnesic client asks the same questions hundreds of times each hour, the questions can become very distressing for staff, families or friends. Alderman and Knight (1997) reported several cases in which the DRL technique was successful in reducing aggressive behaviours. In several of these cases the low rate was dropped in a stepwise fashion until in some cases the final stage becomes a full extinction programme. Interestingly, DRL can reduce some of the frustration and reactions which extinction produces and in a way encourages the staff to think about antecedent techniques in order to gradually reduce the behaviours. Alderman and Knight (1997) reported that these approaches result in less attribution of behaviour to 'between-staff' differences. They also report that staff have the tendency to avoid contact with some aggressive clients, and that by prescribing interactions more closely the interactions become more positive and hence more reinforcing. Another straightforward successful example of treating aggression with DRL involved a young male, 10 years post-injury, who grabbed and kicked passers-by (Hegel and Ferguson 2000). Persel et al. (1997) used a technique of non-contingent reinforcement as a means of enhancing other behavioural approaches for self-injurious behaviour with success.

Recently, Ducharme et al. (2002) have reported the use of errorless training with brain-injured parents and their children. While this technique was aimed at compliance, the effect was to markedly reduce conflict within the family and may also have utility in other brain-injured populations.

Psychopharmacological treatment of aggression can be a valuable adjunct to other approaches. A review of these treatments is beyond the scope of this chapter, but several issues are important with regard to neurobehavioural treatment. Psychopharmacological treatments are used often alongside behavioural treatments, and in the best protocols these interventions are tied to carefully measured behavioural targets. Far too often the effectiveness of a medication is assessed by polling the available staff rather than by using a careful analysis of frequency or intensity measures. Another important aspect of good psychopharmacological treatment is an exit strategy which is tied to behavioural targets. Figure 7.2 illustrates how accepting conventional wisdom regarding the effects of pharmacological agents can be a mistake. This client was assumed to have an affective disorder which required a mood stabilizer, which he had taken for over 10 years. The data strongly raise the hypothesis that much of his physical aggression was iatrogenic (made worse by the treatment).

Generalization and maintenance of behavioural changes is not an area which is particularly well researched with people who have brain injuries. In reviewing approximately 200 articles and books, none was uncovered which focused predominantly on generalization or maintenance. Corrigan and Jakus(1994) recommended the following in skills-oriented approaches:

(a) repeatedly practice targeted skills

(b) use multiple training approaches

(c) practice *in vivo*

(d) assign homework.

In more reinforcement-based approaches the following were recommended:

(a) fade from continuous to intermittent schedules

(b) target naturally reinforced behaviours

(c) teach contingency management to significant others or future carers.

Alderman *et al.* (1995) used a graduated approach which ended with self-monitoring, which also had implications for the generalization of skills.

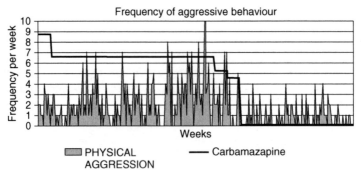

Fig. 7.2 Example of the importance of testing widely held assumptions with individual clients.

Neurobehavioural methods need to be employed responsibly and ethically. Adhering to the doctrine of the least restrictive alternative is important in all treatment approaches. This is important not merely in selecting rehabilitation settings but also when implementing techniques for behaviour change. This doctrine reflects social mores that all individuals are inherently entitled to the least restraint on their freedom. In almost all cases reinforcement programmes should provide extra privileges and activities. They must not impinge upon clients having regular nutritionally balanced meals, having regular exercise, having visitors, having their own space, sleeping in a comfortable bed, or engaging in normal leisure pursuits such as watching television (Kazdin 2001). Avoiding the use of punishment and aversive techniques minimizes most ethical dilemmas in attempts to change behaviour. If this precaution is adhered to, neurobehavioural methods raise no more ethical concerns than most other therapies or treatments.

Summary

Both the assessment and the rehabilitation of aggression in people with neurological impairments are complex endeavours with numerous options. The best practice in systematically addressing aggression involves objectively measuring behaviours, as the human factors in assessing salient behaviours will otherwise present very substantial impediments to objectivity. Performing a careful analysis of behaviour prior to designing a rehabilitation protocol is preferred in all but the most urgent cases. Reliable measurement is at the core of any carefully derived treatment plan. The treatment of aggression can very roughly be divided into the following: antecedent techniques, skills-based approaches, consequential approaches, and biological approaches. Each has in common the need to develop monitoring systems to measure their effectiveness. Skills-based approaches generally take a longer time to show their effect and hence are often used adjunctively with behavioural methods or when the aggression is less intense. Antecedent approaches are important and often require intensive staff or carer training. Understanding and compensating for the cognitive and communication impairments can be crucial to the successful rehabilitation of those with brain injury and aggressive behaviour. Although there is little published research regarding maintenance of behaviour or generalization, attention to this area is an important part of good practice in rehabilitation.

References

Aeschleman, S.R. and Imes, C. (1999). Stress inoculation training for impulsive behaviours in adults with traumatic brain injury. *Journal of Rational-Emotive and Cognitive-Behavioural Therapy*, **17**, 51–64.

Alderman, N. (1996). Central executive deficit and response to operant conditioning methods. *Neuropsychological Rehabilitation*, **6**, 161–86.

Alderman, N. (2003). Contemporary approaches to the management of irritability and aggression following traumatic brain injury. *Neuropsychological Rehabilitation*, **13**, 211–40.

Alderman, N. and Knight, C. (1997). The effectiveness of DRL in the management and treatment of severe behaviour disorders following brain injury. *Brain Injury*, **11**, 79–101.

Alderman, N., Fry, R.K., and Youngson, H.A. (1995). Improvement of self-monitoring skills, reduction of behavior disturbance and the dysexecutive syndrome: comparison of response cost and a new program of self-monitoring training. *Neuropsychological Rehabilitation*, **5**, 193–221.

Alderman, N., Knight, C., and Henman, C. L. (2002). Aggressive behaviour observed within a neurobehavioural rehabilitation service: utility of the OAS-MNR in clinical audit and applied research. *Brain Injury*, **16**, 469–89.

Andrewes, D. (1989). Management of disruptive behaviour in the brain-damaged patient using selective reinforcement. *Journal of Behavior Therapy and Experimental Psychiatry*, **20**, 261–4.

Baguley, I.J., Cooper, J., and Felmingham, K. (2006). Aggressive behavior following traumatic brain injury. How common is common? *Journal of Head Trauma Rehabilitation*, **21**, 45–56.

Bjorkly, S. (2006). Empirical evidence of a relationship between insight and risk of violence in the mentally ill: a review of the literature. *Aggression and Violent Behavior*, **11**, 414–23.

Braunling-McMorrow, D. (1992a). Behavioural rehabilitation. In: *Innovations in head injury rehabilitation* (ed P. Deutsch and K. Fralish). Mathew Bender, New York.

Braunling-McMorrow, D. (1992b). Social skills training for persons with traumatic brain injury. In: *Innovations in head injury rehabilitation* (ed P. Deutsch and K. Fralish). Mathew Bender, New York.

Brower, M.C. and Price, B.H. (2001). Neuropsychiatry of frontal lobe dysfunction in violent and criminal behaviour: a critical review. *Journal of Neurology, Neurosurgery and Psychiatry*, **71**, 720–6.

Carr, E.G. and Durand, V.M. (1985). Reducing behavior problems through functional communication training. *Journal of Applied Behavior Analysis*, **18**, 111–26.

Corrigan, J.D. and Bogner, J.A. (1995). Assessment of agitation following brain injury. *Neurorehabilitation*, **5**, 205–10.

Corrigan, J.D. and Jakus, M.R. (1994). Behavioral treatment. In: *Neuropsychiatry of traumatic brain injury* (ed J.M. Silver, S.C. Yudofsky, and R.E. Hales). American Psychiatric Press, Washington, DC.

Deffenbacher, J.L., Oetting, E.R., Huff, M.E., Cornell, G.R., and Dallager, C.J. (1996). Evaluation of two cognitive behavioural approaches to general anger reduction. *Cognitive Therapy and Research*, **20**, 551–73.

Demark, J. and Gemeinhardt, M. (2002). Anger and its management for survivors of acquired brain injury. *Brain Injury*, **16**, 91–108.

Ducharme, J. (1999). A conceptual model for treatment of externalizing behaviour in acquired brain injury. *Brain Injury*, **13**, 645–68.

Ducharme, J.M., Spencer, T., Davidson, A., and Rushford, N. (2002). Errorless compliance training: building a cooperative relationship between parents with brain injury and their oppositional children. *American Journal of Orthopsychiatry*, **72**, 585–95.

Eames, P. and Wood, R. (1985). Rehabilitation after severe brain injury: a follow-up-study of a behavior-modification approach. *Journal of Neurology, Neurosurgery and Psychiatry*, **48**, 613–19.

Feeney, T.J., Ylvisaker, M., Rosen, B.H., and Greene, P. (2001). Community supports for individuals with challenging behavior after brain injury: an analysis of the New York State Behavioral Resource Project. *Journal of Head Trauma Rehabilitation*, **16**, 61–75.

Fluharty, G. and Glassman, N. (2001). Use of antecedent control to improve the outcome of rehabilitation for a client with frontal lobe injury and intolerance for auditory and tactile stimuli. *Brain Injury*, **15**, 995–1002.

Grafman, J., Schwab, K., Warden, D., Pridgen, A., Brown, H.R., and Salazar, A. M. (1996). Frontal lobe injuries, violence, and aggression: a report of the Vietnam Head Injury Study. *Neurology*, **46**, 1231–8.

Greve, K.W., Sherwin, E., Stanford, M.S., Mathias, C., Love, J., and Ramzinski, P. (2001). Personality and neurocognitive correlates of impulsive aggression in long-term survivors of severe traumatic brain injury. *Brain Injury*, **15**, 255–62.

Greve, K.W., Love, J., Sherwin, E., Stanford, M.S., Mathias, C., and Houston, R. (2002). Cognitive strategy usage in long-term survivors of severe traumatic brain injury with persisting impulsive aggression. *Personality and Individual Differences*, **32**, 639–47.

Hartley, L. (1995). *Cognitive communicative abilities following brain injury*. Thompson Delmar Learning, New York.

Hegel, M.T. and Ferguson, R.J. (2000). Differential reinforcement of other behavior (DRO) to reduce aggressive behavior following traumatic brain injury. *Behavior Modification*, **24**, 94–101.

Hoaken, P.N.S., Shaughnessy, V.K., and Pihl, R.O. (2003). Executive cognitive functioning and aggression: Is it an issue of impulsivity? *Aggressive Behavior*, **29**, 15–30.

Hollander, E., Posner, N., and Cherkasky, S. (2002). Neuropsychiatric aspects of aggression and impulse control disorders. In: *American Psychiatric Publishing textbook of neuropsychiatry and clinical neurosciences* (ed S. Yudofsky and R.E. Hales). American Psychiatric Press, Washington, DC.

Karol, R.L. (2003). *Neuropsychosocial intervention: the practical treatment of severe behavioural dyscontrol after acquired brain injury*. CRC Press, Boca Raton, FL.

Kazdin, A.E. (2001). *Behavior modification in applied settings*. Wadsworth, Belmont, CA.

Khan-Bourne, N. and Brown, R.G. (2003). Cognitive behaviour therapy for treatment of depression in individuals with brain injury. *Neurological Rehabilitation*, **13**, 89–107.

Manchester, D. and Wood, R.L. (2001). Applying cognitive therapy in neuropsycholoical rehabilitation. In: *Neurobehvaioural disability and social handicap folloing traumatic brain injury* (ed R.L. Wood and T.M. McMillan). Psychology Press, Hove.

Medd, J. and Tate, R. (2000). Evaluation of an anger management therapy programme following acquired brain injury: a preliminary study. *Neuropsychological Rehabilitation*, **10**, 185–201.

Meyers, L.H. and Evans, I.M. (1989). *Nonaversive intervention for behaviour problems: a manual for home and community*. Paul H Brooks, Baltimore, MD

Mittenberg, W. and Burton, D.A. (1994). A survey of treatments for postconcussion syndrome. *Brain Injury*, **8**, 429–37.

Novaco, R.W. (1975). *Anger control: the development and evaluation of an experimental treatment*. Lexington Books (DC Health), Lexington, MA.

O'Leary, C.A. (2000). Reducing aggression in adults with brain injuries. *Behavioral Interventions*, **15**, 205–16.

Persel, C.S., Persel, C.H., Ashley, M.J., and Krych, D.K. (1997). The use of noncontingent reinforcement and contingent restraint to reduce physical aggression and self-injurious behaviour in a traumatically brain injured adult. *Brain Injury*, **11**, 751–760.

Ponsford, J. (1995). *Traumatic brain injury rehabilitation for everyday adaptive living*. Lawrence Erlbaum, Hove.

Santor, D.A., Ingram, A., and Kusumakar, V. (2003). Influence of executive functioning difficulties on verbal aggression in adolescents: moderating effects of winning and losing and increasing and decreasing levels of provocation. *Aggressive Behavior*, **29**, 475–88.

Treadwell, K. and Page, T.J. (1996). Functional analysis: identifying the environmental determinants of severe behavior disorders. *Journal of Head Trauma Rehabilitation*, **11**, 62–74.

Wesolowski, M.D. and Burke, W.H. (1994). Behavior managment techniques. In: *Innovations in head injury rehabilitation* (ed P. Deutsch and K. Fralish). Mathew Bender, New York.

Wood, R.L. (1987). *Brain injury rehabilitation: a neurobehavioural approach*. Croom Helm, London.

Wood, R.L. (1990a). Conditioning procedures in brain injury rehabilitation. In: *Neurobehavioural sequelae of traumatic brain injury* (ed R.L. Wood). Taylor & Francis, London.

Wood, R.L. (1990b). Neurobehavioral paradigm for brain injury rehabilitation. In: *Neurobehavioural sequelae of traumatic brain injury* (ed R.L. Wood). Taylor & Francis, London.

Ylvisaker, M. and Feeney, T.J. (1998). *Collaborative brain injury intervention: positive everyday routines*. Singular Publishing, San Diego, CA.

Yody, B.B., Schaub, C., Conway, J., Peters, S., Strauss, D., and Helsinger, S. (2000). Applied behavior management and acquired brain injury: approaches and assessment. *Journal of Head Trauma Rehabilitation*, **15**, 1041–60.

Yudofsky, S., Silver, J., Jackson, W., Endicott, J., and Williams, D. (1986). The overt aggression scale for the objective rating of verbal and physical aggression. *American Journal of Psychiatry*, **143**, 35–9.

Yuen, H.K. and Benzing, P. (1996). Guiding of behaviour through redirection in brain injury rehabilitation. *Brain Injury*, **10**, 229–38.

Zald, D.H. and Kim, S.W. (2001). The orbital frontal cortex. *The frontal lobes and neuropsychiatric illness* (ed S.P. Salloway, P.F. Malloy, and J.D. Duffy). American Psychiatric Press, Washington, DC.

8

Managing anger: a practical approach

Helen O'Neill

Kemsley National Centre for Brain Injury Rehabilitation,
St Andrew's Hospital, Northampton

Introduction

Following brain injury, the experience of anger can often become a particular problem either to the person who has suffered the injury or to those around them. However, there is a disparity between the limited literature on anger and the more extensive references to aggression which can result from anger (Lira *et al.* 1983; McKinlay and Hickox 1988; Uomoto and Brockway 1992; Whitehouse1994; Medd and Tate 2000; Kinney 2001; Manchester and Wood 2001; Denmark and Gemeinhardt 2002; Alderman 2003).

Until recently, anger was usually studied in conjunction with aggression or hostility rather than as an emotion in its own right (O'Neill 2006). Novaco, a major contributor to the techniques of managing problematic anger, noted the dearth of references to the emotion anger when he wrote 'anger is said to be the most talked about but least studied emotion' (Novaco 1978).

This chapter will initially clarify concepts and consider the particular reasons for anger following brain injury, before reviewing treatment options.

Clarifying concepts

The terms anger and aggression are commonly used, yet there is ambiguity concerning their definition. The terms are often used interchangeably. Expressed anger, particularly if accompanied by aggression, has tended to be viewed as a behavioural problem rather than an emotional response (Eames and Wood 1985; Wood and Burgess 1988; Alderman and Burgess 1990). For the purpose of this chapter the following definitions will be used (O'Neill 2006).

Anger refers to a subjective emotional state defined by the presence of physiological arousal and cognitions of antagonism (Novaco 1994). It is a normal emotion having many adaptive features, yet when the frequency, intensity, or duration of anger outweighs its adaptive features, it is said to be dysfunctional (Novaco 1992). Spielberger (1988) divided anger into two types, trait anger (the individual differences of disposition to anger) and state anger (the temporary emotional state arising from frustration or annoyance of the moment). The division was an attempt to separate the personality factors peculiar to individuals from the external factors that could anger any of us.

Aggression refers to overt behaviour, either physical or verbal, that does or could bring harm to another person, object, or system (Eckhardt and Deffenbacher 1995). Barratt (1994) classified aggression broadly into three categories: (1) premeditated or learned aggression, which varies between social groups and cultures; (2) medically related aggression, which may be secondary to illness, including psychopathology; (3) impulsive aggression, which is characterized by a 'hair-trigger' temper. This is a helpful categorization when considering the role of anger in aggression.

It is widely assumed that anger occurs as a result of frustration, perceived threat, or a belief that a personal injustice has occurred (O'Neill 2006). The basic role of the emotion is to convey a message. At best, this is a helpful warning that something is wrong, which then prompts us to communicate and/or solve the problem. At other times anger reflects a distorted or imbalanced appraisal of the situation. The latter is common following a brain injury when cognitive deficits lead to a person's interpreting and dealing with their world differently. Emotions may be magnified and felt more intensely. Beliefs that maintain or justify anger may also be unhelpful (e.g. 'Unless I look strong they won't listen). However, such beliefs may be amenable to modification with therapy.

Novaco's model of anger (Novaco 1994) takes a contextual view and emphasizes on the environmental factors as well as internal processes. Following a brain injury there will be additional variables. The complex and interactive consequences of a brain injury, any of which may be contributing to the presenting emotional and behavioural state, must be considered, for only then can an appreciation of the role of anger be obtained and a full assessment made. Those factors contributing to the experience of anger following brain injury are considered in the following section.

Anger following brain injury

While anger is part of the normal range of human emotional response, brain injury can heighten the experience of anger. This can occur by exacerbating previous characteristics, undermining capacity for self-control, and causing loss of autonomy and social roles.

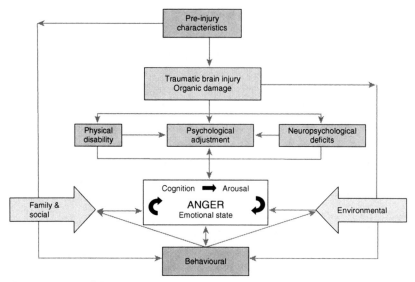

Fig. 8.1 Emotion following traumatic brain injury.

Pre-injury characteristics

Knowledge of the person's pre-injury personality and functional status provides a basis for making judgements about what can be attributed to the brain injury. Age, and hence stage of skill development, at injury will be an important factor, particularly if the injury occurred before adulthood. Pre-injury character traits may be exacerbated and personality characteristics that were considered desirable and empowering before the injury may take on a new direction that can be troublesome for the individual or others. For example, a person who had very high standards of timekeeping, speed, and volume of work may develop a rigid unforgiving style, not respecting any human fallibility and hence becoming prone to intolerance and anger with themselves and/or others. When these pre-trauma expectations and assumptions are coupled with executive disorder, the individual may develop an inflexible concrete style of thinking and find it difficult to solve 'on-the-spot' problems, such as someone being late.

Wood (1989) described premorbid characteristics as being the 'fabric' of behaviour and therefore the 'material' that therapy staff have to work with'. Tate (1998) found evidence that only the severity of the injury, and not the premorbid personality variables, was related to psychosocial functioning. In any case it is important to consider what resources an individual had to deal with problems before their brain injury. Some may have had maladaptive coping strategies such as excessive use of alcohol (MacMillan *et al.* 2002).

Impact of brain injury on anger

Studies concerning the impact of brain lesions have focused on aggressive behaviour rather than the subjective experience of anger. Nevertheless, they suggest that the ability to inhibit or control aggression can be reduced by injury to the frontal or temporal lobes of the brain and to subcortical structures. Brower and Price (2001) report case descriptions which suggest that focal orbitofrontal injury specifically impairs the capacities for social judgement, risk avoidance, and empathy that inhibit inappropriate or reflexive aggression. Grafman and colleagues (Grafman 1989, 1994; Grafman *et al.* 1996) argue that a loss of behavioural control can result from a loss of the inhibition exerted by the orbital frontal lobes over the subcortical limbic structures that regulate aggression and other primitive impulses.

Impulsive aggression has also been associated with damage to the temporal lobes and limbic system. Within the limbic system, the hippocampus and amygdala have been investigated in relation to fear and rage responses (Mark and Ervin 1970; Martinius 1982). Case reports have highlighted damaged limbic structures in patients exhibiting episodic violence. There are case studies of patients in whom previously uncontrolled episodic aggressive outbursts were significantly reduced following surgical removal of tumours affecting the amygdala. (Sachdev and Smith 1992; Bowman 1997).

Physical disability

Actual loss of function, the consequent need for aids and adaptations, and reduced independence often lead the individual to feel resentment and frustration. Sensory loss (hearing, sight, sensation, smell and/or taste, and depth perception) interferes with the way the world is perceived. Patients often consider their body to be unpredictable, particularly if they have developed epilepsy, and feel that they cannot rely on it as they used to. Some actually express strong feelings of hatred about their non-functioning limb or body as it acts as a constant reminder of their loss. Others who appear to have recovered physically report regular pain, distress, and annoyance. Anger is a common component of the emotional experience of chronic pain, and personal management styles may influence outcomes in pain management (Burns *et al.*1998).

Neuropsychological deficits

Poor self-monitoring and self-awareness can fuel a sense of injustice when degrees of supervision are imposed on individuals who see no need for them. Treatment interventions may provoke an increased awareness of cognitive deficits, which can in turn threaten the sense of self (Toglia and Kirk 2000).

Receptive and expressive language deficits may cause frustration, misinterpretation, poor adjustment, and increased dependence (Shammi and Stuss 1999; Alderman *et al.* 2002).

Psychological adjustment

The psychological and personal aspects of adjustment following brain injury are complex and varied (Macniven *et al.* 2003). Pre-injury status and coping styles, attributions about the injury, perceived control over recovery, and the degree of external social support available all contribute to adjustment. A great many patients experience a period of anger at some time during their recovery process.

Role changes and social isolation are recognized as common problems after severe TBI (Wood *et al.* 2005). Both of these can have an adverse effect on self-concept, self-esteem, and feelings of self-worth.

Family and social impact

The trauma of a brain injury affects more than just the injured person. The effect on families has been well documented (Oddy and Herbert 2003). Anger as a reaction to loss and emotional distress may occur in both the injured person and their family. Perlesz and O'Loughlan (1998) showed that relatives reported a reduction in their anger following family counselling, but that this reverted to the original levels at the follow-up 24 months later.

There is a high incidence of relationship breakdown after trauma (Lees 1999, Stilwell *et al.* 1997), and the loss of personal and economic status is a strain for all. It is inevitable that social networks will change. The patient's expectations of the family, and vice versa, may place unrealistic demands on others and lead to emotional distress and frustration.

Environmental factors

Environmental factors influence the patient's emotional response. Time spent in hospital or living in a rehabilitation unit or other communal setting, or simply being physically dependent, can result in the development of an external locus of control (Rotter 1954). However, if patients feel some control over their recovery, this increases self-efficacy and in turn aids recovery (Partridge and Johnson 1989; van den Broek 2005).

Executive dysfunction may lead to decreased tolerance of environmental triggers. Patients frequently describe difficulty in concentrating in busy, noisy, or active surroundings where the demands on attention are complex. For example, performing a task with interruptions or processing information that is delivered rapidly can cause overload and reduced performance, which in turn can feed negative thinking, strong emotional responses, and impulsive reactions.

The state of anger

When anger is triggered it may not always be possible to isolate any one cause. Indeed, it has become clear that emotional reactions are more complex than was once assumed (Teasdale 1997). For example, cognitions may be antecedents, consequences, or part of a reciprocal relationship with emotion.

Following brain injury, emotions are often experienced with greater intensity. For example, a patient explained that when he experienced an emotion he felt that 'his nerves were raw and being scraped by some wire strippers'. He compared his feelings of sadness and anger on seeing a squirrel run over to those experienced when a close relative had died. Such intensity of feeling was incomprehensible to him as he struggled to reconcile this newly felt sensitivity and lability with his former unsentimental values. In this case psychoeducational work helped the patient to appreciate his emotional fragility, and emotional management techniques (described later) enabled him to recover a sense of mastery.

Behavioural reaction

Brain injury and the resulting impairments in executive functioning increase the probability of the occurrence of aggression and violence at lower levels of arousal. This has particular impact on personal relationships (Wood *et al.* 2005) and can be exacerbated by alcohol abuse (Marsh and Martinovich 2006).

Aggression following neurological insult is likely to have multiple causes (Golden *et al.* 1996; Alderman 2003; Cohen *et al.* 2003), and therefore a comprehensive formulation is necessary to understand the meaning, and the maintaining factors, of the behaviour before effective treatment can be devised.

Intervention

If anger leads to challenging behaviour and/or emotional distress it is generally seen as a problem, but the question is—a problem for whom? Requests for treatment may come from another party, such as a spouse or colleague, because they find the behaviours difficult. The intervention will vary depending upon who is suffering or who perceives it as a problem, as well as the stage of recovery.

Ideally, the patient also needs to perceive their anger as a problem and hence be motivated to change or to address the issue by using self-management techniques. When this is not the case, a different approach to management has to be used.

Realistic expectations are necessary depending upon the stage of recovery. Initially, soothing external environmental changes and perhaps medication may be the best ways to help. The role of family members and health professionals will be influenced by the rehabilitation services available and the duration of input (Oddy *et al.* 1996). Family and health professionals may have differing or opposing aims, which can also cause conflict (Oddy *et al.* 1996). Kreutzer *et al.* (2002) suggest that family members can unwittingly worsen problems by giving the person with brain injury very different advice. Hence it is essential for health professionals to acknowledge and respect the family's frustration, distress, and necessary adjustment. Professionals need to work closely with the family, providing brain injury information and an explanation of the rationale behind any of their decisions (Wood *et al.* 2005).

As the patient's self-awareness increases it will be necessary for others to validate their distress, yet provide a sense of hope. Self-help reading matter, both for people who have had a brain injury and for their families, can complement professional input.

Assessment

A full assessment leading to a case formulation will determine the level of treatment input required. A combination of both self-report and observational measures can contribute to this as well as providing the necessary data to assess the efficacy of treatment. The author has found all of the following to be useful:

- archival records and information from significant others
- ABC analysis and observational baseline data
- the Overt Aggression Scale–Modified for Neurorehabilitation (OAS-MNR) (Alderman *et al.* 1997)
- semi-structured interview
- self-report measures such as the Novaco Anger Scale and Provocation Inventory (NAS-PI) (Novaco 2003), the Hospital Anxiety and Depression Scale (HADS) (Snaith and Zigmond 1994), and the Rosenberg Self-Esteem Scale (Rosenberg 1965).

Assessment should also consider basic biological rhythms, as poor sleep patterns may contribute to increased arousal and aggression (Worthington and Melia 2006), together with eating habits, activity levels, fatigue, and pain. It is important to exclude medical reasons for any angry outbursts (Eames and Wood 2003). Uncommonly, outbursts of explosive aggression can arise with little or no trigger; it is important that this is properly evaluated as in some instances it will lead to a diagnosis of episodic dyscontrol syndrome and may respond to treatment with mood-stabilizing anti-epileptic medication (Golden *et al.* 1996; Eames and Wood 2003).

A sense of enquiry will be needed to try and understand the person's anger, its triggers, and its expression. If there is any overt behaviour the following questions should be asked.

- Has it developed as a learned pattern to avoid the interaction or activity associated with rehabilitation, which may evoke pain or fatigue?
- Does it maintain or substantiate a belief of strength or power?
- Is it attention gaining? If so, what is the need underlying this?
- Are there communication needs (Alderman *et al.* 2002)?
- Is there an intolerance of environmental noise or triggers?
- Is the origin of the physiological arousal an anxious thought? For example, 'Oh why can't I do this now? Why's that therapist asked me to do this? She's a silly …' As the cognition changes to a blaming thought, the emotion converts to anger.

Levels of treatment intervention

Working with individuals who have an acquired brain injury has necessitated modifications and additions to the delivery of the original Novaco anger control procedure (Novaco 1993–1994). This is an evidence-based treatment approach now used with a variety of populations. A treatment manual *Managing anger* (O'Neill 1999, 2006), based on this work, evolved to fill a need as a practical resource to assist therapists working with those who have cognitive impairment. The cognitive-behavioural programme includes visual and workbook materials together with necessary techniques to facilitate generalization out of the treatment room and boost clients' self-regulation skills.

Initially, treatment allows the individual to understand the components of anger, how it differs from aggression, and how the two are related. The costs and benefits of anger are discussed to increase motivation to change. The training aims to empower the individual, allowing him/her to become equipped to understand and manage his/her anger arousal. Time is needed to develop a good therapeutic alliance, as this is the basis of successful rehabilitation work (Manchester and Wood 2001; Schonberger *et al.* 2006). van den Broek (2005) emphasizes the importance of client-centred neurorehabilitation and defining goals with the patients.

Many clients are still not able to work in this way but will be able to learn and use components as part of their broader rehabilitation programme. Hence, in order to allow more patients to benefit, two levels of intervention are suggested. Before such interventions are undertaken it is important to consider the role of staff and the impact of such work.

What is different about working with angry people?

For many, this is not a popular area of work. Staff members' own value systems, expectations, judgements, and past experiences will be relevant. However, the emotion anger has a great deal in common with the emotion anxiety. There are biological similarities, but the cognitive content is very different as are the possible behavioural responses. Hence anger is often regarded as a particular emotional problem and the effect it has on others has to be recognized. Anger may evoke judgement, whereas anxiety often evokes concern and empathy. Staff members' anticipatory anxiety may be raised when considering a patient who has a history of aggression and whose potential risks are discussed; this can then skew their attentional focus, their expectations, and sometimes their reactions. It is important that they feel confident in 'listening to reported anger' and using de-escalation techniques (O'Neill 2006). If doing specific CBT work, staff will be exposed to a great deal of anger expressed both orally and in written form in diaries. Therefore, when working in close proximity to clients who are communicating their levels of anger, it is wise to remember that this process can evoke strong feelings within those who are listening. The therapist is no exception to this and, like everyone else, will have his/her own anger triggers. If the therapist either identifies with, or is too distressed by, the anger reported by others, his/her own personal feelings could potentially affect the delivery of treatment and the therapeutic relationship (O'Neill 2006).

Level 1: Preparatory stage of treatment

This first level aims to introduce:

- emotional awareness
- arousal reduction techniques
- self-monitoring
- self-instruction
- the role of strategies.

The role of, and the need for, relaxation training needs to be explained as it is a necessary and central skill to reduce levels of physiological arousal when managing anger. However, it is not an easy task for many people whose arousal levels are rapidly changing and extreme. For example, one client stated: 'I get so intensely angry now and without any warning signs'. Hence this input needs to be coupled with brain injury awareness work to aid understanding of the new patterns of arousal.

Relaxation may be viewed unfavourably by some clients for a variety of reasons (O'Neill 1997). They may have already tried it unsuccessfully, or see it as a sign of weakness or backing down. In the heat of the moment, when experiencing intense anger, they do not want to calm down because they believe the message that their anger is giving them. Another prejudice is that relaxation is only for women in leotards! Hence, when introducing relaxation as a necessary part of managing anger, there is a need to be creative or 'sell its benefits', even to relabel it. Motivation to test out relaxation may be increased by considering both the costs and the benefits of being tense and aroused in contrast with the benefits of being calm (O'Neill 2006).

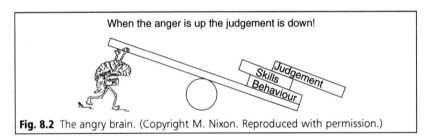

Fig. 8.2 The angry brain. (Copyright M. Nixon. Reproduced with permission.)

It is important to assess whether the person is able to self-monitor changes in their body, and can recognize what it feels like to be calm and relaxed in contrast to being tense and physiologically aroused. This is a necessary step for them before they are able to gauge their level of arousal—a skill they may need to acquire.

In order to allow the person to appreciate the contrast between tension and calm, the following component skills can be introduced.

◆ Calming techniques to accompany activity—soothing music, reduced stimuli, dim lighting, and a calmer environment.

◆ Self monitoring, for example by using a 0–10 or 0–100 scale or a personalized visual thermometer designed with the patient which can also be given the person's name (e.g. Tom's scale). This aims to gain the person's attention, increase self-awareness, encourage ownership, and in turn facilitate self-management.

◆ Strategies to compensate for dysexecutive syndrome and 'sell' the need for routines, for example delivery of external cues such as: 'Tom, what's your mercury level?' Such prompts to monitor are more readily accepted if they are designed with the person rather than being prescribed for the person.

- On The Spot Arousal Reduction (OTSAR) (O'Neill 1997, 1999, 2006): this form of cued relaxation evolved as a way of reducing levels of arousal for people who were not keen to carry out traditional relaxation. It can become a practised technique that can be used easily at times of anger arousal, and can be prompted by a customized script which can be either read or listened to. If the script is to be recorded, it is important to discuss whose voice will be calming and received well in the heat of the moment
- The record of relaxation or OTSAR practice form (O'Neill 2006) to note pre and post levels of arousal in a systematic way and notice trends of improvement.

These skills can be integrated in complementary sessions which reinforce and rehearse techniques (e.g. chill-out sessions, coping with emotions, dealing with feelings) or skill-building groups such as assertiveness and problem-solving.

Behavioural experiments (McGrath and King 2004) can allow the person to collect evidence that high arousal affects both their cognitive functioning and their communication skills. This may then increase self-awareness and motivation to use such calming techniques (Whitehouse 1994). Such experiments can be part of a wider rehabilitation programme and hence involve other members of the team or family. For example, when approaching a long queue, which normally precipitates impatience and agitation, both parties rate their level of arousal, and then self-instruct STOP and use OTSAR. They can then re-monitor to notice any effects of the intervention. Such a routine can become a useful habit in life's frustrating situations.

Other attention-gaining and memorable routines can provide a structure to follow. The following are examples from the treatment manual (O'Neill 2006).

- If you use the P words (plan, pace, prioritorize, prepare, practice) then you won't need to use the F words (fatigue, flustered, forget or swearing!).
- The problem-solving routine for use when anger may be conveying the message that there is a valid problem to solve.

The rehabilitation programme needs to include brain injury awareness work to allow the person to acknowledge, own, and then manage their differences.

Level 2: Managing anger

When the person has sufficient insight and motivation to use self-management skills, specific treatment to help them manage their anger can begin. This uses specific CBT techniques to address anger and anxiety. There is growing recognition that CBT can be used successfully with individuals with anger problems (Lira *et al.* 1983; Uomoto and Brockway 1992; Whitehouse 1994; Montgomery 1995; Medd and Tate 2000; Kinney 2001; Manchester and Wood 2001;

Denmark and Gemeinhardt 2002; Alderman 2003; Eames and Wood 2003; McGrath and King 2004).

Skill training

This stage involves teaching cognitive-behavioural coping techniques that can be used when there is a sense of provocation. The individual is trained to see anger as a warning sign and feel empowered to use the techniques. Because anger involves the way we *think* and *feel*, and what we *do*, the process considers the three components of anger arousal.

Cognitive restructuring

- Self-monitoring and discovering triggers, using a variety of diaries and pictorial worksheets
- Appreciating the power of thoughts
- Modifying attentional focus
- Reappraisal of threat or provocation
- Adjusting expectations of self and others
- Visualization
- Developing self-instruction
- Coping statements
- Reviewing attributions or recurring causal blame
- Changing rigid assumptions—shoulds, oughts, and musts or unhelpful beliefs

An individual's beliefs about anger may need to be identified and re-evaluated if they prevent a desire to change. For example, 'Anger means strength; I must let my anger out' was a strongly held belief by a young man whose physical disability caused anxiety that he was now unable to protect himself. Such beliefs were initially empowering but later unhelpful. There may be a fear of letting go of what seems justified anger: 'If I get calm I'm backing down and he's wrecked my life'.

A pending legal case may trigger and maintain such thoughts. In this case therapy needs to acknowledge the role of anger, yet allow the person to discover that by keeping the anger alive they themselves are suffering, and they deserve better! Hence the functional costs of anger on cognitive functioning and communication need to be appreciated and linked.

Arousal reduction training

- Self-monitoring escalating arousal
- Interrupting this using self-instruction
- Breathing *out* and the relaxation response OTSAR or imagery

Behavioural coping skills

◆ Strategic withdrawal

◆ Planning the task

◆ Using a problem-solving routine

◆ Attending to social skills, assertion and negotiation, or effective expression of angry feelings. There are many reasons why this communication may go wrong (O'Neill 2006) and guidance may be needed from the speech and language therapist.

◆ Modelling and rehearsal of effective coping

Personal action plan

Although all three components of skill acquisition are essential, some clients may require greater emphasis on one aspect of training. The new skills can then be practised in a variety of situations and provide evidence of coping. A record of treatment in the form of an individualized summary and personal action plan (O'Neill 2006) are developed during treatment. This can benefit contributions by both the patient and others involved in their care, and may include any prompts or cues that the patient has given others permission to use. therefore, as the person becomes more effective, they have a wider choice of responses when anger is triggered. This, in turn, encourages increased confidence, reduces fear of losing control, and consequently improves self-esteem levels.

Example of a personal action plan

My anger can cause me and my family a lot of trouble and grief:

◆ At times I get angry; these times are usually when … people question me or when they make me feel stupid, ask me to repeat myself.

◆ I get annoyed if people are late or don't do things properly!

I know I'm angry because I can recognize that:

◆ I am *thinking* … It's happening again! Why don't they f … off!

◆ My body is *feeling* hot and tense, my heart is racing and I grit my teeth

◆ I am *doing* the following things—pacing, swearing and muttering, slamming the door

◆ The reasons I would like to change are: I know I give the wrong impression of myself, it upsets my family and later I mull on it and regret it

So I will try to interrupt or arrest the anger if I:

(1) Think or say this to myself—Take a chill pill! … Was I speaking clearly?

(2) Do a calming breath *out* and then check how my body is feeling. Has the thermometer stopped rising? If not, do more slow breathing.

Now, if there is something to deal with or a problem to solve:

- I will do it calmly and use the P words and *not* the F words!
- Then it is more likely to be Purrrrrrfect!

(O'Neill 2006)

Duration of treatment

Although CBT is commonly and effectively used to treat problem anger, the complications of anger following brain injury require special consideration. Neuropsychological deficiences, including poor attention, memory, learning, problem-solving, reasoning, and self-control, have to be taken into account. Moreover, losses of independence and status are common after brain injury and can act as enduring sources of frustration, bitterness, and anger. Consequently therapy is often protracted and up to four times longer than recommended in the original Novaco treatment procedure (O'Neill 2006). For example, Alderman (2003) noted that more than 40 sessions plus daily checks over a 22-week period were needed with an inpatient. Those treated on an outpatient basis may require up to 16 weekly sessions followed by 12 fortnightly and 12 monthly follow-ups, a total of 40 sessions.

Conclusion

An approach to help clients manage their anger following brain injury has been outlined in this chapter. It is based on a CBT approach using Novaco's seminal work on the management of anger. The need to keep a sense of enquiry in order to gain a full formulation of any problematic anger and related behaviours is emphasized. A number of variables, including premorbid characteristics, may need to be considered in arriving at a comprehensive formulation. Several stages of intervention have been described to accommodate the wide range of needs and abilities of those affected. Intervention needs to be built around the individual, as an 'off-the-peg' approach is rarely successful. Working with anger is an emotive issue for the client, their family, and rehabilitation professionals. The anxieties, value systems, and attitudes of all members of the rehabilitation team need to be considered when working with clients who exhibit difficulties in managing their anger.

References

Alderman, N. (2003). Contemporary approaches to the management of irritability and aggression following traumatic brain injury. *Neuropsychological Rehabilitation*, **13**, 211–40.

Alderman, N. and Burgess, P. (1990). Integrating cognition and behaviour: a pragmatic approach to brain injury rehabilitation. In: *Brain damage and cognition: cognitive rehabilitation in perspective* (ed R. Wood and I. Fussey), pp. 204–28. Taylor & Francis, London.

Alderman, N. Knight, C., and Morgan, C.(1997). Use of a modified version of the Overt Aggression Scale in the measurement and assessment of aggressive behaviours following brain injury. *Brain Injury*, **11**, 503–23.

Alderman, N., Knight, C., and Henman, C. (2002). Aggressive behaviour observed within a neurobehavioural service: utility of OAS-MNR in clinical audit and applied research. *Brain Injury*, **16**, 469–89.

Barratt, E. (1994). Impulsiveness and aggression. In: *Violence and mental disorder: developments in risk assessment* (ed J. Monahan and H. Steadman), pp. 61–79. University of Chicago Press.

Bowman, M.L. (1997). Brain impairment in impulse violence. In: *Impulsivity: theory, assessment, and treatment* (ed C.D. Webster and M.A. Jackson), pp. 117–41. Guilford Press, New York.

Brower, M.C. and Price B.H. (2001). Advances in neuropsychiatry. Neuropsychiatry of frontal lobe dysfunction in violent and criminal behaviour: a critical review. *Journal of Neurology, Neurosurgery and Psychiatry*, **71**, 720–6.

Burns, J., Johnson, B., Devine, J., Mahoney, N., and Pawl (1998). Anger management style and the prediction of treatment outcome among male and female chronic pain patients. *Behaviour Research and Therapy*, **36**, 1051–62.

Cohen, R., Brumm, V., Zawacki, T., Paul, R., Sweet, L., and Rosenbaum, A. (2003). Impulsivity and verbal deficits associated with domestic violence. *Journal of the International Neuropsychological Society*, **9**, 760–70.

Denmark, J. and Gemeinhardt, M. (2002). Anger and its management for survivors of acquired brain injury. *Brain Injury*, **16**, 91–108.

Eames, P. and Wood, R.(1985). Rehabilitation after severe brain injury: a special unit approach to behaviour disorders. *International Rehabilitation Medicine*, **7**,130–3.

Eames, P. and Wood, R. (2003). Episodic disorders of behaviour and affect after acquired brain injury. *Neuropsychological Rehabilitation*, **13**, 241–58.

Eckhardt, C. and Deffenbacher, J. (1995). Diagnosis of anger disorders. In: *Anger disorders: definition, diagnosis and treatment* (ed H Kassinove), pp. 27–49. Taylor & Francis, London.

Golden, C., Jackson, M., Peterson-Rohne, A., and Gontkovsky, S. (1996). Neuropsychological correlates of violence and aggression: a review of the clinical literature. *Aggression and Violent Behaviour*, **1**, 3–25.

Grafman, J. (1989). Plans, actions, and mental sets: managerial knowledge units in the frontal lobes. In: *Integrating theory and practice in clinical neuropsychology* (ed E. Pereman), pp. 93–138. Lawrence Erlbaum, Hillsdale, NJ.

Grafman, J. (1994). Alternate frameworks for the conceptualization of prefrontal lobe dysfunction. In: *Handbook of neuropsychology* (ed F. Boller and J. Grafman), pp. 187–202. Elsevier, Amsterdam.

Grafman, J., Schwab, K., Warden D., Pridgen, A., Brown, H.R., and Salazar, A.M. (1996). Frontal lobe injuries, violence, and aggression: a report of the Vietnam Head Injury Study. *Neurology*, **46**, 1231–8.

Kinney, A. (2001). Cognitive therapy and brain injury: theoretical and conceptual issues. *Journal of Contemporary Psychotherapy*, **31**, 89–102.

Kreutzer, J., Kolakowsky-Hayner, S., Demm, S., and Meade, M. (2002). A structured approach to family intervention after brain injury. *Journal of Trauma Rehabilitation*, **17**, 349–67.

Lees, M. (1999). The social and emotional consequences of severe brain injury: a social work perspective. In: *Rehabilitation of the severely brain injured adult: a practical approach* (2nd edn) (ed G. Muir Giles and J. Clark Wilson), pp. 241–61. Stanley Thornes, Cheltenham.

Lira, F., Carne, W., and Masri, A. (1983). Treatment of anger and impulsivity in a brain damaged patient: a case study applying stress inoculation. *Clinical Neuropsychiatry*, **4**, 159–60.

McGrath, J. and King, N. (2004). Acquired brain injury. In: *Oxford guide to behavioural experiments in cognitive therapy* (ed J. Bennett-Levy, G. Butler, M. Fennell, A. Hackman, M. Mueller, and D. Westbrook), pp.331–48. Oxford University press.

McKinlay, W. and Hickox, A. (1988). How can families help in the rehabilitation of the head injured? *Journal of Head Trauma Rehabilitation*, **3**, 64–72.

MacMillan, P., Hart, R., Martelli, M., and Zasler, N. (2002). Pre-injury status and adaptation following traumatic brain injury. *Brain Injury*, **16**, 41–9.

Macniven, J., Poz, R., Bainbridge, K., Gracey, F., and Wilson, B. (2003). Emotional adjustment following cognitive recovery from 'persistent vegetative state': psychological and personal perspectives. *Brain Injury*, **17**, 525–33.

Manchester, D. and Wood, R. (2001). Applying cognitive therapy in neurorehabilitation. In: *Neurobehavioral disability and social handicap following traumatic brain injury* (ed R. Wood and T. McMillan), pp. 157–74. Psychological Press, Hove.

Mark, V.H. and Ervin, F.R. (1970). *Violence and the brain.* Harper & Row, New York.

Martinius, J. (1982). Homicide of an aggressive adolescent boy with right temporal lesion: a case report. *Neuroscience and Biobehavioural Review*, **7**, 419–22.

Marsh, N. and Martinovich, W. (2006). Executive dysfunction and domestic violence. *Brain Injury*, **20**, 61–6.

Medd, J. and Tate, R. (2000). Evaluation of an anger management therapy programme following acquired brain injury: a preliminary study. *Neuropsychological Rehabilitation*, **10**, 185–201.

Montgomery, G. (1995). A multi-factor account of disability after brain injury: implication for neuropsychological counselling. *Brain Injury*, **9**, 453–69.

Novaco, R.W. (1978). Anger and coping with stress.In: *Cognitive behaviour therapy: research and application* (ed J.P. Foreyt and D.Rathjen), pp.135–73. Plenum Press, New York.

Novaco, R.W. (1992). A contextual perspective of anger with relevance to blood pressure. In: *Personality, elevated blood pressure and essential hypertension* (ed E. Johnson, W. Gentry, S. Julius), pp. 113–132. Hemisphere, Washington, DC.

Novaco, R.W. (1993–1994). *Stress inoculation treatment for anger control: therapist procedures (1993–1994 modifications).* Available from Professor R. Novaco, University of California, Irvine, CA 92717.

Novaco, R.W. (1994). Clinical problems of anger and its assessment and regulation through a stress coping skills approach. In: *Handbook of psychological skill training: clinical techniques and applications* (ed W. O'Donohue and L. Krasner), pp. 320–38. Boston, MA: Allyn & Bacon.

Novaco, R. (2003). *The Novaco Anger Scale and Provocation Inventory (NAS-PI).* Western Psychological Services, Los Angeles, CA.

Oddy, M. and Herbert, C. (2003). Intervention with families following brain injury: evidence-based practice. *Neuropsychological Rehabilitation*, **13**, 259–73.

Oddy, M., Yeomans, J., Smith, H., and Johnson, J. (1996). Rehabilitation. In: *Brain injury and after: towards improved outcome* (ed F.D. Rose and D.A. Johnson), pp 73–95. John Wiley, Chichester.

O'Neill, H.(1997). Relax, when I'm angry? You must be joking. *Therapy Weekly*, 19 June, p. 11.

O'Neill, H.(1999). *Managing anger.* Whurr, London.

O'Neill, H. (2006). *Managing anger* (2nd edn). Whurr, London.

Partridge, C. and Johnson, M. (1989). Perceived control and recovery from stroke. *British Journal of Clinical Psychology*, **28**, 53–60.

Perlesz, A. and O'Loughlan, M. (1998). Changes in stress and burden in families seeking therapy following traumatic brain injury: a follow-up study. *International Journal of Rehabilitation Research*, **21**, 339–54.

Rosenberg, M.(1965). *Society and the adolescent self-image.* Princeton University Press.

Rotter, J. (1954). *Social learning and clinical psychology.* Prentice Hall, Englewood Cliffs, NJ.

Sachdev, P. and Smith, J. (1992). Amygdalo-hippocampectomy for pathological aggression. *Australian and New Zealand Journal of Psychiatry*, **26**, 671–6.

Schonberger, M., Humle, F., and Teasdale, T. (2006). The development of the therapeutic alliance: patients' awareness and their compliance during the process of brain injury rehabilitation. *Brain Injury*, **20**, 445–54.

Shammi, P. and Stuss, D. (1999). Humour appreciation: a role of the right frontal lobe. *Brain*, **122**, 657–66.

Snaith, R. and Zigmond, A. (1994). *HADS: Hospital Anxiety and Depression Scale.* NREF Nelson, Windsor.

Spielberger, C (1988). *Manual for the State Trait Anger Expression Inventory.* Psychological Assessment Resources, Odessa, FL.

Stilwell, J., Hawley, C., Stilwell, P., Davies, C., and Fletcher, J. (1997). *National Traumatic Brain Injury Study Draft Report.* Centre for Health Services Studies, University of Warwick.

Tate, R. (1998). 'It is not only the kind of injury that matters, but the kind of head'. The contributions of premorbid psychosocial factors to rehabilitation outcomes after severe traumatic brain injury. *Neuropsychological Rehabilitation*, **8**, 1–18.

Teasdale, J. (1997). The relationship between cognition and emotion: the mind-in-place mood disorders. In: *Science and practice of cognitive therapy* (ed D. Clark and C. Fairburn), pp. 67–93. Oxford University Press.

Toglia, J. and Kirk, U. (2000). Understanding awareness deficits following brain injury. *Neurorehabilitation*, **15**, 57–70

Uomoto, J. and Brockway, J. (1992). Anger management training for brain injured patients and their family members. *Archives of Physical Medicine and Rehabilitation*, **73**, 674–9.

van den Broek, M. (2005). Why does neurorehabilitation fail? *Journal of Head Trauma Rehabilitation*, **20**, 464–73.

Whitehouse, A. (1994). Applications of cognitive therapy with survivors of head injury. *Journal of Cognitive Psychotherapy*, **8**, 141–60.

Wood, R. (1989). A salient factors approach to brain injury rehabilitation. In: *Models of brain injury rehabilitation* (ed R. Wood and P. Eames), pp. 75–99. Chapman & Hall, London.

Wood, R. and Burgess, P. (1988). The psychological management of behaviour disorders following brain injury. In: *Rehabilitation of the severely brain damaged adult* (ed I. Fussey and G. Giles), pp. 43–68. Croom Helm, London.

Wood, R., Liossi, C., and Wood, L. (2005). The impact of head injury neurobehavioural sequelae on personal relationships: preliminary findings. *Brain Injury*, **19**, 845–51.

Worthington, A. and Melia, Y. (2006). Rehabilitation is compromised by arousal and sleep disorders: results of a survey of rehabilitation centres. *Brain Injury*, **20**, 327–32.

9

The impact of executive function impairments on communication

Sinead Corkery and Mandy Fairweather

Brain Injury Rehabilitation Trust, York and Milton Keynes

Human communication is a highly evolved social activity which allows us to communicate beyond our immediate need. It enables us to discover others and ourselves and achieve things through a myriad of relationships that could not be achieved alone. Executive functions can play a major role in this level of sophisticated communication, and disruption in these functions can have devastating effects on the quality of a human life.

In this chapter we discuss areas of communication affected by executive functions, outline assessment of these communication skills, and explore possible treatment approaches to support rehabilitation of these skills. Clinicians working with people who have executive dysfunction will no doubt have examples to support the descriptions within this chapter but it maybe useful to consider the scenario shown in the box before we begin.

Nigel

It's Saturday morning and you're off to do some shopping. On your way you meet your old friend Clare. You've known her for many years and you have a lot in common. You are always happy to see her. You stop for a chat and talk about what you have been up to. Clare talked about what she'd been doing but she spoke so quickly, and the kids were chatting away, that you found it difficult to follow. At one point you think Clare hasn't realized everything you have been up to but she eventually she gets it. Her kids are adorable and getting big. Overall it was a really nice chat and you were pleased to see her. You both agree to call to arrange a night out.

Clare

You're out with your family on Saturday morning. You're in a real rush, as you have to drop some information off for work before getting the kids to swimming class. Just before you are about to leave town you bump into your old friend Nigel. Nigel sustained a head injury in a car accident about 10 months ago. You notice that Nigel has seen you because he has stopped, although he hasn't said anything. You greet him and ask how he is. Nigel begins to talk about some of things he has been up to. His conversation jumps all over the place and you ask him some questions to try to understand better. However, Nigel just repeats the same information as before and you are none the wiser. The only information you have clearly followed is about a party he went to and that is because he has told you about it three times. In fact at one point Nigel goes into explicit details of his romantic liaison at the party—right in front of your kids. The poor kids, they keep trying to hide behind you because Nigel keeps touching their faces even though they clearly don't like it. He talks for a long while even though you have tried to indicate you're in a rush. You literally have to start walking away before he gets the hint. You are glad to have seen him but talking with him is hard work. He mentioned going out but you indicated that you were busy and weren't sure. Your friendship has changed since his accident and you have avoided going out with him.

This scenario describes one interaction with two very different subjective outcomes. Although fictional, this communicative interaction could have been written within a variety of contexts, and the features of Nigel's communication style will not be unfamiliar to those who work with people who have an acquired brain injury and subsequent impairments of executive function. Executive functions are usually associated with the frontal lobes, specifically the prefrontal cortex. It is important to note that other language disorders are related to the frontal lobe regions but are not specifically dysexecutive and therefore will not be discussed here (Alexander 2002). There are two distinct and contrasting presentations of executive function impairments that are useful to keep in mind when working with people with communication difficulties. Mesulam (2002) describes two main subtypes of frontal lobe syndrome, both resulting in executive dysfunction but presenting with very different clinical pictures. The first is associated with damage to the dorsolateral regions of the prefrontal cortex, associated with activation, control, and regulation of internal drives. Individuals are observed to show loss of initiative, creativity, and concentration power, appearing apathetic and with reduced emotional range. This presentation can also be described as frontal abulic syndrome (Mesulam 2002). Luria (1970, 1973) also describes the characteristic of reduced spontaneous output and impoverished propositional language in 'dynamic aphasia' in the absence of naming, reading repetition (and in some cases grammatical or syntactical) difficulties. Robinson *et al.* (1998) explore this further, describing how the prepositional output becomes more impoverished with increasing number of competing response options. For example, the individual J.T. performed better on phrase generation with sentences where there were few options for completion (e.g. 'The man bought a sandwich and…') and failed on sentences where there were multiple competing responses (e.g. 'The man ate a sandwich and…'). An executive controlling system would normally address this conflict of competing responses. The second key frontal syndrome involves orbitofrontal lesions resulting in disruption of intellectual regulation of behaviour and cognition (McDonald 1993). Here, individuals such as Nigel can be described as having frontal disinhibition syndrome, with increased behaviours that appear to lack judgement, insight, and foresight. They may also be impulsive, labile, aggressive, and perseverative, and appear not to learn from experience (Ylvisaker *et al.* 2005). Neither syndrome is associated with primary deficits in cognitive domains, including language, but they do play an executive role in successful communication.

Ylvisaker and Szekeres (1989) identify several features of executive function that influence communication. These include self-awareness, goal-setting, planning, self-direction and initiation, self-inhibition, self-evaluation, and flexible problem-solving. Communication breakdown due to impairment of executive function is difficult to categorize into neat components because of the complex interactions between core linguistic abilities (receptive and expressive), non-linguistic cognitive, abilities and higher-order executive functions (Hinchliffe *et al.* 1998). Communication difficulties resulting from executive dysfunction are strongly interrelated, and no one area is independent of another, but an attempt will be made to look at how executive dysfunction can affect key areas—comprehension of extended language, social competence, discourse, and indirect communication. We will also explore possible interventions to increase successful communication

Areas of communication affected by executive function

Comprehension

During the opening interaction Nigel had difficulty following all the information that Clare provided during their conversation. It is not uncommon for individuals with TBI to describe a feeling of being overwhelmed by information. When processing incoming written or verbal language, the executive system allocates the necessary resources according to the needs of the situation. When following extended material the executive system is responsible for controlling and allocating attentional resources, target selection, inference control, switching between tasks, and error monitoring to help an individual to sustain his/her attention and focus and shift attention to different aspects when necessary (Rios *et al.* 2004). The capacity of the executive attention system is seen as limited, and non-routine activities require more effortful/strategic processing than the processing of information in more routine/automatic tasks. As extended language is generally used to convey more complex or novel information, it will utilize this system extensively. A significant component of these executive processes is working memory (Park *et al.* 1999). Baddeley (1992) describes working memory as a limited capacity that allows for the storage and manipulation of information. Several authors describe holding information 'online' or 'in mind' (Petrides 1994; Goldman-Rakic 1995) so that it can be manipulated, monitored, and reorganized. Hartley (1995) describes how working memory is involved in organizing of data to allow more efficient learning, control of interference and the development of strategies for storage and retrieval. Cabeza and Nyberg (2000) describe how the prefrontal areas are seen as being involved in the encoding and retrieval of information and Burgess and Robertson (2002) suggest that people with problems of working memory will have difficulties tracking incoming information and comparing various aspects of the data. When extended passages of verbal or written material are presented, the information must be processed for meaning, organized, encoded, stored, and retrieved, prioritizing key ideas, identifying essential and non-essential details, and revising the organization as the incoming material evolves. If people experience difficulties in organizing incoming information, they may be unable to see the relevance of what is being said or detect the real intent behind it because of impairments in integrating the data. Those with organizational impairments or difficulty integrating incoming information, such as long sequential instructions and rapidly spoken narratives, may be unable to detect the main theme or condense information usefully.

These difficulties can have repercussions on several areas of participation, including following instructions, conversations, or utilizing data within the work, home, and social environments. Rapid topic change within conversation can further hinder the ability to 'keep up' because of overall slowed processing (Hartley 1995). Conversations require regular reference to what has already been said, and this is disrupted if people experience processing difficulties due to impairments of executive function. Working memory is necessary to integrate incoming information with existing knowledge and guide the interpretation of evolving conversations. Because of variable levels of awareness the individual's response to these difficulties is not always predictable. Burgess and Robertson (2002) found that 17 per cent of patients reported that they had problems with lack of insight, compared with 39 per cent of their caregivers. For example, clients have been observed to report that their communication partner is not making themselves clear, recognizing that they are not following everything that is being said but believing that the problem is external to them. On another occasion a man with executive dysfunction was observed to nod repetitively as if to indicate he had understood, and only revealed that he was having difficulties following conversation with those that he felt he could trust.

Interpretation and use of social communication

Nigel clearly experiences difficulties in understanding Clare's perception of the situation. He is unable to pick up on clues that his communication is not fully successful and shows little attempt to repair or adapt his style. This breakdown occurs verbally (explicit details of his romantic encounter) and non-verbally (excessive touching of the children's faces). Cicerone and Tanenbaum (1997) describe how disorders of executive function can affect several areas of ability necessary for social interactions. They argue that in communication it is necessary:

(1) to predict the effect of communication;

(2) to understand that a communication partner may have an alternative perspective;

(3) to recognize other people's reactions to communication;

(4) to modify communication accordingly.

For successful communication each stage needs to be 'active' at any one time, rather than a linear progression through the steps, which further increases the demands on executive functions. Even before an individual activates multilevel executive functions, i.e. organizing both incoming verbal and non-verbal information, they can experience difficulties within more specific domains. McDonald and Flanagan (2004) found that many individuals with TBI, particularly those with frontal lobe pathology, have difficulty in recognizing all basic emotions. A possible explanation for changes in communication and the breakdown of interaction quality and relationships could be impaired theory of mind (ToM), i.e. the ability to understand others' emotions, motivations, and thoughts and to understand their behaviour accordingly (Bibby and McDonald 2005). Henry et al. (2006) recognize that deficits in ability to infer mental state can have serious implications for social functioning. In Henry's study, performance on an executive function test (verbal fluency) and ToM recognition were significantly related. Although it is still unclear whether executive impairments lead to poor performance on measures of ToM, or that both ToM and executive function depend on the same or interrelated neuroanatomical systems, it can be surmised that mental flexibility and self-regulation (including inhibition) are essential when considering situations from another perspective. A member of staff accompanying a client to a hospital waiting room observed her say the following to anyone who sat near her during the visit: 'Hello I'm B. Are you married? I am. I'm married to V. We make love every other day. Have you children? I do...'. McDonald and Flanagan (2004) looked at the ability of people with TBI to assess the speaker's emotions and beliefs (first-order ToM), what the speaker intended their conversational partner to believe (second-order ToM), and whether remarks were a lie or sarcastic retorts. If individuals had problems judging basic emotions, they would experience difficulties assessing more subtle emotions during conversation. However, intact or reduced capacity to assess basic emotions was not an indicator of second-order ToM abilities, although ability to understand the speaker's intentions (second-order ToM) was closely linked to abilities to comprehend conversational inference such as sarcasm.

McDonald and Pearce (1998) note that 'Patients with executive impairments are less likely to make non-conventional, socially effective requests that address possible obstacles to listener compliance than non-brain-damaged counterparts'. In other words, because of the contextual constraints and poor inferential reasoning, requests were less sensitive to the needs of the listener and fewer strategies were used by brain-injured subjects to win over the listener, for example asking to stay at a friend's house without offering an incentive (such as bringing food and drink).

Bond and Godfrey (1997) identified that subjects with TBI were perceived to be less socially rewarding because of changes in their social behaviour. They describe one such change as a reduction in the number of prompts that people with TBI use during conversation. The role of prompting is seen as focusing the conversation on the listener and creating opportunities for them to talk about themselves (e.g. asking open-ended questions). In fact, people with TBI were found to dominate turn-taking, and the fewer prompts those with TBI used, the more their communication partner initiated. As TBI subjects use fewer prompts than controls, they do not encourage their communication partner to talk about themselves or their interests, reinforcing the perception of egocentricity and creating imbalance in roles. Nigel demonstrated this behaviour in the vignette above, and Hartley (1995) also describes individuals who talk excessively about their feelings and own experiences. Snow and Douglas (2000) found that there were difficulties in initiating and maintaining topics of conversation, pushing the responsibility for successful communication onto the communication partner.

Narratives and conversational discourse

At a non-interactive narrative level, Coelho *et al.* 1995 noted a correlation between executive problems and story telling (complete/incomplete episodes) in adults with TBI. Hartley and Jenson (1991) found that, after severe TBI, individuals presented with fragmented discourse because of less productive and less efficient speech (reduced content, longer utterances, and fewer cohesive ties). At an interactive level the demands on executive functions increase as an individual has to exchange information in a much more dynamic realm than when setting and executing a plan for a non-interactive narrative. Conversations are naturally an important aspect of relationships, and we can see that Clare found it difficult to follow Nigel's discourse and found that he talked excessively and the topic 'jumped all over the place'. Grice's model of conversational practice (Grice 1978) describes how speakers cooperate and expect cooperation when conversing with each other, following four maxims of quantity, quality, relevance, and manner. McDonald (1993) found that subjects with TBI found it difficult to speak in a manner that was clear and unambiguous, presenting as confused and disorganized, and had difficulties monitoring quantity, either saying too much or too little.

Alexander (2002) described 'unelaborated conversational output with restricted capacity for complex discourse procedures' after damage to the anterior left frontal region and, in contrast, 'discourse deficit with dilapidated organization and socially inappropriate or frankly confabulatory output' after right lateral and anterior frontal damage. These disorders are not seen as aphasic in nature but stem from the reduced ability to use action plans to assemble complex functional language. McDonald (1993) hypothesized that verbose, repetitive, and uninformative narrative could suggest failure to detect an appropriate endpoint and inability to terminate output even at the completion of a communication plan. Coelho *et al.* (1995) noted that individuals with traumatic brain injuries succeed at word or sentence level (possibly as more linguistically based) but struggle when attempting to impose structure and organization within their narratives (more cognitive-based skills), resulting in reduced overall organization and poor progression of logical ideas within narratives. Errors of sequencing and focus on inappropriate tangents may also be due to failure to monitor performance (McDonald 1993). Van Leer and Turkstra (1999) suggested that disruption in cohesion (linking meaning across sentences using cohesive markers, e.g. 'and', 'but', 'however') can lead to a breakdown in functional communication. Impairments of organization alone can lead to problems sequencing information, word-retrieval problems, and imprecise language. All the above will affect the person's ability to contribute meaningfully in situations such as those where detailed explanation is required, and the communicative partner will have to exert more effort to follow the conversation. Even when Clare has to request clarification in an attempt to understand Nigel, he is unable to revise and adapt his output to repair the breakdown.

Abstract, ambiguous, and indirect communication

Our interactions are littered with abstract language and with subtle and ironic uses of verbal and non-verbal communication. After injury to the frontal lobes, comprehension can be disrupted by a tendency to be concrete or understand at a superficial level (McDonald 1993) and responses may be bound to the most concrete aspects of the information given (McDonald and Pearce 1996). Snow and Douglas (2000) found that people often had difficulty in interpreting or using indirect communication such as sarcasm. Verbal irony often includes sarcasm that can be used to convey positive intent, i.e. 'banter' as well as more negative indirect speech acts. During these indirect acts of communication the intended meaning is the opposite to, or different from, the literal meaning that has been stated (Haverkate 1990). This also can be conveyed non-verbally, for example smiling during a tedious situation when the intent is to convey frustration not happiness. The process involved in the comprehension of sarcasm is complex and not fully understood, but McDonald and Pearce (1996) report that evidence continues to support the theory that the literal meaning is identified first and alternative meanings subsequently.

Consider the following scenario involving a client with executive dysfunction who experienced difficulties accessing the figurative meaning of metaphors during testing. During a naturalistic conversation a member of staff was observed to say 'Don't cry over spilt milk', whereupon the client lifted up his coffee cup to look below it, stating, 'I haven't spilt any milk'. Although the client had only accessed the literal meaning, the staff member interpreted his concrete statement as a purposeful attempt at humour. In turn, the client was completely unaware of any alternative meaning and interpreted his communicative partner as joking that he had spilt milk.

Another example of difficulties with flexibility and more abstract interpretation involves a female client who had sustained TBI and had resultant executive difficulties. Her young children would frequently attempt to engage their mother in make-believe play. Her response to their interaction was to deny the existence of the pretend items they used in their play, using slight reprimands, e.g. 'No there aren't any swamps in here. You're not wet. Stop being silly.' When staff discussed the concept and benefits of make-believe play with her later, she was unable to see the event from the perspective of her children, although she recognized their need for that type of play. At the time of the event she was unable to access an alternative abstract meaning for the play and displayed 'concreteness' in her interpretation.

Assessment

Traditionally, cognitive communication assessment has been made up of a battery of tests of cognitive and language function amongst others. This approach aims to help health professionals determine areas of weakness that require input and areas of strength that can help compensate for impairments. More recently, there has been a move towards assessment of functional outcome, looking particularly at outcome in real-life situations and mainte-nance of gains in the longer term. Clinicians select tests to answer specific clinical questions, namely: Is there a problem and what are its characteristics? What are the everyday implications for that person and might treatment help? Therapists working with clients with dysexecutive difficulties often use both standardized and non-standardized assessment tools to answer those questions. Turkstra et al. (2005) listed the tests that met validity and reliability criteria (as set by the US Agency for Health Care Policy Research) for use with those with cognitive communication disorders. These included the Behaviour Rating Inventory of Executive Function (BRIEF) (Gioia et al. 2000), the Communication Activities of Daily Living (CADL-2) (Holland et al. 1999), the Western Aphasia Battery (Kertesz 1982), and the Test of Language Competence (extended) (Wiig and Secord 1989). They noted the lack of tests developed specifically to assess the communication of those with cognitive communication disorders.

The person with executive dysfunction often requires an individualized assessment process as few published assessments cover the spectrum of poten-tial communication impairments. The clinician may need to use a number of measures to obtain detailed information on particular areas. For example, subtests within the Measure of Cognitive-Linguistic Abilities (Ellmo et al. 1995) or Discourse Comprehension Test (Brookshire and Nicholas 1993) measure ability to process incoming information. The Awareness of Social Inference Test (McDonald et al. 2002) examines interpretation and use of social language and ambiguity. A discourse analysis procedure such as that described by Coelho (1999) can inform the clinician as to how executive deficits affect conversation. These are just a few of the more commonly used assessments in this field. Clinicians may form additional conclusions from the client's performance on tests measuring specific aspects of executive function. For example, the Controlled Oral Word Association Test (assesses verbal fluency Spreen and Benton 1977). The DEX Questionnaire within the Behavioral Assessment of Dysexecutive Syndrome (BADS) (Wilson *et al.* 1996) can highlight difficulties that the client is experiencing with communication.

However, as is clear in the vignette at the beginning of this chapter, communication deficits stemming from dysexecutive dysfunction are often subtle yet disabling in everyday life, and so the clinician needs to determine the person's overall level of communicative competence in the contexts relevant to them. Anderson *et al.* (2000) note the inconsistency between performance on tests and everyday functioning, describing this difference as 'both an important diagnostic indicator as well as a major challenge in the evaluation of persons with prefrontal dysfunction'. Observation of a client in a range of everyday situations can allow the clinician to analyse the antecedents and outcomes around various communication acts. In settings that undertake client observation and record antecedents, behaviours, and consequences (ABC recordings), it is also possible to obtain information from many sources (carers, professionals, family). Body and Parker (1999) point out how this can improve others' awareness of communication and brain injury as well as provide insight into the client in his/her differing life roles. Interview and self-rating tools, such as the La Trobe Communication Questionnaire (Douglas *et al.* 2000), provide further insight as to the client's perception of their level of function. Ylvisaker *et al.* (2002) advocate 'collaboration' with the individual and other professionals to reduce over-testing and inefficiency. This approach encourages joint identification of the questions that need to be answered before planning intervention.

Coelho *et al.* (2005) conclude that non-standardized real-life assessment procedures should complement language and neuropsychological testing when aiming to determine ability and plan intervention. They support the use of 'collaborative, contextualized hypothesis testing' and make a number of useful recommendations regarding discourse analyses and the influence of context on assessment.

How do we help people who present with communication difficulties arising from executive dysfunction?

Despite the amount written about the nature of communication difficulties arising from executive dysfunction, less has been written about their remediation. There are no prescriptive formulas. However, some approaches have more evidence to support them than others. For example, approaches using applied behavioural analysis have a greater body of evidence than the comparatively newer approach of positive behaviour supports, although Ylvisaker *et al.* (2005) report significant movement towards the latter since 2000. Success very much depends on a formulation of the individual's characteristics, including the impact of mood, behaviour, social history, psychosocial well-being, beliefs and values, insight, and other cognitive impairments. In fact, there are so many variables within this population that even two clients with similar cognitive or behavioural profiles may respond differently to an intervention. However, finding an intervention that works successfully with the client is one of the features that make this work so interesting. The aim of interventions is not to 'cure' the executive impairment but to facilitate increased participation in a functional domain. Although knowledge of the executive impairment is necessary, most evidence is found for approaches that address the communication disability. In this chapter we will explore not only interventions that look at eliciting change from the individual with executive difficulties, but also interventions that look for change from the communication partner and the environment.

General considerations

Ideally, the client should always be involved when identifying their goals for communication. Reduced self-awareness and self-monitoring after brain injury results in many clients experiencing difficulties in redefining their strengths and weaknesses. Because of this they often set goals that relate to their pre-injury skills. This is a common phenomenon—for example, the person with severe dysarthria who wants to work in a call centre or the person with disorganized and tangential language who wants to teach evening classes. Although it is not helpful to encourage unrealistic goals, neither is it helpful to negate a person's aims. It would be hard for anyone to be told that they could no longer fulfil a role important to their sense of self such as being a husband, mother, teacher, or musician, especially if they still truly believe they can do so.

Sometimes helping a client to identify smaller goals towards their wider aim allows them to explore their strengths within a personally meaningful framework. For example, the woman who wants to teach evening classes could be asked to prepare and plan a small section of a client group session on a topic of her choice. If this goal is met with resistance, e.g. 'I can already do that', she should not be immediately told that she can't or that she needs to practice. Instead, acknowledgement of the person's beliefs allows the person to feel listened to and therefore more in control. Sometimes the person can be persuaded that they will actually be helping the staff member and the group, rather than 'performing' or being 'tested' on skills. It is more useful to work in 'real-life' situations where the communication difficulties occur, as generalization of skills can be limited (Ylvisaker and Feeney 1998).

Goals often need to be prioritized within this population, as there can be more than one component of their communication that will need to be supported. Sometimes it will be clear which feature of their communication is having the greatest impact on their lives and therefore should be addressed first, for example a client who cannot inhibit asking personal questions, therefore making themselves vulnerable and socially isolated. However, other considerations need to be taken into account, as the 'greatest' problem may not lead to the greatest success, which may lead to an individual failing early on in their rehabilitation. Therefore it may be more beneficial to work on smaller but more achievable goals at first in order to build a sense of success with an individual who may initially be resistant to input (Burgess and Robertson 2002). Cicerone and Tanebaum (1997) worked with a 38-year-old woman, SAL. One of the most troublesome components was identified as her lack of insight into her difficulties, and therefore this area was prioritized. She experienced difficulties inhibiting behaviour, but when given verbal and video feedback appeared to adapt her behaviour in the presence of the camera and was able to correct and produce appropriate responses in these situations. However, the skills did not generalize beyond these sessions. It was also noted that she became increasingly angry and depressed when she was given feedback, and her resistance to treatment increased. Another individual might have responded well to the intervention, but it is important to be vigilant to such adverse responses and to the potential impact on their general well-being.

Most of all it is important to stay positive and to feed back the successes of an individual's communication. If realistic feedback is balanced with feedback concerning the person's strengths, the person, who is frequently in a situation of frustration, can see how things can work and be more motivated to problem-solve in less successful areas. When working with staff members who need training and guidelines to support an individual's communication, it is important to allow the individual to participate as much as possible. If a client can be actively involved in writing their own support programmes and training staff, it can increase their ownership of interventions as well as helping them evaluate their profile of post-injury skills more realistically.

Self-monitoring training

Traditionally, this approach looks at an individual's behaviour, but it can be applied to communication skills, particularly those in the social domain. Alderman *et al.* (1995) have used this approach in several areas including repetitive use of a particular topic in discourse. They describe five key stages of intervention.

1. Record a baseline of target communication 'behaviour'.

2. Spontaneous self-monitoring: provide the person with a counting device (e.g. mechanical clicker) and ask them to keep a record of how many times they demonstrate the target communication behaviour, while continuing to carry out an activity to focus attention elsewhere.

3. The person is expected to self-monitor while carrying out an activity, but this time staff prompt when communication behaviour is observed but not recorded. This is done in order to increase the accuracy of an individual's self-monitoring.

4. External cues are withdrawn but subjects are rewarded if their self-monitoring is within a given range of the therapist's recording. By increasing the criteria to achieve the reward, the individual's accuracy of self-monitoring is improved.

5. The final stage looks at encouraging the individual to inhibit the target communication behaviour. Here the person is rewarded if they have not exhibited the communication behaviour for a given period of time.

This approach addresses increased 'problem' behaviours, such as excessive touch and interrupting, but does not support individuals who present with reduced behaviours, such as lack of initiation or reduced verbal output. It can extinguish, or at least reduce, 'inappropriate' communication, but not replace it. It does not help the client develop alternative forms of communication; rather, it increases awareness of, and therefore inhibits, communication that is not viewed as successful. One individual experienced difficulties with aspects of his non-verbal communication. This included excessive touching and difficulties monitoring proxemic variations according to social norms, despite understanding the principals of whom you should and should not hold tightly or put your arm around. For the authors the most success and generalization has occurred when monitoring can take place in a variety of settings and activities within an individual's life.

Positive behavioural supports

Ylvisaker and Feeney (1998) explored several positive support strategies including 'positive setting events', 'momentum', and 'scaffolding'. First, they describe investigating the setting events that occur prior to an activity in order to optimize outcome. This can include the internal states of the person (cognition, physical and emotional state, and perception of task meaningfulness and difficulty) as well as the more traditional antecedent analysis of external factors (recent positive or negative interactions, environmental stressors such as noise, crowding, presence of specific 'preferred' people, and time of day. Positive setting events increase the likelihood of success in an activity and include rest, nutrition, exercise, orientation, understanding of a task, feelings of competence and control, recent success, and meaningful activity.

Positive behaviour momentum refers to the impact of success on further motivation to tackle harder and more challenging activities. If an individual experiences failure in an activity they are more likely to withdraw from further attempts, but if they experience success then they are likely to be motivated to continue. Ylvisaker and Feeney (1998) outline this in detail, describing how difficult tasks should be addressed within the setting of achievable successful activities. Burgess and Robertson (2002) also recommend consideration of the precise demands of a situation where impairment occurs. If a client feels that every time they work with their therapist they experience failure and/or have these failures highlighted, that client is likely to want to withdraw—fearing failure. On the other hand, if the client feels that they are succeeding at some level, they are more likely to feel that they have some control, influence, and potential to succeed, and therefore have more motivation to work on more difficult components.

Too frequently in life and in care settings, people are not given feedback on their successes. This is not to say that people do not need support to focus on areas that can be improved; it is more about the balance of supporting and helping them to see their successes as well as more difficult areas of their communication. For example, our client who experiences difficulties inhibiting inappropriate comments may work on these in a real social context and his strengths (e.g. good initiation, turn-taking) would be reflected upon as well as his weaknesses.

Another positive support is introducing meaningful activities so that they are achievable but not patronizing. Ylvisaker and Feeney (1998) emphasize that these situations should not be artificial, but meaningful real-life tasks, though finding activities that are intrinsically rewarding is not always easy. Sometimes identifying the correct level for individuals can be difficult, but it is essential in order to maintain their motivation to work. Hartley (1995) describes how individuals can be strongly supported to experience success initially (e.g. external structure, prompts, assistance), and as they learn within the activity the supports can be gradually reduced. Supports can also include cueing prior to a problematic situation. Ylvisaker and Feeney (1998) describe this as 'scaffolding' where the scaffolding is not seen as fixed but flexible and adaptable to the person's needs. Much of their 'collaborative and apprenticeship project-focused' work can allow the systematic withdrawal/reinstatement of supports within a meaningful framework.

Self-rating

This approach can be used for many components of communication (e.g. discourse skills, social competence), and can be used to encourage the use of strategies. Ylvisaker and Feeney (1998) used a 1–10 rating scale that is completed by the client and by supporting staff as a post-evaluation of executive components of an activity. Again, evaluation should be of specific components and not just general categories (e.g. rating of 'initiation' of conversations rather than rating 'conversational skills') so that the client can understand what they are working on. Some self-rating approaches look at prediction of performance versus actual performance within a task in order to increase self-awareness and therefore the ability to monitor their skills. Turner and Levine (2004) discuss how this approach may be most useful for people in the early stages after their injury or whose cognitive deficits mean that they are unable to benefit from higher-level educational input about the brain and specific difficulties related to injury. Again, this approach should be used within the context of success by rating 'What went well?' as well as rating targeted communicative behaviour. If the task is too difficult, self-rating can be a very negative experience for the client. It is important to build up slowly so that an individual can experience success on the ratings. Goals should be specific, measurable, and achievable. Video recording can be used to aid more realistic prediction and actual performance rating (Cicerone and Tanenbaum 1997).

Interpersonal process recall

One of the articles cited as evidence of successful intervention for increasing social communication skills is Helffenstein and Wechsler (1982). During this study individuals were given 20 hours of interpersonal process recall (IPR), which consisted of the following stages (Struchen 2005).

(1) videotaped interaction with client and conversational partner.
(2) structured review of the taped interactions with feedback from the participant, conversational partner, and therapist.
(3) development of an alternative skill.
(4) modelling of the skill.
(5) rehearsal.

After intervention, professional staff and independent observers who were not aware of the intervention rated individuals' specific interpersonal skills as significantly improved compared with controls. Those who received IPR also reported significant reduction in anxiety levels and improved self-concept. Ylvisaker et al. (2005) outlined the practice of social communication in the actual situations in which they would occur with the additional support of video self-modelling. However, because the ability to review and evaluate one's self from video footage requires many cognitive processes, some individuals with executive impairment will be unable to engage in this intervention to the necessary level.

External cues

As described earlier, some people experience reduced initiation after TBI. Core skills may be intact but the individual cannot spontaneously use them. Sohlberg *et al.* (1988) worked with an individual who presented with reduced initiation of interactions and reduced range of affect. Giving an external cue (e.g. intermittently placing a visual cue card in front of the person), enabled the subject to increase their initiation of verbal interactions successfully. However, once the external cue was removed the level of initiation dropped again, albeit above the baseline level. Perhaps this intervention showed only limited generalization because it did not address the individual's self-monitoring at any level. The functional benefits of such an intervention may be limited but could perhaps be used in conjunction with self-rating so that an individual experiences success before moving on to an intervention that helps address their own self-monitoring.

Communication partners

Rather than seeing the problem and the solution coming from the individual with the brain injury, the solution can be sought within those who communicate with the client (Ylvisaker *et al.* 2005). The social model of disability focuses on the impact of the environment and how factors within the environment can act as barriers to an individual's success in carrying out their life roles (Finkelstein and French 1993). Kagan (1999) has worked with people who have aphasia to create communication in 'real-world' situations using supported conversation for adults with aphasia (SCA). Although people with communication difficulties caused by executive impairments present a very different clinical picture from those with aphasia, the approaches used in supported conversation (SC) can help in several areas. People who experience processing difficulties and problems integrating information and eliciting main themes and ideas can benefit from SC as it can augment 'online' processing of incoming information as well as help individuals to access information from previous conversations. Putting visual supports in place can enhance working memory as they are more 'permanent' than verbal language alone. Visual supports can help organize and structure expressive output. This approach looks at creating opportunities and means of communication and how these can be generated through conversational partners rather than independently from the client. The responsibility for successful communication is shared by both partners, rather than focusing on the client using strategies independently. This approach is useful, as the communication partner learns generic skills that can be utilized with many people rather than specific approaches only relevant to one individual. Kagan (1999) designed training for conversation partners covering four modules (below). In the original article the content focuses on supporting aphasia, but additional points have been added to support those who experience communication problems arising from impairments of executive function.

- **Conceptual/motivational** This module outlines SC and how it can have an impact on a person's conversation, for example showing a videoed interaction between a client and conversational partner without and then with SC.

- **Technical** This looks at the techniques that can be used in SC. It notes the importance of acknowledging and revealing clients' competencies. Competencies can be revealed by supporting comprehension (using gesture, written keywords, drawing, and specific resource materials to support the topic, allowing time to process information), supporting expression (using yes–no or fixed-choice questions, allowing time to respond, providing means of response), and clarifying responses (using written, pictorial, or key verbal information to summarize, reflect, clarify, and expand on what has been communicated). When working with people with executive problems it is important not to overload an individual with the complexity, rate, duration, or amount of material that is provided. When using SC it is sometimes useful to establish conversation on one key area or topic before expanding or introducing additional aspects. Clients, even with different modes of support, may experience difficulties holding several ideas and lose track of what has been discussed previously. By identifying their capacity to process information during SC you can gauge how much to cover during each interaction. All these techniques are used simultaneously to permit the natural flow of an interaction and allow adult conversation.

- **Integrative role play** Role-play scenarios covering a variety of situations are presented. For example, some interactions are based on the necessity to exchange specific content, while others are more about the quality of the social interaction. Therefore people can experience successful interactions without having to follow all the information.

- **Evaluation exercise** The trainees are provided with pre-recorded videotaped interactions and asked to rate the conversational partner's skills on a nine-point scale. This is done in order to aid self-reflection and rating in non-threatening situation.

The *Pictographic communication resource manual* (Kagan *et al.* 1996) covers basic yes–no questions right up to topics like case conferences and informed consent. Rayner and Marshall (2003) trained volunteers working with people with aphasia, and found that even those with many years of experience showed increased knowledge and quality of interaction with their clients after training, and that those with aphasia also gained in levels of participation. There have been no studies using this approach with people with TBI, but many of the core features are similar to the communication competencies checklist for rehabilitation staff working with people with TBI (Ylvisaker and Feeney 1998). Kagan (1999) indicated that when one person within an individual's environment uses SC, there can be a cascading effect as more people see success, resulting in increased motivation to use it. Ylvisaker *et al.* (2005) also highlighted the importance of supporting communication competence in an individual's everyday communication partners.

Conclusion

Executive functions contribute significantly to a host of communication skills, from receptive and expressive language skills to overall social competence. There are many theories and models of how executive processes are activated during communication and how a breakdown in these processes can result in a myriad of communication difficulties for the individual. Working with people who have communication difficulties resulting from impairments of executive function can be a challenging, fascinating, and rewarding process. Assessment should identify impairments but also guide the team towards functional outcomes that reflect the reality of an individual's life. There is evidence supporting interventions that can change the individual's communication from 'within' as well as interventions that look at supporting the individual using positive external supports and training of communication partners. Specific interventions cannot be prescribed; rather, each person needs ongoing evaluation of goals and interventions so that their rehabilitation programme evolves and develops. An approach that works for one client may not work for another, but a positive and collaborative approach will optimize success and an individual's involvement, sense of worth, and control within the rehabilitative process.

References

Alderman, N., Fry, R.K., and Youngson, H.A. (1995). Improvement of self-monitoring skills, reduction of behaviour disturbance and dysexecutive syndrome: comparison of response cost and a new programme of self-monitoring training. *Neuropsychological Rehabilitation*, 5, 193–221.

Alexander, M.P. (2002). Disorders of language after frontal lobe injury: evidence for the neural mechanisms of assembling language. In: *Principles of frontal lobe function* (ed D. Stuss and R. Knight), pp. 8–30. Oxford University Press, New York.

Anderson, S.W., Damasio, H., Tranel, D., and Damasio, A.R. (2000). Long-term sequelae of prefrontal cortex damage acquired in early childhood. *Developmental Neuropsychology*, **18**, 281–96.

Baddeley, A. (1992) Working memory. *Science*, **225**, 556–9.

Bibby, H. and McDonald, S. (2005). Theory of mind after traumatic brain injury. *Neuropsychologia*, **43**, 99–114.

Body, R. and Parker, M. (1999). The use of multiple informants in the assessment of communication after brain injury. In: *Communication disorders following traumatic brain injury* (ed S. McDonald, L. Togher, and C. Code), pp.147–74. Psychology Press, Hove.

Bond, F. and Godfrey, H. (1997). Conversation with traumatically brain-injured individuals: a controlled study of behavioural changes and their impact. *Brain Injury*, **11**, 319–29.

Brookshire, R. and Nicholas, L. (1993). *Discourse Comprehension Test*. BRK, Minneapolis, MN.

Burgess, P.W. and Robertson, I.H. (2002). Principles of rehabilitation of frontal lobe function. In: *Principles of frontal lobe function* (ed D. Stuss and R. Knight), pp. 557–72. Oxford University Press, New York.

Cabeza, R. and Nyberg, L. (2000). Imaging cognition. II:Aan empirical review of 275 PET and fMRI studies. *Journal of Cognitive Neuroscience*, **12**, 1–47.

Cicerone, K. and Tanenbaum, L. (1997). Disturbance of social cognition after traumatic orbitofrontal brain injury. *Archives of Clinical Neuropsychology*, **12**, 173–88.

Coelho, C.A. (1999). Discourse analysis in traumatic brain injury. In: *Communication disorders following traumatic brain injury* (ed S. McDonald, L. Togher, and C. Code), pp. 55–79. Psychology Press, Hove.

Coelho, C.A., Liles, B., and Duffy, R. (1995). Impairments of discourse abilities and executive functions in traumatically brain-injured adults. *Brain Injury*, **9**, 471–7.

Coelho, C., Ylvisaker, M., and Turkstra, L.S. (2005). Nonstandardized assessment approaches for individuals with traumatic brain injuries. *Seminars in Speech and Language*, **26**, 223–41.

Douglas, J., O'Flaherty, C.A., and Snow, P.C. (2000). Measuring perceptions of communicative ability: the development and evaluation of the La Trobe communication questionnaire. *Aphasiology*, **14**, 251–68.

Ellmo, W.J., Graser, J.M., Krchnavek, E.A., Calabrese, D.B., and Hauck, K. (1995) *Measure of Cognitive-Linguistic Abilities (MCLA)*. Speech Bin, Norcross, GA.

Finkelstein, V. and French, S. (1993). Towards a psychology of disability. In: *Disabling barriers—enabling environments* (ed J. Swain, V. Finkelstein, S. French, and M. Oliver), pp 26–33. Sage, London.

Gioia, G.A., Isquith, P.K., Guy, S.C., and Kenworthy, L. (2000). *Behaviour Rating Inventory of Executive Function*. Psychological Assessment Resources, Odessa, FL.

Goldman-Rakic, P.S. (1995). Architecture of the prefrontal cortex and central executive. *Annals of the New York Academy of Science*, **769**, 212–20.

Grice, H.P. (1978). Further notes on logic and conversation. In: *Syntax and semantics: pragmatics* (ed P. Cole), pp.113–28. Academic Press, New York.

Hartley, L. (1995). *Cognitive-communication abilities following brain injury: a functional approach*, pp. 44, 49, 126. Singular Publishing, San Diego, CA.

Hartley, L. and Jenson, P. (1991) Narrative and procedural discourse after closed head injury. *Brain Injury*, **5**, 267–85.

Haverkate, H. (1990). A speech act analysis of irony. *Journal of Pragmatics*, **14**, 77–109.

Helffenstein, D.A. and Wechsler, F.S. (1982). The use of interpersonal process recall (IPR) in the remediation of interpersonal and communication skill deficits in the newly brain injured. *Clinical Neuropsychology*, **4**, 139–43.

Henry, J.D., Phillips, L.H., Crawford, J.R., Ietswaart, M., and Summers, F. (2006). Theory of mind following traumatic brain injury: the role of emotion recognition and executive dysfunction. *Neuropsychologia*, **44**, 1623–8.

Hinchliffe, F.L., Murdoch, B.E., and Chenery, H.J. (1998). Towards a conceptualization of language and cognitive impairments in closed head injury: use of clinical measures. *Brain Injury*, **12**, 109–32.

Holland, A., Frattali, C., and Fromm, D. (1999). *Communicative activities of daily living* (2nd edn). Pro-Ed, Austin, TX.

Kagan, A. (1999). Supported conversation for adults with aphasia: methods and resources from training conversation partners. *Aphasiology*, **12**, 816–30.

Kagan, A., Winckel, J., and Shumway, E. (1996). *Pictographic communication resources manual*. Aphasia Centre, North York, Toronto.

Kertesz, A. (1982). *Western Aphasia Battery*. Psychological Corporation, San Antonio, TX.

Luria, A.R. (1970). *Traumatic aphasia*. Mouton, The Hague.

Luria, A.R. (1973). *The working brain: an introduction to neuropsychology*. Penguin Books, Harmondsworth.

McDonald, S. (1993). Viewing the brain sideways? Frontal versus right hemisphere explanations of non-aphasic language disorders. *Aphasiology*, **7**, 535–49.

McDonald, S. and Flanagan, S. (2004). Social perception deficits after traumatic brain injury: interaction between emotion recognition, mentalizing ability and social communication. *Neuropsychology*, **18**, 572–9.

McDonald, S. and Pearce, S. (1996). Clinical insights into pragmatic theory: frontal lobe deficits and sarcasm. *Brain and Language*, **53**, 81–104.

McDonald, S. and Pearce, S. (1998). Requests that overcome listener reluctance: impairment associated with executive dysfunction in brain injury. *Brain and Language*, **61**, 88–104.

McDonald, S., Flanagan, S., Kinch, J., and Rollins, J. (2002). *The Awareness of Social Inference Test (TASIT)*. Thames Valley Test, Bury St Edmunds.

Mesulam, M.M. (2002).The human frontal lobes: transcending the default mode through contingent encoding. In: *Principles of frontal lobe function* (ed D. Stuss and R. Knight), pp. 8–30. Oxford University Press, New York.

Park, N.W., Moscovitch, M., and Robertson, I.H. (1999). Divided attention impairments after traumatic brain injury. *Neuropsychologia*, **37**, 1119–33.

Petrides, M. (1994). Frontal lobes and working memory: evidence from investigations of the effects of cortical excisions in nonhuman primates. In: *Handbook of neuropsychology*, Vol 9 (ed F. Boler and J. Grafman), pp. 59–82. Elsevier, Amsterdam.

Rayner, H. and Marshall, J. (2003). Training volunteers as conversation partners for people with aphasia. *International Journal of Language and Communication Disorders*, **38**, 149–64.

Rios, M., Perianez, J.A., and Munoz-Cespedes, J.M. (2004). Attentional control and slowness of information processing after severe traumatic brain injury. *Brain Injury*, **18**, 257–72.

Robinson, G., Blair, J., and Cipolotti, L. (1998). Dynamic aphasia: an inability to select between competing verbal responses. *Brain*, **121**, 77–89.

Snow, P. and Douglas, J. (2000). Conceptual and methodological challenges in discourse assessment with TBI speakers: towards an understanding. *Brain Injury*, **14**, 397–415.

Sohlberg, M.M., Sprunk, H., and Metzelaar, K. (1988). Efficacy of an external cueing system in an individual with severe frontal lobe damage. *Cognitive Rehabilitation*, **6**, 36–41.

Spreen, F.O. and Benton, A.L. (1977). Manual of instructions for the Neurosensory Centre Comprehensive Examination for Aphasia. British Columbia, Canada: University of Victoria.

Struchen, M.A. (2005). Social communication interventions. In: *Rehabilitation for traumatic brain injury* (ed W.M. High, A.M. Sander, M.A. Struchen, and K.A. Hart), pp. 88–117. Oxford University Press, New York.

Turkstra, L.S., Coelho, C., and Ylvisaker, M. (2005). The use of standardized tests for individuals with cognitive-communication disorders. *Seminars in Speech and Language*, **26**, 215–22.

Turner, G. and Levine, B. (2004). Disorders of executive functioning and self-awareness. In: *Cognitive and behavioural rehabilitation: from neurobiology to clinical practice* (ed J. Ponsford), pp.224–68. Guilford Press, New York.

Van Leer, E. and Turkstra, L. (1999). The effect of elicitation task on discourse coherence and cohesion in adolescents with brain injury. *Journal of Communication Disorders*, **32**, 327–49.

Wiig, E. and Secord, W. (1989). *Test of Language Competence—expanded edition*. Psychological Corporation, San Antonio, TX.

Wilson, B.A., Alderman, N., Burgess, P.W., Emslie, H., and Evans, J.J. (1996). *Behavioural Assessment of the Dysexecutive Syndrome (BADS)*. Thames Valley Test, Bury St Edmunds.

Ylvisaker, M. and Feeney, T. (1998). *Collaborative brain injury intervention: positive everyday routines*, pp. 161–223. Singular Publishing, San Diego, CA.

Ylvisaker, M. and Szekeres, S.F. (1989). Metacognitive and executive impairments in head-injured children and adults. *Topics in Language Disorders*, **9**, 34–49.

Ylvisaker, M., Hanks, R., and Johnson-Greene, D. (2002). Perspectives on rehabilitation of individuals with cognitive impairment after brain injury: rationale for reconsideration of theoretical paradigms. *Journal of Head Trauma Rehabilitation*, **17**, 191–209.

Ylvisaker, M., Turkstra, L., and Coelho, C. (2005). Behavioural and social interventions for individuals with traumatic brain injury: a summary of the research with clinical implications. *Seminars in Speech and Language*, **26**, 256–67.

10

Physiotherapy approaches with people with executive disorders

Peter Zeeman

Centre for Rehabilitation of Brain Injury, University of Copenhagen, Denmark

The executive system: living up to minimum requirements

It has been suggested that humans evolved as hunter–gatherers who needed to store food in times of plenty so that they could meet their energy requirements and avoid starvation in times of famine (Neel 1962). In the modern world, sedentary man has constant food accessibility and the so-called 'thrifty gene' leads us to become unhealthily obese through lack of exercise. Fortunately, our species is equipped with executive abilities which, in theory, can override our propensity to overeat and under-exercise. Ideally, our frontal lobes should play the role of the super-ego and tell us to restrict calorie intake in accordance with decreasing calorie expenditure or, conversely, to increase calorie expenditure to counter excess dietary calories.

Unlike other mammals that are prone to the detrimental effects of being overfed and deprived of exercise, *Homo sapiens* has the executive capacity to plan ahead, inhibit or initiate behaviour, and revise plans that are already formulated, and thus potentially has the ability to ward off health hazards. However, innate laxity and social conventions often get the better of the endeavours of the frontal lobes to adjust behaviour in time, as evidenced by the epidemic increase in lifestyle-related diseases.

People who sustain brain injuries are often at a double disadvantage. They may have motor deficits which make exercising even harder and they may have executive deficits. If an ever-increasing number of people find it virtually impossible to take adequate exercise and maintain a stable weight, any executive disorder arising from acquired brain injury (ABI) will act as a further impediment to meeting the recommended daily quota of exercise, i.e. a minimum of 30 minutes of moderate-intensity exercise per day and 1–2 hours of moderate- to high-intensity exercise per week. Experts unanimously advocate a minimum weekly leisure time calorie expenditure of 2000 kcal (8400 kJ), preferably at an intensity exceeding 6 kcal/minute. Those who have suffered a brain injury resulting in difficulties with impaired self-awareness, modulating behaviour, initiating and inhibiting, planning, and structuring their time are even less likely than the rest of us to engage in adequate levels of exercise, In addition, an ABI may result in motor sequelae that prevent physical activity at any intensity but the lowest. For those with less severe motor impairment, slower movement patterns and fatigability will lead to lower calorie expenditure per minute.

Physical consequences of ABI

People suffering from stroke are far more likely to sustain severe physical disability than those with traumatic brain injury (TBI). Three months after stroke, 20 per cent of patients remain wheelchair-bound, and approximately 70 per cent walk at reduced velocity and capacity (Bohannon et al. 1988). Common long-term physical consequences after stroke include hemiparesis leading to varying degrees of loss of volitional movement patterns, muscle strength and dexterity, muscular endurance, and speed, as well as balance and efficient motor planning. Although very few TBI patients continue to remain wheelchair-bound, there was little change in mobility between 2 and 5 years after injury in a sample of TBI patients (Olver et al. 1996). Five years after injury, 41 per cent continued to have difficulties with activities requiring higher-level balance skills, such as running and jumping. Sixty-seven per cent of the sample reported that they fatigued more easily on physical exertion than prior to their accidents. Common long-term physical consequences after TBI include epilepsy, dizziness, headaches, and visual difficulties at 5 years after injury (Olver et al. 1996). Other physical consequences are ataxia, dyscoordination, and motor-sequencing problems, as well as sequelae after fractures. All these physical consequences of stroke and TBI lead to impaired mobility and reduce not only the overall level of physical activity, but also the muscular and cardiovascular intensity with which every single physical activity throughout every single day is performed.

Although the extremities contralateral to the side of the lesion are usually referred to as the affected side, there is evidence that the side ipsilateral to the lesion is also affected to some extent. The acute effects of hemiparesis and impaired balance are often exacerbated by an ensuing period of prolonged hospitalization where not only fatigue and post-injury depression, but also inadequate rehabilitation resources contribute to additional decline in strength and endurance. With more hours spent lying in bed or sitting than was the case premorbidly, and with the only active periods of the day being defined and structured by the therapist in charge, it is no wonder that patients tend to become very dependent on their therapists, and that many patients come to look upon rehabilitation as a matter for specialists rather than as an area where they can play a very responsible role by simply boosting the process through their own level of activity.

In an ongoing study conducted at the Centre for Rehabilitation of Brain Injury (CRBI) in collaboration with the Copenhagen Muscle Research Centre (CMRC), muscle biopsies taken from hemiplegic stroke and TBI patients have proved to differ significantly on the affected side compared with the less affected side. The preliminary results show an overall tendency towards a breakdown in muscle fibre symmetry, size, and distribution on the affected side. In the largest muscles (i.e. the leg muscles), endurance is essential for standing and walking, and so a high percentage of enduring fibre types I and IIa is crucial for normal endurance and safety. However, the research at the CRBI has demonstrated that the shift in fibre types is reversible to a significant degree if the patients engage in heavy progressive resistance training three times a week for a 12-week period. Not only does this kind of training improve the strength of the affected muscles, the peak rate of force development (RFD), and the twitch peak torque (i.e. the neural ability to produce a full muscle contraction quickly), but the acquired strength translates into significantly improved walking speed and gait quality.

The advantages of exercise and goals of physical rehabilitation after ABI

The ultimate goal of any rehabilitation process must always be to bring about optimum restoration of function, thus permitting the patient to revert to independent living and regular physical activity with as little assistance as possible. A retrospective study by Gordon *et al.* (1998), in which 240 individuals with TBI (64 exercisers and 176 non-exercisers) and 139 control individuals without a disability (66 exercisers and 73 non-exercisers) were compared on scales measuring disability, handicap, depression, and self-perceived symptoms categorized as cognitive, concluded that not only were the TBI exercisers significantly less depressed than the non-exercisers, but they also perceived themselves as having significantly fewer cognitive problems and significantly better health status than the TBI non-exercisers. This finding was despite the fact that there were no differences between the two TBI groups on measures of disability and handicap. Significantly more cerebral lesion patients than cranial fracture patients found emotional control more difficult, as well as having increased difficulties with memory and concentration, maintenance of leisure time interests, and general life satisfaction (Engberg and Teasdale 2004). Minimizing the sense of loss of leisure time interests and social integration through attainable and easily appreciable physical improvements is a very effective way of boosting self-efficacy.

Many studies (e.g. Weiss *et al.* 2000; Teixeira-Salmela *et al.* 2001) have clearly demonstrated that high-intensity muscle strengthening and physical conditioning are superior to more conventional physiotherapy, not only in terms of earlier discharge, but also in terms of attaining better functional performance outcome. Many physiotherapists and occupational therapists have had reservations about resistance exercise, and many still do. Reputedly, weight training cannot transfer to functional improvements and is thought to exacerbate hypertonia and provoke abnormal movement patterns. These fears have proved to be groundless in a large number of studies, many of which are cited in a very thorough review article (Patten *et al.* 2004). Intensity is of vital importance, and this also applies to the increasingly popular techniques of treadmill training with or without body weight support (Hesse *et al.* 2001; Pohl *et al.* 2002). The question no longer seems to be which physiotherapy approach is the most effective, but how to maintain functional outcome levels over time after discharge.

The sedentary threat

Many people with ABI have a potential for improved mobility, ranging from independent ambulation and/or increased walking velocity and capacity to regaining the ability to run. The prerequisite for achieving such improvements is to challenge the cardiorespiratory and musculoskeletal systems at levels where the challenge actually makes a difference. However, this prerequisite is not always evident to therapists and caregivers, let alone to the patients themselves. Consequently, almost all rehabilitation of motor function is carried out at a submaximal level, where the termination of a rehabilitative session is defined by the therapist running out of time rather than the patient reaching his/her limit and needing to rest. Cardiorespiratory training without the use of a heart rate monitor will leave both therapist and the patient in the dark with regard to the level of exertion, and will not supply vital and motivating information about a lower heart rate and energy expenditure during a given activity as a result of the beneficial effect of intensive cardiovascular training. Strength or resistance training without prior knowledge of maximal strength defined as 1 RM (one repetition maximum) will be diluted to simple programmes of certain sets of exercises repeated a certain number of times, not because this is the very best the patient can do this day, but because the number of repetitions fits into the regimen or the time frame for the rehabilitation session. Exercises tend to be repeated in series of three sets of 15 repetitions because this number has become ingrained in physiotherapy. If patients doing 3 × 15 repetitions were asked to do two or three times as many repetitions, many would easily be able to do so, but precisely for that reason the exercise cannot be defined as actual strength training (Patten *et al.* 2004). If a given exercise can be performed well more than eight to ten times it begins to lose its strengthening effect. The more repetitions that can be performed in one set, the smaller is the gain in actual strength. This is common knowledge in athletics and in any serious strength training programme for healthy individuals, but apparently does not apply in most physiotherapy approaches for neurological patients. In the absence of basic knowledge of their cardiovascular and muscular performance levels, and lacking the necessary resources to remedy potentially remediable deficits, many brain-injured individuals run the risk of spiralling downwards in what can be termed a 'vicious circle of inactivity' (Figure 10.1).

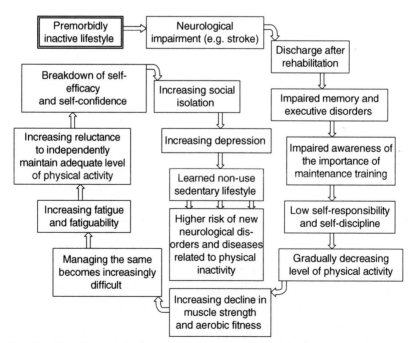

Fig. 10.1 The vicious circle of inactivity. A premorbidly inactive lifestyle may lead to stroke which, in turn, may lead to an even lower level of physical inactivity, thus further increasing the risk of new neurological disorders and other diseases related to physical inactivity.

Although first coined by Edward Taub (Knapp *et al.* 1958) to describe the tendency of hemiplegic patients not to use the affected upper extremity, the term 'learned non-use' is equally applicable to non-use of the cardiovascular system, cognitive faculties, and social skills, as well as of meaningful leisure-time activities and language. Faced with the punishing experiences of unsuccessful attempts to perform at the premorbid level, many people with ABI resign themselves to inactivity or even apathy in domains where they used to be active and engaged.

Benefits of physical activity: relevance to rehabilitation

Data from animal studies have indicated that exercise promotes brain vascularization, neurogenesis, and neuronal survival, and helps to resist brain insult (reviewed by Cotman and Berchtold 2002). There is also a positive relation between exercise and levels of brain-derived neurotrophic factor (BDNF), a protein with neurotrophic and neuroprotective properties which may be linked to brain plasticity (Cotman and Berchtold 2002). The levels of neurotransmitters, such as serotonin and dopamine, are also increased as a result of exercise (e.g. Blomstrand *et al.* 1989).

The research on humans is consistent with the results of the animal studies that provide evidence of the beneficial effects of exercise on cognitive functioning. In a meta-analysis of longitudinal intervention studies in adults over the age of 55, Colcombe and Kramer (2003) reported that fitness training in older adults increased performance on different cognitive tasks by an average of 0.5 SD compared with control groups. Executive control tasks appeared to benefit the most from the exercise. Frontal regions of the brain may be more likely to show improvements with exercise. Deficits in executive functioning, together with decreased processing speed and a decline in short-term memory, are among the most common cognitive consequences of TBI. Therefore it follows that exercise has the potential to promote brain repair in patients with brain injury, and in fact evidence of cognitive improvements following motor enrichment after brain injury has been found in both animal and human studies (reviewed by Kleim *et al.* 2003).

Physical activity is probably the domain where appreciable improvements can be achieved most rapidly in brain injury rehabilitation. Given the many difficulties that face both therapists and patients in the long process of establishing a therapeutic alliance and compliance that can pave the way for awareness, insight, and adaptation to a new life, it is often an advantage to embark on this process by exploiting the latent possibility of increased endurance, strength, and mobility. A general feeling of well-being leading to improved mood and malleability can often be observed after a physical training session where the brain-injured person really challenges the cardiorespiratory system and consequently becomes out of breath and begins to sweat. Nevertheless, brain-injured persons are very rarely seen to sweat or pant during physiotherapy.

People with acquired brain injury, and especially those with executive disorders, will often seem reluctant to put in an effort during rehabilitation. Where this is compounded by problems with drive, alertness, and initiative, cognitive-behavioural rehabilitation methods have been shown to be effective in increasing engagement in physical therapy (Worthington et al. 1997). Often, however, executive disorders such as lack of initiative, distractibility, and impulsivity are misinterpreted as a lack of motivation. While in some rare instances this may be true, what has been put down to lack of motivation on the part of the patient can often be traced back to the therapist who has failed to be sufficiently motivating or has omitted to explain the purpose and goal of the activity. If a patient does not see the relevance of an activity during a rehabilitation session, the cognitive and executive difficulties may be to blame, but the reason may just as well be that the activity lacks the intensity to result in any of the beneficial after-effects of physical exertion. The greater the difficulties with attention, concentration, and memory, the greater is the need for charting all training results in order to ensure cooperation with regard to an effort level that exceeds that of the previous session and to ensure motivation for improving performance. Adhering to a chart and exerting oneself to reach a preset goal that has been set by oneself and the therapist in conjunction can be very helpful in curbing impulsivity and staying on the track. This will be described in greater detail later in this chapter.

The ultimate goal of physiotherapy after ABI

Successful physical rehabilitation should endeavour to arrest the patient's gradual descent down the spiral by addressing all domains that are prone to the development of learned non-use. Skilful performance of any motor task has as a prerequisite adequate muscle strength and cardiovascular endurance. Without these fundamental physiological capacities the motor task in question will be doomed to meet with failure, poor performance, or early interruption. Given the limited resources available for rehabilitation of people with ABI, the more time spent on skill acquisition, avoidance of excessive tone, stretching, and other elements of conventional physiotherapy (e.g. Bobath-oriented Neurodevelopmental Treatment (NDT), Movement Science, and Proprioceptive Neuromuscular Facilitation (PNF)), the less time will be available to address the fundamental issues of strengthening and conditioning. Unless the patient is an athlete or has other previous experience from intensive training, it is very unlikely that he/she will have the courage to challenge dogma and to demand a training regime that focuses on cardiorespiratory conditioning and progressive resistance training, both of which are crucial in countering the deleterious effects of immobilization. Therapists and patients alike may rejoice in improved task performance, but many therapists know only too well that the correct performance of a task is short-lived to the point where the patient will revert to his/her compensatory strategy or inactivity as soon as the therapist's back is turned. Although this phenomenon is often referred to as lack of motivation or insight on the part of the patient, the truth of the matter may very well be that what the patient actually lacks is muscle strength and cardiovascular endurance to maintain 'correct' movement patterns for more than a brief period.

Tests and assessments

Apart from obvious research purposes, using relevant physical tests and assessments serves the dual purpose of motivating the patient to improve performance while at the same drawing the therapist's attention to resources and deficits in a quantifiable way.

Given the wide range of physical sequelae that can be observed in the wake of ABI, validated and reliable tests may not be available or applicable in all cases. Simple basic tests of fitness, endurance, strength, and walking speed that are easy to administer and reproduce offer patients and therapists a common ground for motivation, a good working alliance, and patient compliance. Without knowledge of the initial baseline levels of the above parameters, neither patient nor therapist will have any objective measure of functional gains, and consequently they will invariably resort to subjective and anecdotal interpretations of subtle improvements that may have qualitative relevance, but hardly ever reflect the concomitant quantitative improvements.

While relevant for research purposes and in the overall assessment of outcome, scales such as the Functional Independence Measure (FIM) (Keith et al. 1987), the Motor Assessment Scale (MAS) (Carr et al. 1985), the Fugl-Meyer Scale (Fugl-Meyer et al. 1975), the Berg Balance Scale (Berg et al. 1989), and the Action Research Arm Test (ARAT) (Lyle 1981), to name but a few, are all validated and reliable but are far too complex to be interpreted by patients and therefore are unsuitable for enhancing patient motivation. Testing and charting progress made in the number of times one can perform sit-to-stand, the time it takes to dress, the number of flights of stairs that can be climbed in, say, 5 minutes, or the maximum walking speed are far more likely to challenge the patient and to produce the incentive to put in an extra effort.

Relevant physiotherapeutic tests in brain injury rehabilitation

$VO_{2\,max}$ or cardiorespiratory endurance can be estimated in most neurological patients by using the submaximal 'Åstrand stationary bicycle test' (Åstrand and Rhyming 1986). Some patients may be so deconditioned that even the lowest workload allowed in this test (50 W) leads to exhaustion before reaching a steady state heart rate. Other patients cannot reach the required minimum steady state heart rate because of β-blockers. In both instances, the Borg Rating of Perceived Exertion (RPE) (Borg 1962) can offer valuable informa- tion with regard to the interpretation of the test result. A high correlation exists between a person's perceived exertion (range 6–20) multiplied by 10 and their steady-state heart rate during physical activity (Borg et al. 1987). If a person's maximum heart rate has been lowered by medication and therefore does not reflect the observable level of exertion (i.e. the person is panting and sweating whilst the heart rate remains low), the perceived exertion rating may provide a fairly good estimate of what the heart rate would have been during the same activity had it not been for the medication. For example, if a person's RPE is 15, then it may be assumed that the heart rate would have been approximately 150 beats/minute, although the heart rate monitor is showing 110 beats/minute.

Strength and endurance can be assessed by using a modified version of the Harvard Step Test where any change in the number of steps taken during 5 minutes as well as any drop in the total amount of heart beats counted after completion of the test will indicate improved strength and endurance. The official version of the Harvard Step Test can rarely be administered since it requires the subject to climb up and down a high step or box (usually 40 cm for women and 50 cm for men) 30 times per minute for 5 minutes, without any support. However, if a lower step height, fewer steps per minute, and support are allowed, almost anyone who can stand with support can perform the test.

Maximum walking speed can be measured with the 6-minute walk test (Guyatt et al. 1985) and compared with reference values for healthy subjects (Enright and Sherrill 1998), and with the 10-metre walk test (Wade 1992), which, although it overestimates walking speed (Dean et al. 2001), gives a very good impression of the fastest safe walking speed over short distances.

Grip strength can be evaluated with the Jamar dynamometer and compared with reference values for healthy subjects (Bohannon *et al.* 2006). Manual dexterity can be assessed with the Grooved Pegboard Test with reference values for healthy subjects (Ruff *et al.* 1993). With a little ingenuity, simple tests can be devised and charted for any physical impairment.

Brain injury rehabilitation at the CRBI

The Centre for Rehabilitation of Brain Injury (CRBI) at the University of Copenhagen was founded by Dr Anne-Lise Christensen in 1985. Since then, it has expanded considerably, but it still offers a neuropsychologically based holistic interdisciplinary 4-month outpatient rehabilitation programme for adults with ABI, followed by an 8-month follow-up period, the aim of which is return to education or gainful employment at some level. The day programme caters for people aged between 17 and 65 years. The programme is highly individualized, and can be extended from 4 to 6 or 8 months at a lower intensity if fatigue is an impediment to full-day attendance. As an integral part of the programme all patients (who are called students at the CRBI) are assigned to physiotherapy in accordance with their requirements. Prior to entering the programme, all students undergo a thorough neuropsychological investigation and a thorough examination by a special education teacher. Students with aphasic or dysarthric difficulties are also examined by a speech and language pathologist. All students are also required to undergo a 2-hour physiotherapeutic examination in which conventional tests play a negligible role since these tests are unable to provide new information, and because it is important from the very first meeting between student and therapist to stress the fact that the physiotherapeutic intervention at the CRBI emphasizes strenuous training rather than treatment. For the same reason, all sessions involving physical rehabilitation are called physical training, rather than physiotherapy or treatment.

Physiotherapy approaches at the CRBI: the initial examination

All rehabilitation must begin with thorough assessment. Conventional physiotherapeutic tests of abnormal tone and reflexes, reduced range of motion (ROM), compensatory movement patterns, adverse neural dynamics, etc. cannot supply any information pertaining to the present level of fitness and strength.

The physiotherapeutic examination at the CRBI always begins with an interview of 30–45 minutes, the purpose of which is to map self-perceived physical sequelae including pain, fatigue, etc., previous and present treatment, premorbid and present level of physical activity, and present wishes and goals. The next part of the physical examination (in order of administration) focuses on:

- resting blood pressure and heart rate
- enquiry into blood lipids
- prescription medication
- smoking and dietary habits
- grip strength
- dexterity
- dynamic balance
- body weight and calculation of BMI
- $VO_{2\,max}$ or cardiorespiratory endurance
- overall strength and endurance
- maximum walking or running speed.

All results of the examination are discussed with the student. Getting the student engaged in realistic goal-setting begins with conveying information and feedback at whatever level is permitted by his/her cognitive status. At the initial examination almost all students have poor endurance and strength, and suffer from fatigue and fatiguability as well as elevated blood pressure despite medication. Consequently, special attention is given to feedback regarding cardiorespiratory endurance and strength findings. These are presented candidly yet empathically with reference to official best-practice guidelines and outcome data from previous students at the CRBI. The physiotherapist describes the student's potential for improvement and the likely impact of such improvements on successful return to employment, independence in activities of daily living (ADL), and meaningful leisure-time activities including safe and independent ambulation. Most students are surprised at their low levels of endurance, which are already evident during the 6–9 minutes sub-maximal bicycle test and even more during the modified Harvard Step Test. Their spontaneous reaction is often that they have not been this much out of breath since their brain injury. Another common reaction is one of frustration at having been allowed to decline so dramatically during acute and post-acute rehabilitation. This mixture of surprise and frustration forms the ideal basis for setting goals and, if necessary for compliance, drawing up a contract with the student. Two to four days after the initial test, many students still experience delayed onset muscle soreness (DOMS) from the unaccustomed and strenuous activities and this serves as a lingering reminder of the goals set.

All initial tests are repeated at the end of the rehabilitation programme.

Two different physical interventions at the CRBI

People referred to the CRBI for rehabilitation fall into two categories:

- those referred for more specific purposes, e.g. speech and language, individual psychotherapy, or intensive gait training
- those referred for full participation in the interdisciplinary day programme.

The CRBI gait rehabilitation programme

People with significantly impaired gait or no independent ambulation can be offered an intensive 12 week gait rehabilitation programme either as a pre-programme or, if they do not meet the inclusion criteria for the full programme (e.g. because of age or substantial cognitive deficits), as a purely physiotherapeutic intervention. The 12-week gait programme consists of five weekly 90-minute sessions that take place in the CRBI gait lab. The structure and progression of this programme (Figure 10.2) has been developed in collaboration with researchers at the CMRC. Although drawing on inspiration from existing literature on body-weight-supported treadmill training (BWSTT), the CRBI model differs from other similar programmes not only in the duration of each session, but also in its highly structured use of high-intensity progressive resistance training (PRT) for the affected lower extremity. Every session begins with approximately 30 minutes of BWSTT at continuously increasing speed and incline gradient, with gradually deceasing harness support. On Mondays and Wednesdays the next hour is scheduled for high-intensity cardiorespiratory training in various machines, and on Tuesdays, Thursdays, and Fridays PRT is on the schedule. The PRT machines are equipped with visual feedback with regard to range of motion, movement speed, immediate watt-output for each repetition and average watt-output for each set. All training results are saved on individual USB memory keys which, after transfer of training results to the computer, are re-programmed for the following day. In this way, all machines are re-programmed for new adjustments and challenges. To ensure optimum engagement, the students undergo various gait tests every Monday, and they are given printouts which graphically illustrate their progress as well as relevant training results. Since many of those participating in this intervention are more cognitively impaired and have more executive disorders than students in the full CRBI day programme, a very rigid structure is essential to ensure motivation and compliance. Several students in this group have been wheelchair-bound for up to 2 years, and if the goal is to regain the ability to transfer and walk independently and safely, albeit usually with a cane or walker and wearing an ankle–foot orthosis, there is

The CRBI G.A.I.T. Program – 1½ hours per day for 60 days				
Cardiorespiratory and functional training Tests	BWSTT + progressive resistance training 3 × 12 reps	Cardiorespiratory and functional training	BWSTT + progressive resistance training 3 × 12 reps	BWSTT + progressive resistance training 3 × 12 reps
Week 2				
Cardiorespiratory and functional training Tests	BWSTT + Progressive resistance training 3 × 10 reps	Cardiorespiratory and functional training	BWSTT + Progressive resistance training 3 × 10 reps	BWSTT + Progressive resistance training 3 × 10 reps
Compliance rating	**Week 3**			
Cardiorespiratory and functional training Tests	BWSTT + progressive resistance training 4 × 8 reps	Cardiorespiratory and functional training	BWSTT + progressive resistance training 4 × 8 reps	BWSTT + Progressive resistance training 4 × 8 reps
Week 4 - Theme week				
BWSTT + stair climbing Tests	BWSTT + gait training	BWSTT + stair climbing	BWSTT + gait training	BWSTT + Walkathon (as far as possible in 30 mins)
Week 5				
Cardiorespiratory and functional training Tests	BWSTT + Progressive resistance training 4 × 8 reps	Cardiorespiratory and functional training	BWSTT + Progressive resistance training 4 × 8 reps	BWSTT + Progressive resistance training 4 × 8 reps
Week 6				
Cardiorespiratory and functional training Tests	BWSTT + Progressive resistance training 4 × 8 reps	Cardiorespiratory and functional training	BWSTT + progressive resistance training 4 × 8 reps	BWSTT + progressive resistance training 4 × 8 reps
Week 7				
Cardiorespiratory and functional training	BWSTT + progressive resistance training 12,10,10,8 reps	Cardiorespiratory and functional training	BWSTT + progressive resistance training 12,10,10,8 reps	BWSTT + progressive resistance training 12,10,10,8 reps
Week 8				
Cardiorespiratory and functional training Tests	BWSTT + progressive resistance training 10,8,8,8,6 reps	Cardiorespiratory and functional training	BWSTT + progressive resistance training 10,8,8,8,6 reps	BWSTT + progressive resistance training 10,8,8,8,6 reps
Week 9				
Cardiorespiratory and functional training Tests	BWSTT + progressive resistance training 8,6,6,6,4 reps	Cardiorespiratory and functional training	BWSTT + progressive resistance training 8,6,6,6,4 reps	BWSTT + progressive resistance training 8,6,6,6,4 reps
Week 10 - Theme week				
BWSTT Tests	BBWSTT + gait training	BWSTT + progressive resistance training 8,6,6,6,4 reps	BWSTT + gait training	BWSTT + Walkathon
Compliance rating	**Week 11**			
Cardiorespiratory and functional training Tests	BWSTT + progressive resistance training 10,8,8,6 reps	Cardiorespiratory and functional training	BWSTT + progressive resistance training 10,8,8,6 reps	BWSTT + progressive resistance training 10,8,8,6 reps
Week 12				
Cardiorespiratory and functional training Tests	BWSTT + progressive resistance training 8,6,6,4 reps	Cardiorespiratory and functional training	BWSTT + progressive resistance training 8,6,6,4 reps	BWSTT + progressive resistance training 8,6,6,4 reps
Week 13				
Final tests at the CRBI, EMG, KinCom and biopsies				

Fig. 10.2 The highly structured schedule of the 12-week CRBI Gait Rehabilitation Programme comprising high-speed body weight support treadmill training (BWSTT) and high-intensity cardiorespiratory training with heavy progressive resistance training for the more affected lower extremity.

no time for discussing intensity, duration, or choice of equipment. To ensure generalization, two theme weeks are interspersed in the 12-week programme in which students practise stair climbing, outdoor walking, riding a tricycle, and various leisure-time activities at the CRBI as well as in their home environment.

Physical training as part of the interdisciplinary day programme

The conclusions from the initial physiotherapeutic examination as well as all test results and ensuing recommendations and goals are written into a report that is shared with the other members of the rehabilitation staff at the weekly staff meeting, where a highly individualized rehabilitation schedule is pieced together and revised whenever necessary.

In the day programme, the bulk of physical training takes place in a well-equipped public fitness centre located at a nearby four-star hotel. Apart from the obvious advantage of gaining access to state-of-the-art equipment, this location also offers the students the possibility of leaving the patient role. Training in a non-clinical setting after a prolonged period of hospitalization greatly boosts students' self-efficacy, once they have overcome their initial reservations with regard to displaying their physical impairments in public. The greatest advantage of using cardiorespiratory and strengthening equipment lies in the possibilities of challenging the students physically to a far greater extent than would be possible without such equipment. Ordinary stair climbing, for example, would never be able to challenge a hemiplegic person as much as training on a Stair Master. The slowness and awkwardness of movement, the tendency to shift function to the less affected side, and the insecure balance of many hemiplegic persons slow down all movement patterns to a degree where neither heart rate nor muscle strength are challenged effectively.

According to the severity of their physical and cognitive difficulties, students are assigned to one to three weekly training sessions at the fitness centre. Each session lasts for 2 hours including the walk to and from the gym and time for changing clothes and showering, leaving the average student an effective training time of 1½ hours. Students train in groups of two to six and are always accompanied by one or two physiotherapists.

Charting training results to ensure continuous progress

The greater the executive disorder the more important it is to organize, time, and chart the routines before and after the actual training, since time spent in the locker room, for example, can seriously encroaches on effective training time. Students are encouraged to time themselves, and examples of distractibility in dressing, for example, can be used in other domains to exemplify latency in reaction to cognitive tasks (e.g. in the cognitive group at the CRBI or during work trials). Once dressed, the students are required to find their personal folder in the ring binder, take out previous training charts, secure them on a clip board, and add a new training chart (Figure 10.3) on which they write their name and the date. After having copied their weight from the previous training session into the appointed space, they weigh themselves and write their current weight in the space below. By consulting last session's chart, they can fill in the spaces for kilos lifted last time and their highest calorie expenditure ever. Since every training session presupposes an improvement in intensity and output, high, but realistic, goals should be formulated for expected weight lifted and calorie expenditure in the current session, taking into account remaining training time and any comments in the previous session's remarks and plans for the next training session. It goes without saying that almost all students require assistance with the preliminary work with the chart, but entering and comparing data and setting goals are essential to many persons with executive disorders and impaired memory, not only in their rehabilitation process, but also in most other aspects of their lives.

The individual training protocols of the students focus on impacting on whatever elements of strengthening and conditioning are deemed most relevant for optimum restoration of function. By comparing previous training results, such as effort level, lifted weight, and number of repetitions, with the present output, it is the student's responsibility to improve all output within the same 1½-hour time frame. At the end of each training session, all lifted weight in kilos and all expended calories are summed and entered in the spaces below the goals set for the session. With the assistance of a physiotherapist or another student, the students are required to fill in the spaces entitled 'Comments and remarks with regard to today's training session' and 'Plans for next training session'. These two spaces require meta-cognitive processes since reasons for non-fulfilment are usually cognitive rather than physical.

To encourage competition not only with oneself but also with one's peers, high-score charts and graphs of calorie expenditure are drawn up by a physiotherapist or by one of the students at regular intervals.

The charts used for the physical training sessions can be used as templates for any physical rehabilitation session at any level, either acute or post-acute. It is merely necessary to substitute activities and output measures. As mentioned earlier, measures of physical progress and outcome that can be charted include anything measurable from, at the lowest level, the time it takes to walk from bed to bathroom or the number of times sit-to-stand can be performed safely in 1 minute, to, at the highest level, the time it takes to run a certain distance or the number of flights of stairs that can be climbed.

Progressive resistance training - Arms

Machine no./name	Side	Kilos	Reps	Total kilos
Pulley high pos *Pull in/down*	Right			
	Left			
Pulley high pos *Pull out/down*	Right			
	Left			
Pulley low pos. *Pull in/up*	Right			
	Left			
Pulley low pos. *Pull out/up*	Right			
	Left			
7 Chest Press	Both			
	Right			
	Left			
Seat:				
38 Low Row	Both			
Seat:	Right			
Chest:	Left			
18 Lat. Mach.	Both			
	Right			
3 Shoulder Press	Both			
	Right			
Seat:	Left			

Progressive resistance training - Legs

Machine no./name	Side	Kilos	Reps	Total kilos
8 Leg Press	Both			
Seat:	Right			
	Left			
9 Leg Extension	Both			
Seat:	Right			
Roller:	Left			
10 Leg Curl	Both			
Seat:	Right			
Roller:	Left			
Grand total kilos				

Name		Body weight last time	
Date		Body weight today	
Lifted kilos last time		Highest cal. expenditure ever	
Goal for lifted weight		Goal for calorie expenditure	
Lifted weight today		Calorie expenditure today	

Comments and remarks with regard to today's training session

Plans for next training session

Cardiorespiratory training

	Programme	Distance	HR	Level	Time	Calories
Bicycle *Seat:*	Programme	Distance	HR	Level	Time	Calories
Stair Master	Programme	Distance	HR	Level	Time	Calories
Tread-mill	Programme	Distance	HR	% Kph	Time	Calories
Skiing machine	Programme	Distance	HR	Level	Time	Calories
Arm cycle *Bilateral Uni-lat. Seat:*	Programme	Distance	Arm length	Level	Time	Calories
Rowing machine	Programme	Distance	Watts	Level	Time	Calories
Grand total calories						

Fig. 10.3 Excerpt from full training chart.

Goal attainment scaling

In more severe executive disorders, training charts may not ensure the desired progress. In such cases, awareness and motivation can be enhanced by supplementing charts and graphs by goal attainment scaling (GAS). This is a process in which important outcomes are selected in collaboration with individual subjects, and the changes in those outcomes are measured over time. The usual approach for GAS is to use a standard question format for each item and allow the individual to select a preset number of areas of importance (usually three or more). Generally, a list of choices is provided, and the number to be selected is fixed to maintain standardized answers without being too restrictive. To measure the outcomes for each area, a grade scale is used with a minimum of five choices. The units used for the scale may vary depending on the use, but some common examples are from 'much less than expected' (value −2) to 'much more than expected' (value +2), from 'strongly disagree' to 'strongly agree', and from 'very much worse' to 'very much better'.

Summary

Lack of sufficient physical activity has become a universal health threat. Together with the unprecedented availability of food accessible to an ever-increasing number of sedentary people, this inactivity has led to the pandemic of 'diabesity' and other inactivity-related diseases. Insufficient physical activity poses a double threat to people with ABI and/or executive disorders. Not only will a sedentary lifestyle, due to motor sequelae as well as impaired initiative and planning, tend to worsen the physical consequences of the brain injury and thus further reduce mobility and health, but it will also tend to exacerbate the tendency to become increasingly socially isolated. To counter this vicious circle, physiotherapists, and indeed all professionals engaged in rehabilitation and support of brain-injured individuals, should incorporate physical activity into every rehabilitation curriculum or programme. To ensure compliance and carry-over, the activities chosen must be meaningful and accord with the brain-injured person's goals.

Conclusions

Physiotherapists and other groups of professionals dealing with brain-injured individuals may have been motivated to choose their profession by a wish to 'do good', to care for human beings who suffer, in short to put their empathic side to use. Although patients thrive on empathy, therapists should bear in mind that persons with executive disorders are impaired in precisely those domains that are so crucial for initiating and maintaining a regular level of physical activity. Therapeutic empathy does not preclude a high intensity of physical training. At all times, the therapist should remember that he/she possesses the executive faculties that are impaired in the patient and should provide whatever drive, incentive, and structure the patient lacks. Physical exertion and challenge, combined with scrupulous charting of results, continuous progression, and competition with oneself or peers, will often be seen by the patient as more meaningful, rewarding, and fun than submaximal physical activities which, in the short run, only lead to non-discernible improvements but not to fatigue, victory, or improved mood.

References

Åstrand, P.O. and Rhyming, I. (1954). A nomogram for calculation of aerobic capacity (physical fitness) from pulse rate during submaximal work. *Journal of Applied Physiology*, **7**, 218–21.

Berg, K., Wood-Dauphinée, S., Williams, J.I., Gayton, D. (1989). Measuring balance in the elderly: preliminary development of an instrument. *Physiotherapy Canada*, **41**, 304–11.

Blomstrand, E., Perrett, D., Parrybillings, M., and Newsholme, E.A. (1989). Effect of sustained exercise on plasma amino-acid concentrations and on 5-hydroxytryptamine metabolism in 6 different brain-regions in the rat. *Acta Physiologica Scandinavica*, **136**, 473–81.

Bohannon, R., Andrews, A.W., and Smith, M.B. (1988). Rehabilitation goals of patients with hemiplegia. *International Journal of Rehabilitation Research*, **11**, 181–3.

Bohannon, R.W., Peolsson. A., Massy-Westropp, N., Desrosiers, J., Bear-Lehman, J. (2006). Reference values for adult grip strength measured with a Jamar dynamometer: a descriptive meta-analysis. *Physiotherapy*, **92**, 11–15.

Borg, G. (1962). Physical performance and perceived exertion. *Studia Psychologica et Paedagogica*, **2**(11).

Borg, G., Hassmén, P., and Lagerström, M. (1987). Perceived exertion related to heart rate and blood lactate during arm and leg exercise. *European Journal of Applied Physiology*, **56**, 679–85.

Carr, J.H., Shepherd, R.B., Nordholm, L., and Lynne, D. (1985). Investigation of a new motor assessment scale for stroke patients. *Physical Therapy*, **65**, 175–80.

Colcombe, S. and Kramer, A.F. (2003). Fitness effects on the cognitive function of older adults: a meta-analytic study. *Psychological Science*, **14**, 125–30.

Cotman, C.W. and Berchtold, N.C. (2002). Exercise: a behavioral intervention to enhance brain health and plasticity. *Trends in Neurosciences*, **25**, 295–301.

Dean, C.M., Richards, C.L., and Malouin, F. (2001). Walking speed over 10 metres overestimates locomotor capacity after stroke. *Clinical Rehabilitation*, **15**, 415–21.

Engberg, A.W. and Teasdale, T.W. (2004). Psychosocial outcome following traumatic brain injury in adults: a long-term population-based follow-up. *Brain Injury*, **18**, 533–45.

Enright, P.L. and Sherrill, D.L. (1998). Reference equations for the six-minute walk in healthy adults. *American Journal of Respiratory and Critical Care Medicine*, **158**, 1384–7.

Fugl-Meyer, A.R., Jääskö, L., Leyman, I., Olsson, S., and Steglind, S. (1975). The post-stroke hemiplegic patient: a method for evaluation of physical performance. *Scandinavian Journal of Rehabilitation Medicine*, 7, 13–31.

Gordon, W.A., Sliwinski, M., Echo, J., McLoughlin, M., Sheerer, M., and Meili, T.E. (1998). The benefits of exercise in individuals with traumatic brain injury: a retrospective study. *Journal of Head Trauma Rehabilitation*, 13, 58–67.

Guyatt, G.H., Sullivan, P.J., Thompson, P.J., *et al.* (1985). The six-minute walk: a new measure of exercise capacity in patients with chronic heart failure. *Canadian Medical Association Journal*, 132, 919–23.

Hesse, S., Werner, C., Paul, T., Bardeleben, A., and Chaler, J. (2001). Influence of walking speed on lower limb muscle activity and energy consumption during treadmill walking of hemiparetic patients. *Archives of Physical Medicine and Rehabilitation*, 82, 1547–50.

Keith, R.A., Granger, C.V., Hamilton, B.B., and Sherwin, F.S. (1987). The Functional Independence Measure: a new tool for rehabilitation. *Advances in Clinical Rehabilitation*, 1, 6–18.

Kleim, J.A., Jones, T.A., and Schallert, T. (2003). Motor enrichment and the induction of plasticity before or after brain injury. *Neurochemical Research*, 28, 1757–69.

Knapp, H.D., Taub, E., and Berman, A.J. (1958). Effect of deafferentation on a conditioned avoidance response. *Science*, 128, 842–3.

Lyle, R.C. (1981). A performance test for assessment of upper limb function in physical rehabilitation treatment and research. *International Journal of Rehabilitation Research*, 4, 483–92

Neel, J. (1962). Diabetes mellitus: a 'thrifty' genotype rendered detrimental by 'progress'? *American Journal of Human Genetics*, 14, 352–3.

Olver, J.H., Ponsford, J.L., and Curran, C.A. (1996). Outcome following traumatic brain injury: a comparison between 2 and 5 years after injury. *Brain Injury*, 10, 841–8.

Patten, C., Lexell, J., and Brown, H.E. (2004). Weakness and strength training in persons with poststroke hemiplegia: rationale, method, and efficacy. *Journal of Rehabilitation Research and Development*, 41, 293–312.

Pohl, M., Mehrholz, J., Ritschel, C., and Rückriem, S. (2002). Speed-dependent treadmill training in ambulatory hemiparetic stroke patients. *Stroke*, 553–8.

Ruff, R.M. and Parker, S.B. (1993). Gender- and age-specific changes in motor speed and eye–hand coordination in adults: normative values for the Finger Tapping and Grooved Pegboard Tests. *Perceptual and Motor Skills*, 76, 1219–30.

Teixeira-Salmela, L.F., Nadeau, S., McBride, I., and Olney, S.J. (2001). Effects of muscle strengthening and physical conditioning training on temporal, kinematic and kinetic variables during gait in chronic stroke survivors. *Journal of Rehabilitation Medicine*, 33, 53–60.

Wade, D.T. (1992). *Measurement in neurological rehabilitation*. Oxford University Press, New York.

Weiss, A., Suzuki, T., Bean, J., and Fielding, R.A. (2000). High intensity strength training improves strength and functional performance after stroke. *American Journal of Physical Medicine and Rehabilitation*, 79, 369–76.

Worthington, A., Williams, C., Young, K., and Pownall, J. (1997) Re-training gait components for walking in the context of abulia. *Physiotherapy Theory and Practice*, 13, 247–56.

11

Rehabilitation of everyday living skills in the context of executive disorders

Andrew Worthington and Jackie Waller

Introduction

It says much about the complexity of executive functions that scientists and clinicians can agree on their importance for daily living without being able to reach a consensus on what the term means. In daily life we take for granted executive skills that allow us to initiate an activity, stop, consider the impact on others, think again, try something a different way, switch priorities, or retrace our steps to see where we went wrong, making a mental note for future reference. We recognize that executive functions are related to intelligence, and yet intelligence is little comfort when faced with a loss of executive control over behaviour. Indeed, for many years the absence of apparent intellectual deficits associated with disease or injury to the prefrontal region contributed to its relative neglect by investigators (Benton 1991).

Executive functions evolved to help us adapt to a complex social world, and some scientists believe that the relatively recent emergence of the prefrontal region, with all its elaborate complexity and mystique, renders it particularly vulnerable to disruption. It has been described as having a low functional breakdown threshold (Goldberg 2001) and executive disorder is a fairly common, if non-specific, sign of cerebral dysfunction. Yet the impact of executive disorder can be debilitating, an effect that cannot be encapsulated wholly by a profile of test scores or behavioural changes. Executive dysfunction undermines capacity for independent living like no other form of cognitive disorder, striking at the heart of personal autonomy. Both professionals and families bear daily witness to the devastating impact that such disorders can have on everyday living.

This chapter is concerned with the importance of executive functions for independence and well-being, and to that end it is concerned with functional outcomes, i.e. the extent to which intervention improves a person's functioning in the real world. Worthington (2005) argued that interventions for disorders of executive functioning should be socially as opposed to statistically significant and should have personal relevance for the individual (rather than the therapist). We believe that interventions targeted at everyday activities can simultaneously be theoretically informed, practical, and meaningful. With this aim in mind this chapter is written for all practitioners concerned with improving the quality of life for their clients by promoting greater independence in daily activities.

Executive function and daily activities

Rehabilitation outcomes are generally less favourable in the context of persistent executive deficits, whether measured on cognitive tests (Hanks *et al.* 1999) or indicated by behaviour (Cope *et al.* 1991). Frequently a person has difficulty in resuming their former lifestyle because of problems in carrying out ordinary activities of daily life. However, it is important to be clear about what we mean by such activities because terminology is used inconsistently. When psychologists talk about behaviour a distinction needs to be made between largely instinctive or reflex acts (which do not concern us here), very familiar or routine activities (sometimes referred to as over-learned), and new or unfamiliar tasks. The crucial difference is between routine tasks and so-called non-routine tasks, because executive skills are not generally utilized in the performance of routine actions. Most actions become routine with practice as the need for monitoring and reflection reduces and a skill is acquired. Hence the experienced car driver differs from the novice in being able to hold a conversation while driving in busy traffic. This is because routine tasks require less effort, or processing resources, than new or more difficult tasks, thereby freeing attention and other resources for a secondary task. Amongst the characteristics of skilled performance in rehabilitation described by Wood and Worthington (2001), the means of learning through experience is the most important. This is the basis by which many tasks become routine, even complex behavioural sequences such as preparing a meal for a dinner party. However, such tasks initially require considerable planning and monitoring during their execution. As novelty and difficulty are the basis for the recruitment of executive skills, it follows that the first casualty of an executive disorder will be tasks thus characterized rather than the more familiar activities of daily life. Hence when conducting assessments clinicians need to consider carefully whether the functional context is appropriate for the kind of investigation being undertaken. Failure to appreciate this distinction can result in insensitive evaluations and false-negative diagnostic errors.

For example, routine activities do not generally require planning, and therefore an impairment in the formation of plans may well not manifest when observing a person making coffee in the manner that they have done for many years.

Of course daily life does not consist of single tasks that are either entirely routine or novel, as we are often faced with multiple demands for attention. As demand for greater 'attentional effort' increases, performance should change in response, a mechanism mediated by increased prefrontal cholinergic activity (Sarter et al. 2006). However this process has its limits. When more than one task requires effort, we face competition for attentional resources and, inevitably, something has to give as we cannot perform two effortful activities simultaneously as well as we could do either in isolation (Norman and Bobrow 1976). Multi-tasking recruits many specialized regions within the frontal lobes and neighbouring areas that are involved in forming intentions, planning, monitoring, and memory retrieval (Burgess 2000; Burgess et al. 2000). Executive dysfunction can disrupt this process at several levels, and a skilled therapist needs to disentangle the many potential reasons why a person who can carry out single tasks might struggle when required to multi-task.

The ability to multi-task gets easier as we become used to it because, as activities become routine, we develop motor programs for skilled performance which can be allowed to run more or less unsupervised. This involves posterior as well as frontal brain regions, including the parietal lobe (Castiello et al. 1999) and cerebellum (Imamizu et al. 2000). However, although we can carry out familiar tasks without the need for constant self-monitoring, we rely on executive processes to maintain control over our actions, a mechanism described by Scheibel et al. (2007, p. 36) as the 'active maintenance of patterns of neural activity associated with internal representation of goals and the means to achieve them'. This requires the facility to inhibit responses to irrelevant stimuli, a process which often happens automatically until affected by frontal lobe damage (Sumner et al. 2007). Subsequently some patients become aware of the inappropriateness of their actions but report being powerless to stop the behaviour. Conversely, the problem may be less to do with response suppression than an inability to initiate appropriate activity. Pachalska et al. (2002) referred to these different behavioural manifestations of executive disorder as acting without thinking and thinking without acting.

Rehabilitation of executive function in daily tasks

There is now good evidence that rehabilitation programmes that specifically target social and functional skills can provide significant gains in terms of discharge placement (Eames *et al.* 1995; Wood and Worthington 1999), levels of supervision, and productive occupation (Seale *et al.* 2002; Worthington *et al.* 2006). These programmes create a behavioural mileu in which the environment temporarily substitutes for internal executive control mechanisms. Effective management of executive dysfunction in a functional context requires a sensitive method of assessment and careful consideration of the appropriate intervention in order to address specific executive disorders.

Assessment methods

Increasingly it is argued that, more than any other domain of cognition, executive skills demand a functional approach to assessment, with tools specifically designed to reflect situations encountered in daily life, from multi-tasking to social interaction (Manchester *et al.* 2004; Burgess *et al.* 2006). This is not necessarily true (Stuss 2007) but it is frequently a useful means of examining how executive deficits may present in the real world. Structured neuropsychological tests have their place in rehabilitation planning (Bennett 2001), but they are often insensitive or have limited predictive validity (Chaytor and Schmitter-Edgcombe 2003; Odhuba 2005). Retesting is a particular concern when evaluating executive functions as it becomes difficult if not impossible to test the ability to respond to novelty. This problem is shared by the so-called ecologically valid tests such as the Behavioural Assessment of Dysexecutive Syndrome (BADS) battery (Norris and Tate 2000). A more promising approach is the development of loosely structured real-world tasks that incorporate aspects of multi-tasking such as the development of the Multiple Errands task (Shallice and Burgess1991; see also Knight *et al.* 2002 and Chapter 6, this volume). Questionnaires or rating scales such as the DEX (from the BADS battery) or the Behaviour Rating Inventory of Executive Function (Gioia *et al.* 1996) can be used and may highlight discrepancies between self-appraisal and evaluation by others, but it should be remembered that they are all subjective measures and vulnerable to bias.

Another method of evaluation is to ask people to describe how they would carry out an activity. This assesses whether people retain the conceptual ability to formulate a goal and plan of action. Damage to prefrontal regions disrupts this ability and often steps are recalled out of sequence or missed out altogether (Sirigu *et al.* 1995). However, this may not reflect how a task would actually be performed, as the presence of real objects may serve as cues to action (Zalla *et al.* 2001). Although very familiar acts, such as making a cup of tea, may be thought to have little executive loading, performance may be compromised by executive deficiencies (e.g. the distracting presence of irrelevant objects). Moreover, Schwartz and others (Schwartz and Buxbaum 1997;

Schwartz 2006; Humphreys *et al.* 2001) have proposed that executive dysfunction can undermine even fairly routine activities if the underlying knowledge base for such activities is also compromised, rendering the task more reliant on executive control. Finally, there is a wide range of techniques for observing behaviour in real time which can be adapted for specific tasks and objectives. Space precludes further discussion here, but these methods have been reviewed as measures of process (Wood and Worthington 2001) and outcome (Wood and Worthington 1999).

Rehabilitation methods

Different notions of executive function may suggest different kinds of intervention (Burgess and Robertson 2002), but few of these have been put to the test. Worthington (2003) proposed a pragmatic three-stage framework within which diverse behavioural and cognitive disorders could be encompassed, reflecting a breakdown at one of the three core stages of action planning, initiation, and regulation. Most techniques used to promote the execution of daily activities involve either intensive training (practice) on specific tasks or the adoption of compensatory strategies, especially external aids, although some so-called meta-cognitive techniques are promising (reviewed by Alderman and Burgess 2003; Evans 2003). However, these terms for different interventions are not mutually exclusive, and do not necessarily relate to proven mechanisms of action (Worthington 2005).

Certain cognitive rehabilitation methods target underlying cognitive impairments in anticipation of producing transferable gains in real-world skills. However, this is difficult to achieve with the heterogeneity of executive functions. For example, many attempts to train attention such as Attention Process Training (Park *et al.* 1999) or Attention Control Training (McMillan *et al.* 2002) result in practice effects on training tasks but no generalizable outcomes. However, practice effects can be exploited at a functional level. Training people to carry out specific activities through graded repetitive practice (sometimes known as functional skills training) is widely used in rehabilitation and is particularly effective for individuals with severe executive disorder. The addition of self-prompting or verbal commentary to a task both provides a focus of attention and reinforces the role of language in promoting self-regulation of behaviour (Wood and Worthington 2001; Worthington and Wood, 2008).

External aids have also been widely used in functional contexts because of their versatility. For example, prompting checklists can be tailored to suit specific tasks and particular deficits (Burke *et al.* 1991). Levine *et al.* (2000) demonstrated beneficial use of a goal-oriented checklist for meal preparation in a woman with executive problems following encephalitis. Six months after training she was largely self-prompting, suggesting that she had internalized many of the cues in the checklist. Additionally, external aids such as an electronic pager (Evans *et al.*1998; Emslie *et al.* 2007) or SMS text message (Pijnenborg *et al.* 2007) have proved effective in prospective memory tasks, where people have to remember to do something at a particular time. \

Cueing has also been used to good effect in facilitating meta-cognitive skills. Meta-cognition (knowledge about knowledge) is the ability to know something about our abilities and limitations and is involved in the learning and execution of skilled performance. These include the important executive abilities of abstraction, planning, and self-monitoring. Once a skill has been acquired, meta-cognitive processes determine when and how it will be employed (see Figure 11.1 for an illustrative therapy training model).

While it is obviously important to carry out a sensitive assessment to try to identify why a person is having difficulty with a task, one cannot simply go on investigating and not try to intervene. A properly conceived and evaluated intervention can sometimes illuminate the nature of a difficulty as much as any assessment tool. For instance, apparent deficiency in a complex activity may simply reflect absorption in one component of the task, in which case introducing task interruptions can itself be helpful. It is not necessary for such interruptions to provide an explicit cue for action. For example a prospective memory task—remembering to carry out an activity—can be facilitated by a text message simply stating 'Stop' (Fish *et al.* 2007; see also Chapter 5,

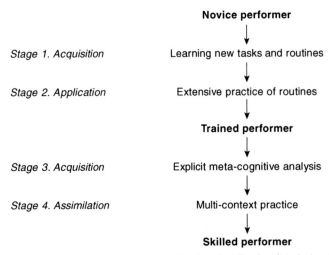

Fig. 11.1 A meta-cognitive approach to learning in rehabilitation (Birnboim 1995).

this volume). This has implications for multi-tasking where external prompts offer the best means to date of helping people to manage two or more tasks. The problem is that, although it is possible experimentally to train brain-injured people to predict when a change between two different tasks is impending (endogenous task shifts), so that they are better able to switch between the two (Stablum *et al.* 2007), this does not help people who have to decide for themselves when to switch between tasks (exogenous task shifts). However, external prompting may also help here. Manly *et al.* (2002) demonstrated that an intermittent auditory stimulus was associated with improved performance on a multi-tasking exercise. The authors speculated that this was because the sound drew attention away from the current task, thereby providing 'a window in which evaluation of actions against the goal is more likely to occur…' (Manly *et al.* 2002, p. 280).

Meta-cognitive interventions are potentially the most beneficial in the rehabilitation of everyday living skills because, when successful, they remove the need to train people on individual tasks. Skills should generalize to new activities which share common features. Therefore much effort is expended in trying to teach people with executive disorders key strategic skills, such as problem-solving, with varying degrees of success (e.g. Fox *et al.* 1989; von Cramon *et al.* 1991; Rath *et al.* 2003; Marshall *et al.* 2004). The difficulty is that executive disorders often preclude strategies learned in one (usually clinical) setting being spontaneously transferred to everyday life. This highlights a potential circularity in this approach, as therapists often use methods which require meta-cognitive skills (e.g. the ability to generalize problem-solving principles) in order to train such skills. Attempts have been made to train attentional control, for instance using dual-task exercises (Stablum *et al.* 2000) or targeting working memory (Sammer *et al.* 2006) or a putative central executive (Serino 2006), without producing any reliable functional benefits. There is currently much debate about the extent to which cognitive rehabilitation should be undertaken in context as opposed to in a classroom or on training tasks (see discussion in Schutz and Trainor (2007)). With executive disorders, specific training in generalization is probably the key to successful transfer of skills, as demonstrated by Cicerone and Wood (1987) in their therapy for planning deficits. More recent evidence suggests that asking people to recall similar activities that they have previously undertaken may improve the planning of new tasks, possibly by facilitating access to autobiographical cues (Hewitt *et al.* 2006).

The social aspect of executive function is often neglected in interventions which target specific tasks. Yet most forms of everyday problem-solving occur in a social context, and evidence suggests that social and psychological factors may underlie some aspects of poor problem-solving and self-regulation (Rath *et al.* 2004). In their own rehabilitation unit, the present authors have run a very successful leisure group with severely brain-injured adults for a number of years, utilizing a problem-solving framework. Constructive use of time is a significant problem for many people with executive disorders. The aim of our group programme is to develop skills in time management, planning, and problem-solving in real time by focusing on participation in productive activity between and after therapy sessions. The key is to avoid paper exercises, except perhaps at the outset in order to introduce basic principles, and to focus on application of the principles in practice—learning by doing rather than declarative learning. A core component of our problem-solving group is the social element which provides realism and peer support, thereby helping to address a multitude of factors contributing to poor problem-solving in daily life.

In the next section we describe an example of an individualized rehabilitation intervention focusing on amelioration of disability associated with executive dysfunction.

Case A: morning routine programme

Background

A is a 24 year old woman who was diagnosed with tuberculous meningitis in December 2000; in 2001 she was fitted with a ventricular shunt following secondary hydrocephalus. She was left with significant cognitive and behavioural disorder. She was also was clinically obese and had low stamina for physical activity. A lived with her parents and sister, but relations were strained, with A reporting feeling frustrated and 'caged in' owing to long periods of time in the house. A's behaviour at home was disinhibited, impulsive, and both verbally and physically aggressive. In April 2005, as family breakdown became imminent, she was admitted for residential rehabilitation.

Assessment

Neuropsychological testing revealed impairments consistent with a dysexecutive profile of neurobehavioural disability. She was impulsive during testing and had difficulty self-monitoring on the more complex tasks. Her verbal and performance measures on the Wechsler Adult Intelligence Scale III (WAIS-III) were extremely low. She had particular difficulties on tasks sensitive to processing speed, seemingly unable to comprehend and recall relevant information about a task. Short-term memory (digit span and spatial span) was impaired, as was narrative recall, primarily because of poor attention to detail and impaired sustained attention. She scored poorly on tasks sensitive to cognitive flexibility and abstract reasoning. Discourse rating using the Measure of Cognitive–Linguistic Abilities scale (MCLA) was also poor, with the main difficulties being in the organization and fluent delivery of conversation.

In a functional context A's key behaviours were non-compliance (68 per cent of all challenging behaviours) and verbal aggression (13 per cent), much of which was associated with an unwillingness to get up, wash, and dress in the morning. A took 2½ to 3 hours to complete her morning routine. She was easily distracted, lost track of the overall task, and had a tendency to perseverate. She was also unaware of how such a long routine limited her participation in other activities. Typically, although A could recognize inappropriate conduct after the event, she was unable to regulate her emotions when the incident was occurring.

Theoretical formulation

A's behaviour could be conceptualized in different ways using theories which emphasize different aspects of the executive system. Thus working memory models of executive function (e.g. Petrides 1994) would attribute A's problems to a deficit in retaining information in her memory long enough to guide behaviour. However, A was able to recount the instructions she had been given, and therefore this unitary account seems inadequate. According to Duncan's goal-neglect theory of frontal lobe function, many patients fail in tasks because they lose track of their intended objective (Duncan *et al.* 1996). Certainly there were times when A appeared to have forgotten what she was supposed to be doing despite environmental cues, which suggests that she may either have lost sight of her internalized goal or lost the ability to evaluate her actions in terms of whether they were achieving her objective. Of course, the key phrase here is 'her objective' because a task objective is not the same as a personal objective (although these are often assumed to be theoretically equivalent). In other words, a therapist may be trying to encourage someone to shower (a task objective) which directly conflicts with their client's reluctance to get out of bed (their personal goal). In A's case it would be naive to presume that she was suffering from 'goal neglect' unless she expressed high levels of motivation for getting washed and dressed and distress when she failed to do so (which she emphatically did not).

In fact, goal conflict would be a more accurate term to characterize her behaviour, and one model in particular, the Supervisory Attentional System (Shallice and Burgess 1991), has proved useful in suggesting what may occur when goals are mutually incompatible. One way of conceptualizing A's distractibility and perseveration is that they are signs of poor inhibitory control over actions (behavioural schemas) triggered by the environment. Hence objects in the environment stimulate particular responses, which she is unable to prevent and, moreover, has difficulty inhibiting once triggered. In addition, A's own reluctance to engage in the task from the outset also has to be considered. It was hypothesized that she had developed alternative action schemas consistent with a more immediate goal (that of staying in bed) and that, even when out of bed, these behaviours competed with the actions being encouraged by the therapist. Some of these counter-productive schemas were situation specific (such as turning off the shower), but others, like her propensity for aggression, were less context bound. Therefore a successful intervention would need to substitute more appropriate goal-oriented actions for her current behavioural repertoire. However, it proved difficult to manager her aggression in this specific context, the explanation being that this behaviour occurred in multiple situations and was frequently being 'rehearsed.' It was considered that her aggression needed additional intervention using a competency-based problem-solving approach to replace this readily activated schema with an alternative schema based on coping skills.

Rehabilitation goals

In terms of her morning routine the objectives for her first 3 months were:

- completion within 75 minutes
- a 25 per cent reduction in non-compliance and aggression over the 3-month period (knowing that any new intervention would probably provoke more challenging behaviour initially).

Intervention

The following intervention was planned and coordinated by her occupational therapist with support in its implementation from rehabilitation support workers.

- The task was divided into three sections and a positive reinforcement programme was introduced with rewards contingent upon completion of each stage.
- The first stage was for A to complete getting out of bed and ready for her shower in 20 minutes or less.
- The second stage involved A completing her shower in 30 minutes or less.
- The final stage involved A getting dried, dressed, and groomed in 25 minutes or less.

◆ Staff gave A a great deal of encouragement and positive feedback through-out the activity. Her performance was recorded on a star chart, with one star awarded for each stage successfully achieved within the appropriate time. A had the opportunity to earn 21 stars a week. If she earned a mini-mum of 15 then she received a larger, more socially reinforcing, weekly reward of her choice, such as a trip out.

◆ In addition, A attended anger-management, feedback, and problem-solving sessions to help her to identify precipitants to her aggression and to learn coping strategies to deal with her frustrations.

◆ A also attended a weekly relaxation session to learn techniques to reduce frustration.

Outcome

After 3 months A's average time to complete her morning routine was 80 minutes although, when focused, she could get washed and dressed within 45 minutes. This enabled her to participate in early morning therapy activities. She enjoyed these greatly, particularly those off the unit, which were an important aspect in improving her quality of life. The objective of a 25 per cent reduction in non-compliant and aggressive behaviour was exceeded. On admission she averaged five major aggressive episodes each week compared with 1.5 episodes per week after 3 months of intervention.

Although A did not return to live with her parents because of the nature of her challenging behaviour (which was easily triggered in the volatile home environment), she continued to make further progress in her morning routine as well as in other everyday living tasks. She was transferred to a supported residential facility for longer-term care where such structured functional rehabilitation could continue.

Conclusions

Ultimately, all rehabilitation is concerned with daily living skills, as it is generally considered to involve reducing the impact of disease and disability on daily life (Ward and McIntosh 2003). Rehabilitation of executive deficiencies is a particular challenge because most everyday living skills rely to some degree on executive control. However, there is a growing range of techniques, reviewed in this chapter, which occupational therapists and others can utilize in addressing the impact of executive disorder on everyday tasks.

Clinicians, families, and commissioners of services should also note that these methods are effective many years after injury, producing meaningful functional gains and improving quality of life long after most therapists will have stopped treating patients. The key to continued functional progress is the implementation of specific interventions within a system or milieu which promotes continued learning (comprising a trinity of contingent feedback, consistency, and structure).

This is true before rehabilitation has commenced, where time since injury may be less important in determining outcome than how that time has been spent (Eames *et al.* 1996). Moreover, once in a rehabilitative environment there is really no theoretical endpoint to the progress that can be made. As a result of a functional retraining approach, Parish and Oddy (2007) reported significant progress in daily living skills made by four adults 11–36 years post-injury residing in a continuing (slow-stream) rehabilitation facility.

Finally, surprising levels of functional performance can sometimes be found in the home environment when it mimics the prosthetic world of the rehabilitation unit. This is well illustrated by Wood and Rutterford's (2004) report of a man with severe executive dysfunction 18 years post-head injury. This man underwent examination on the Multiple Errands Test as one of the original three cases reported by Shallice and Burgess (1991), suffering from what the authors called strategy application disorder. When assessed in 1988 he showed a superior intellect and satisfied most tests of executive function, yet he performed poorly on the multi-tasking Multiple Errands Test. When re-examined on a similar task in 2002 his performance, although improved, was far from flawless. Between these two assessments 14 years apart he had lived mostly with his parents and subsequently married. He had secured work as a barman, but could only deal with one order at a time and was still prone to mishandling money. He remained quick-tempered and vulnerable to fatigue. He lacked initiative and purpose in life. The authors concluded that he functioned as well as he did because his wife and family provided a supportive framework 'to develop social habits patterns and self-care routines that limit the social handicap often associated with this type of neurobehavioral disability'.

References

Alderman, N. and Burgess, P.W. (2003). Assessment and rehabilitation of the dysexecutive syndrome. In: *Handbook of neurological rehabilitation* (ed R.J. Greenwood, M.P. Barnes, and T.M. McMillan), pp. 387–402. Psychology Press, New York.

Bennett, T.L. (2001). Neuropsychological evaluation in rehabilitation planning and evaluation of functional skills. *Archives of Clinical Neuropsychology* **16** 237–253.

Benton, A.L. (1991). The prefrontal region: its early history. In: *Frontal lobe function and dysfunction* (ed H.S. Levin, H.M. Eisenberg, and A.L. Benton), pp. 3–32. Oxford University Press, New York.

Birnboim, S. (1995). A metacognitive approach to cognitive rehabilitation. *British Journal of Occupational Therapy*, **58**, 61–4.

Burgess P.W. (2000). Strategy application disorder: the role of the frontal lobes in human multitasking. *Psychological Research*, **63**, 279–88.

Burgess, P.W. and Robertson, I.H. (2002). Principles of the rehabilitation of frontal lobe function. In: *Principles of frontal lobe function*, (ed D.T. Stuss and R.T. Knight), pp. 557–72. Oxford University Press, New York.

Burgess, P.W., Veitch, E., de Lacy Costello, A., and Shallice, T. (2000). The cognitive and anatomical correlates of multitasking. *Neuropsychologia*, **38**, 848–63.

Burgess, P.W., Alderman, N., Forbes, C., *et al.* (2006). The case for the development and use of 'ecologically valid' measures of executive function in experimental and clinical neuropsychology. *Journal of the International Neuropsychological Society*, **12**, 194–209.

Burke, W.H., Zenicus, A.H., Wesolowski, M.D., and Doubleday F (1991). Improving executive function disorders in brain-injured clients. *Brain Injury*, **5**, 241–52.

Castiello, U., Bennett, K.M., Egan, G.F, Tochon-Danguy, H.J., Kritikos, A., and Dunai, J. (1999). Human inferior parietal cortex programs the action class of grasping. *Journal of Cognitive Systems Research*, **2**, 22–30.

Chaytor, N. and Schmitter-Edgcombe, M. (2003). The ecological validity of neuropsychological tests: a review of the literature on everyday cognitive skills. *Neuropsychology Review*, **13**, 181–97.

Cicerone, K.D. and Wood, J.C. (1987). Planning disorder after closed head injury: a case study. *Archives of Physical Medicine and Rehabilitation*, **68**, 111–15.

Cope, D.N., Cole, J.R., Hall, K.M., and Barkan, H. (1991). Brain injury rehabilitation: analysis of outcome in a post-acute rehabilitation system. Part 2: Subanalyses. *Brain Injury*, **5**, 127–39.

Duncan, J., Emslie, H., Williams, P., Johnson, R., and Freer, C. (1996). Intelligence and the frontal lobe: the organisation of goal-directed behaviour. *Cognitive Neuropsychology*, **30**, 257–303.

Eames, P.G., Cotterill, G., and Kneale, T.A. (1995). Outcome of intensive rehabilitation after severe brain injury: a long-term follow up study. *Brain Injury*, **10**, 631–50.

Emslie, H., Wilson, B.A., Quirk, K., Evans, J.J., and Watson, P. (2007). Using a paging system in the rehabilitation of encephalitic patients. *Neuropsychological Rehabilitation*, **17**, 567–81.

Evans, J.J. (2003). Rehabilitation of executive deficits. In: *Neuropsychological rehabilitation: theory and practice* (ed B A Wilson), 53–70. Swets & Zeitlinger, Lisse.

Evans, J.J., Emslie, H, and Wilson, B.A. (1998). External cueing systems in the rehabilitation of executive impairments of action. *Journal of the International Neuropsychological Society*, **4** 399–408.

Fish, J., Evans, J.J., Nimmo, M., *et al.* (2007). Rehabilitation of executive dysfunction following brain injury: 'content-free' cueing improves everyday prospective memory performance. *Neuropsychologia*, **45**, 1318–30.

Fox, R.M., Martella, R.C., and Marchand-Martella, N.E. (1989). The acquisition, maintenance and generalisation of problem-solving skills by closed head-injured adults. *Behavior Therapy*, **20**, 61–76.

Gioia, G.A., Isquith, P.K., Guy, S.C., and Kenworthy, L. (1996). *Brief Rating Inventory of Executive Function*. Psychological Assessment Resources, Lutz, FL.

Goldberg, E. (2001). *The executive brain*. Oxford University Press, New York.

Hanks, R.A., Rapport, L.J., Millis, S.R., and Deshpande, S.A. (1999). Measures of executive functioning as predictors of functional ability and social integration in a rehabilitation sample. *Archives of Physical Medicine and Rehabilitation*, **80**,1030–7.

Hewitt, J., Evans, J.J., and Dritschel, B. (2006). Theory driven rehabilitation of executive functioning: improving planning skills in people with traumatic brain injury through the use of an autobiographical episodic memory cueing procedure. *Neuropsychologia*, **44**, 1468–74.

Humphreys, G.W., Forde, E.M.E., and Riddoch, M.J. (2001). The planning and execution of everyday actions. In: *The handbook of cognitive neuropsychology* (ed B.Rapp), pp. 565–89. Psychology Press, Philadelphia, PA.

Imamizu, H., Miyauchi, S., Tamada, T., *et al.* (2000). Human cerebellar activity reflecting an acquired internal model of a new tool. *Nature*, **403**, 192–5.

Knight, C., Alderman, N., and Burgess, P.W. (2002). Development of a simplified version of the multiple errands test for use in hospital settings. *Neuropsychological Rehabilitation*, **12**, 231–55.

Levine, B., Robertson, I.H., Clare, L., *et al.* (2000). Rehabilitation of executive functioning: an experimental–clinical validation of Goal Management Training. *Journal of the International Neuropsychological Society*, **6**, 299–312.

McMillan, T.M., Robertson, I.H., Brock, D., and Chorlton, L. (2002). Brief mindfulness training for attentional problems after traumatic brain injury: a randomised control treatment trial. *Neuropsychological Rehabilitation*, **12**, 117–25.

Manchester, D., Priestley, N., and Jackson, H. (2004). The assessment of executive functions: coming out of the office. *Brain Injury*, **18**, 1067–81.

Manly, T., Hawkins, K., Evans, J., Woldt, K., and Robertson, I.H. (2002). Rehabilitation of executive function: facilitation of effective goal management on complex tasks using periodic auditory alerts. *Neuropsychologia*, **40**, 271–81.

Marshall, R.C., Karow, C.M., Morelli, C.A., Iden, K.K., Dixon, J., and Cranfill, T.B. (2004). Effects of interactive strategy modelling training on problem-solving training by persons with traumatic brain injury. *Aphasiology*, **18**, 659–73.

Norman, D.A. and Bobrow, D.G. (1976). On the analysis of performance operating characteristics. *Psychological Review*, **83**, 508–10.

Norris, G. and Tate, R.L. (2000). The Behavioural Assessment of the Dysexecutive Syndrome (BADS): ecological, concurrent and construct validity. *Neuropsychological Rehabilitation*, **10**, 33–45.

Odhuba, R.A. (2005). Ecological validity of measures of executive functioning. *British Journal of Clinical Psychology*, **44**, 269–78.

Pachalska, M., Kurzbauer, H., Talar, J., and MacQueen, B.D. (2002). Active and passive executive function disorder subsequent to closed head-injury. *Medical Science Monitor*, **8**, 1–9.

Parish, L. and Oddy, M. (2007). Efficacy of rehabilitation for functional skills more than 10 years after extremely severe brain injury. *Neuropsychological Rehabilitation*, **17**, 230–43.

Park, N.W., Proulx, G.B., and Towers, W.M. (1999). Evaluation of the Attention Process Training programme. *Neuropsychological Rehabilitation*, 9, 135–54.

Petrides, M. (1994). Frontal lobes and working memory: evidence from investigations of the effects of cortical excisison in nonhuman primates. In: *Handbook of neuropsychology*, Vol 9 (ed F. Boller and J. Grafman), pp. 59–82. Elsevier, Amsterdam.

Pijnenborg, G.H.M., Withaar, F.K., Evans, J.J., van den Bosch, R.J., and Brouwer, W.H. (2007). SMS text messages as a prosthetic aid in the cognitive rehabilitation of schizophrenia. *Rehabilitation Psychology*, 52, 236–40.

Rath, J.F., Simon, D., Langenbahn, D.M., Sherr, R.L., and Diller, L. (2003). Group treatment of problem-solving deficits in outpatients with traumatic brain injury: a randomised outcome study. *Neuropsychological Rehabilitation*, 13, 461–88.

Rath, J.F., Langenbahn, D.M., Simon, D., Sherr, R.L., Fletcher, J., and Diller, L. (2004). The construct of problem solving in higher level neuropsychological assessment and rehabilitation. *Archives of Clinical Neuropsychology*, 19, 613–35.

Sammer, G., Reuter, I., Hullmann, K., Kaps, M., and Vaitl, D. (2006). Training of executive functions in Parkinson's disease. *Journal of the Neurological Sciences*, 248, 115–19.

Sarter, M., Gehring, W.J., and Kozak, R. (2006). More attention must be paid: the neurobiology of attentional effort. *Brain Research Reviews*, 51, 145–60.

Scheibel, R.S., Newsome, M.R., Steinberg, J.L., *et al.* (2007). Altered brain activation during cognitive control in patients with moderate to severe traumatic brain injury. *Neurorehabilitation and Neural Repair*, 21, 36–45.

Schutz, L.E. and Trainor, K. (2007). Evaluation of cognitive rehabilitation as a treatment paradigm. *Brain Injury*, 21, 545–57.

Schwartz, M.F (2006). The cognitive neuropsychology of everyday action and planning. *Cognitive Neuropsychology*, 23, 202–21.

Schwartz, M.F. and Buxbaum, L.J. (1997). Naturalistic action. In: *Apraxia: the neuropsychology of action* (ed L.J.G. Rothi and K.M. Heilman), pp. 269–89. Psychology Press, Hove: Psychology Press.

Seale, G.S., Caroselli, J.S., High, W.M., Jr, Becker, C.L., Neese, L.E., and Scheibel, R. (2002). Use of the Community Integration Questionnaire (CIQ). to characterise changes in functioning for individuals with traumatic brain injury who participated in a post-acute rehabilitation programme. *Brain Injury*, 16, 955–67.

Serino, A. (2006). A rehabilitative program for central executive deficits after traumatic brain injury. *Brain and Cognition*, 60, 213–14.

Shallice, T. and Burgess, P. (1991). Higher-order cognitive impairments and frontal lobe lesions in Man. In: *Frontal lobe function and dysfunction* (ed H.S. Levin, H.M. Eisenberg, and A.L. Benton), pp. 125–38. Oxford University Press, New York.

Sirigu, A., Zalla, T., Pillon, B., Grafman, J., Agid, Y., and Dubois, B. (1995). Selective impairments in managerial knowledge following pre-frontal cortex damage. *Cortex*, 31, 301–16.

Stablum, F., Umilta, C., Mogentale, C., Carlan, M., and Guerrini, C. (2000). Rehabilitation of executive deficits in closed head injury and anterior artery aneurysm patients. *Psychological Research*, 63, 265–78.

Stablum, F., Umilta, C., Mazzoldi, M., Pastore, N., and Magon, S. (2007). Rehabilitation of endogenous task shift processes in closed head injury patients. *Neuropsychological Rehabilitation*, **17**, 1–33.

Stuss, D.T. (2007). New approaches to prefrontal lobe testing. In: *The human frontal lobes* (ed B.L. Miller and J.L. Cummings), pp. 292–305. Guilford Press, New York.

Sumner, P., Nachev, P., Morris, P., *et al.* (2007). Human medial frontal cortex mediates unconscious inhibition of voluntary action. *Neuron*, **54**, 697–711.

von Cramon, D.Y., Matthes-von Cramon, G., and Mai, N. (1991). Problem solving deficits in brain-injured patients: a therapeutic approach. *Neuropsychological Rehabilitation*, **1**, 45–64.

Ward, C.D. and McIntosh, S. (2003). The rehabilitation process: a neurological perspective. In: *Handbook of neurological rehabilitation* (2nd edn) (ed R.J. Greenwood, M.P. Barnes, T.M. McMillan, and C.D. Ward), pp. 15–28. Psychology Press, Hove.

Wood, R.L. and Rutterford, N.A. (2004). Relationships between measured cognitive ability and reported psychosocial activity after bilateral frontal lobe injury: an 18 year follow-up. *Neuropsychological Rehabilitation*, **14**, 329–50.

Wood, R.L. and Worthington, A.D. (1999). Outcome in community rehabilitation: measuring the social impact of disability. *Neuropsychological Rehabilitation*, **9**, 505–16.

Wood, R.L. and Worthington, A.D. (2001). Neurobehavioural rehabilitation: a conceptual paradigm. In: *Neurobehavioural disability and social handicap following traumatic brain injury* (ed R.L. Wood and T.M. McMillan), pp. 107–131. Psychology Press, Hove.

Worthington, A. (2003). The natural recovery and treatment of executive disorders. In: *Handbook of clinical neuropsychology* (ed P.W. Halligan, U. Kischka, and J.C. Marshall). Oxford University Press, New York.

Worthington, A. (2005). Rehabilitation of executive deficits: effective treatment of related disabilities. In: *Effectiveness of rehabilitation of cognitive deficits* (ed P.W. Halligan and D.T. Wade), pp. 257–267. Oxford University Press, New York.

Worthington, A. and Wood, R.L. (2008). Rehabilitation of behaviour disorders. In: *Psychological approaches to rehabilitation after traumatic brain injury* (ed A.D. Tyerman and N. King), pp. 227–259. Blackwell, Oxford.

Worthington, A.D., Matthews, S., Melia, Y., and Oddy, M. (2006). Cost–benefits associated with social outcome from neurobehavioural rehabilitation. *Brain Injury*, **29**, 947–57.

Zalla, T., Plaissiart, C., Pillon, B., and Grafman, J. (2001). Action planning in a virtual context after prefrontal cortex damage. *Neuropsychologia*, **39**, 759–70.

12

Vocational rehabilitation and executive disorders

Andy Tyerman

Community Head Injury Service, Buckinghamshire
Primary Care Trust

Introduction

Return to work is critical to quality of life for people with acquired brain injury (ABI), yet only a minority of those with more severe injury return to previous or alternative employment. Whilst a multitude of factors affect return to work after ABI, difficulties with executive function are of crucial importance.

Executive functions are required for effective problem-solving, planning and organization, self-monitoring, initiation, error correction, and behavioural regulation (Evans 2008). They 'enable a person to determine goals, formulate new and useful ways of achieving them, and then follow and adapt this proposed course in the face of competing demands and changing circumstances, often over long periods of time' (Burgess and Alderman 2004). Cicerone and Fraser (2000) stress how executive difficulties interfere with a person's ability to function without supervision and note that it is not uncommon to see a dissociation between intact ability to describe a procedure or social response and impaired ability to perform the response. This can create the false impression that the client is either unwilling to respond appropriately or non-compliant, which has obvious implications for the workplace. Turner and Levine (2004) note that people with executive dysfunction may only return to rehabilitation services after months or years of a downward spiral in their social or vocational lives, having been unable to meet the demands of unstructured environments.

Executive difficulties are likely to have a particular impact on jobs that require high levels of planning, problem-solving, abstract reasoning, organizational, and management skills. However, they also have a general limiting effect because of clients' reduced awareness of their vocational restrictions and the capacity to monitor and manage them effectively in the workplace. As a result clients may be unaware of their difficulties at work and struggle to improve work performance in response to feedback. Executive difficulties may also restrict ability to sustain work late after ABI, to adapt to change within a job role, and to refine coping strategies. Those required to seek alternative employment also tend to seek, but then struggle with, jobs consistent with their pre-injury qualifications and experience, not taking due account of their restrictions post-injury.

In the Working Out programme, a specialist brain injury vocational rehabilitation programme run by the Community Head Injury Service, Buckinghamshire Primary Care Trust, in the UK (Tyerman *et al.* 2008), the following vocational difficulties are commonly observed for people with executive dysfunction.

- For those returning to previous employment:
  - reduced awareness and insight into the effects of brain injury and difficulties in recognizing their vocational implications
  - difficulties in accepting the need for and/or initiating/implementing agreed plans for return to work
  - unreliable timekeeping because of difficulty in making/executing effective travel plans
  - poor performance/delivery in the job despite appearing to have retained the requisite aptitudes and skills
  - difficulties in planning, prioritizing, and organizing work (e.g. time-keeping and meeting deadlines)
  - rigidity and inflexibility with regard to job roles and work practices
  - poor monitoring of job performance and limited self-management of difficulties
  - difficulties in modifying strategies in response to changes in job role/duties
  - difficulties in work relationships with supervisors, colleagues, and/or customers
  - lack of awareness of impact of own work performance/behaviour on colleagues
  - poor judgement and/or control of social behaviour in the workplace
  - disputes with managers (e.g. about the existence or cause of difficulties at work).

- For those required to seek alternative employment:
  - inappropriate job selection—not taking into account or underestimating restrictions
  - poor structuring and judgement about the content of job applications

- inappropriate job interview behaviour
- difficulties in learning and adapting strategies to the new job.

In this chapter the importance of executive function in return to work after ABI and the implications for vocational rehabilitation are reviewed, drawing on experience from the Working Out programme.

Vocational outcome and executive dysfunction

There is extensive research on vocational outcome after traumatic brain injury (TBI). In a North American multi-centre study, employment was less than half pre-injury levels at successive follow-up after inpatient rehabilitation, ranging from 17 to 25 per cent overall and under 40 per cent even for those previously employed (Sander *et al.* 1996). Furthermore, many of those who return to work experience 'job instability' (Kreutzer *et al.* 2003). In an Australian rehabilitation follow-up, 33 per cent of those employed prior to injury were employed full-time and 9 per cent part-time at 2 years (Ponsford *et al.* 1995). However, 32 per cent of those employed at 2 years were no longer employed at 5 years (Olver *et al.*1996). Furthermore, only 29 per cent of those at school at the time of injury were employed.

In an early UK neurosurgical follow-up study only 29 per cent were employed at 2–7 years, compared with 86 per cent prior to injury (Brooks *et al.* 1987). In a more recent study of all hospital admissions in Glasgow (Thornhill *et al.* 2000), those considered 'unfit for work' rose from 16 per cent pre-injury to 32 per cent at 1 year follow-up, with a third of those employed at injury considered unfit for work. After severe TBI, those considered 'unfit for work' rose from 13 to 56 per cent. Outcome from neurorehabilitation centres in the UK has also been disappointing in the past. For example, only 36 per cent of those admitted to the Wolfson Medical Rehabilitation Centre in Wimbledon were in full-time employment at 2-year follow-up, with most working in a reduced capacity (Weddell *et al.*1980). When seen again at 7 years, some had progressed to jobs comparable to pre-injury but none of those unemployed at 2 years had since found work (Oddy *et al.* 1985). Such studies highlight the need for specialist vocational rehabilitation. Even with specific advice and support on return to work, a successful return was achieved by only 38 per cent in Cambridge, with another 28 per cent having attempted but failed to do so (Johnson 1987). At 10-year follow-up work status had not changed for most participants (82 per cent)— 34 per cent employed full-time, 10 per cent part-time, 6 per cent in sheltered work, and 50 per cent unemployed (Johnson 1998).

Neuropsychological impairment has long been linked with poor vocational outcome. Cognitive impairment (including executive difficulties such as cognitive inflexibility and problem-solving) as early as 1 month post-injury was reported to differentiate between those in and out of work at 1 year (Fraser *et al.* 1988). In a long-term follow-up Brooks *et al.* (1987) found that those in work had fewer cognitive difficulties and also fewer problems emotionally/behaviourally. Numerous studies have since reported a link between neuropsychological function and vocational outcome (e.g. Ryan *et al.* 1992; Ip *et al.* 1995; Girard *et al.* 1996; Sander *et al.* 1997; Teasdale *et al.* 1997; Cattelani *et al.* 2002; Simpson and Schmitter-Edgecombe 2002). However, a relationship between neuropsychological test results and vocational outcome has not always been found (e.g. Johnstone *et al.* 1999, 2003; Tyerman and Young 1999; McCrimmon and Oddy 2006).

Price and Baumann (1990) highlight the difficulties for people with ABI in their work behaviour—in 'work conformance' (mainly relating to social judgement, inappropriate behaviour and communication), 'task orientation' with poor work persistence and need for close supervision (partly due to poor recognition of mistakes), and poor 'work tolerance'. 'Job separation' (i.e. loss of job) for people with ABI in supported employment has been attributed to the following: poor work skills (25.0 per cent), insufficient motivation to work (20.3 per cent), aberrant/inappropriate behaviour (23.5 per cent), external factors (20.3 per cent), and economic lay-offs (10.9 per cent). People with ABI were noted to be far more likely than other groups (i.e. learning disabilities, mental illness or cerebral palsy) to be separated from work due to aberrant or inappropriate behaviour (Kregel *et al.* 1994).

The importance of executive function was supported by a meta-analysis of studies of work status after TBI (Crepeau and Scherzer 1993). Although many predictors and indicators were found to be only weakly or moderately related to work status, the correlation between executive dysfunction (i.e. planning, organization, verification, and lack of flexibility) and unemployment (0.49) was amongst the highest and most reliable. It was suggested that rehabilitation programmes need to emphasize improving executive function and flexibility. Ownsworth and McKenna (2004) also found that executive function was among the factors associated most consistently with employment outcome after TBI. The aspects of executive functioning identified included concept formation, divided and selective attention, mental flexibility, mental programming, and planning. It was recommended that vocational interventions focus on meta-cognitive as well as emotional and social environmental factors.

The role of self-awareness has attracted particular attention. Ben-Yishay *et al.* (1987) identified improvements in self-awareness, discipline, and regulation of emotional responses as one of the principal sources of successful vocational outcome, together with increased effectiveness in functional application of information-processing abilities and improvements in patients' acceptance of their existential situation. In a further study, Ezrachi *et al.* (1991) report that capacity for acceptance is the single most potent variable in determining capacity to benefit from rehabilitation and return to work. As well as self-appraisal, awareness and acceptance were identified as crucial, with a need for interventions to enhance self-awareness and active acceptance. Scherer *et al.* (1998; 2003) report a positive relationship between self-awareness and favourable employment outcome, and advocate interventions to improve self-awareness. Wise *et al.* (2005) report a similar relationship and advocate the use of standardized measures of self-awareness to identify those that may benefit from additional intervention.

A number of models of brain injury vocational rehabilitation have been developed over the last 25 years. A few selected models are outlined in the next section.

Models of vocational rehabilitation after brain injury

Positive outcomes are reported for ABI vocational programmes in the USA, with around two-thirds of patients returning to employment using various models of vocational rehabilitation.

The New York University Head Trauma Program has three phases:

(1) remedial intervention, focusing on cognitive remediation, self-awareness, and social skills

(2) guided voluntary occupational trials under the guidance/supervision/tutoring of a vocational counsellor

(3) assistance with work placements (finding suitable work, job familiarization, and, when needed, initial adjustments to the new work environment).

Of 94 people with very severe injuries, 56 per cent were placed in competitive work and 23 per cent in sheltered work at 6 months with outcome holding up well at 3 years (Ben-Yishay *et al.* 1987).

A 'coordinated model' of service delivery at the Mayo Medical Centre, Minnesota, integrates medical and vocational services through a brain injury nurse coordinator and a brain injury vocational coordinator. Key elements of the vocational coordinator role include integrating vocational goals into core rehabilitation, assessing vocational readiness, developing comprehensive return-to-work plans, providing vocational counselling and evaluation, linking with local work rehabilitation centres, adjustment to disability counselling, on-the-job evaluation, education for employers, and follow-up/support (Buffington and Malec 1997). Of 138 participants assisted through this approach, 80 per cent were in community-based employment (56 per cent with no support) a year after initial placement (Malec and Moessner 2006).

The supported placement model at Virginia Medical College is character-ized by on-site training, counselling, and support by a job coach. The model has four phases:

(1) job placement—matching job needs to abilities/potential, encouraging communication, travel arrangements/training, and analysing the job environment

(2) job site training (skills acquisition, time-keeping, reducing inappropriate behaviour, communication) and advocacy (orientation to the workplace, communication with coworkers, parents, and care workers, and counselling about work behaviours)

(3) ongoing assessment—evaluation from supervisor and client

(4) job retention and follow-along—regular on-site visits, phone calls, reviews of supervisor evaluations, client progress reports, and parent/caretaker evaluations (Wehman *et al.*1988).

Of 43 people with severe TBI, over 70 per cent were placed in competitive employment at 6 months after an average of 290 hours of intervention at a cost of $6000–12 000 per person (Wehman *et al.* 1993).

A cost–benefit analysis of the Work Reentry Program at Sharp Memorial Rehabilitation Center, San Diego, CA, indicated that brain injury vocational programmes are cost–effective. This programme combines elements of work rehabilitation (vocational evaluation, simulated work samples, work hardening, 'work adjustment experience', vocational counselling, and job seeking/keeping skills) with supported placements (including provision for an on-site job coach and an off-site adjustment/support group). Total operational costs over 5 years were on average $4377 per person. However, taking into account taxes paid and savings in state benefits, the average payback period was just 20 months for individuals who would otherwise most likely face a lifetime of unemployment and dependence on public assistance (Abrams *et al.* 1993).

Therefore positive outcomes and cost-effectiveness have been demonstrated for brain injury vocational rehabilitation programmes, with evidence from Israel as well as the USA confirming long-term benefits (Groswasser *et al.* 1999; Wehman *et al.* 2003).

Brain injury vocational rehabilitation in the UK

In the past very few people with ABI in the UK received vocational rehabilitation. In a recent survey 62 per cent of neurological rehabilitation services report that they address vocational issues and, whilst only 8 per cent provide specialist vocational rehabilitation, most refer on to vocational services (Deshpande and

Turner-Stokes 2004). Of the 36 services identified, some are specialist brain injury vocational programmes, some are brain injury services with an added vocational element, and some are generic vocational, educational, or training providers that accept people with ABI. Few services are able to meet the full range of vocational need and many areas have no access to such specialist provision.

The complex vocational needs of people with ABI require close collaboration between brain injury services, Jobcentre Plus, Social Services, and vocational providers, yet such joint working is very patchy. Recent inter-agency guidelines (BSRM/JCP/RCP 2004) provide specific guidelines for a coordinated inter-agency approach to vocational assessment and rehabilitation after ABI and a framework for joint review and development of local service provision. Recognizing the limited provision in the UK, a specific quality requirement on 'Vocational Rehabilitation' is included in the National Service Framework for Long-term Conditions (Department of Health 2005). This states that:

> People with long-term neurological conditions are to have access to appropriate vocational assessment, rehabilitation and ongoing support to enable them to find, regain or remain in work and access other occupational and educational opportunities.

The evidence-based markers of good practice stress the need for a coordinated multi-agency approach, a greater focus on identifying and addressing vocational needs within local rehabilitation services, availability of specialist vocational rehabilitation programmes, and routine monitoring of vocational outcomes.

To date, few NHS brain injury services have developed brain injury vocational rehabilitation programmes but some work in partnership with vocational providers. Jobcentre Plus (part of the Department for Work and Pensions) recognizes brain injury as an area of specialist provision with a National Framework for Contracting for Brain Injury Work Preparation. This covers job-finding behaviour development needs, occupational decision-making needs, and job-keeping behaviour development needs (BSRM/JCP/RCP 2004). In 2003 there were 13 Jobcentre Plus contracted specialist brain injury work preparation providers in the UK. Whilst two of these programmes are NHS-based, most are in the independent or voluntary sector (e.g. Rehab UK). Two examples of UK brain injury vocational rehabilitation programmes will be outlined.

The Working Out programme (Tyerman *et al.* 2008) is run by the Community Head Injury Service, Buckinghamshire Primary Care Trust, with joint working with Jobcentre Plus through a specialist brain injury work preparation contract. The programme comprises four interlinked phases: vocational assessment, work preparation, voluntary work trials, and long-term supported placements. It combines elements of brain injury rehabilitation (e.g. brain injury education, occupational therapy, and individual and group cognitive rehabilitation/psychological therapy) with elements of vocational rehabilitation (e.g. work preparation group, community vocational activities, individual project work, vocational counselling, voluntary work trials, supported placements, and placement support groups). The original project was evaluated for a consecutive series of people with severe TBI (median post-traumatic amnesia (PTA), 42 days) who had been unable to establish or re-establish themselves in employment post-injury. (At the time of injury 62 per cent were in full-time employment, 29 per cent in education, and 9 per cent unemployed.) Outcomes on completion of the programme were encouraging (paid employment/vocational training, 50 per cent; permitted work/voluntary work, 35 per cent; adult education/further rehabilitation, 12.5 per cent; unoccupied, 2.5 per cent) and well maintained at 1- and 2-year follow-up (Tyerman and Young 2000). Ongoing programme outcomes in 2007 were as follows: paid employment/vocational training, 64 per cent; permitted work/voluntary work/adult education, 20 per cent; referral for further rehabilitation/treatment, 5 per cent; unoccupied, 2 per cent; disengaged, 9 per cent).

The Rehab UK programmes contain two elements: a centre-based pre-vocational phase of intensive cognitive rehabilitation and an *in situ* vocational trials phase (Murphy *et al.* 2006). The pre-vocational phase is spread over 12 weeks with sessions carried out in groups of 8–12 clients. The second phase consists of voluntary work placements—sourced, overseen, and monitored by job coaches. The job coaches encourage clients to use compensatory strategies, fine-tune strategies according to the demands of work tasks, provide employers with information and advice on ABI, and collaborate in exploring and providing workplace adjustments. Outcomes are reported for people with ABI, mainly TBI (62 per cent), of whom 92 per cent had a PTA greater than 24 hours, or cerebrovascular accident (22 per cent), across the three Rehab UK sites (Murphy *et al.* 2006). (At the time of injury 70 per cent were employed, 19 per cent were students, and 11 per cent were unemployed.) Programme outcomes were as follows: paid competitive employment, 41 per cent; voluntary work, 16 per cent; mainstream education and training, 15 per cent; discharge to other services, 15 per cent; withdrew from programme, 13 per cent.

Executive difficulties and vocational rehabilitation

The assessment and management of executive difficulties has been the subject of several recent reviews (Callaghan 2001; Burgess and Alderman 2004; Turner and Levine 2004; Gordon *et al.* 2006; see also Chapter 4, this volume). The specific management of reduced awareness has been addressed by several authors (Langer and Padrone 1992; Prigatano 2005; Bach and David 2006; Fleming and Ownsworth 2006). How can executive difficulties best be managed within vocational rehabilitation?

Assessment of executive function is a key component of vocational evaluation after ABI. The role of neuropsychological evaluation in vocational planning has been reviewed in depth by Uomoto (2000). Whilst it is argued that neuropsychological evaluations can be of assistance in making better decisions about jobs and appropriate job tasks, it is acknowledged that they have predictive limitations. Therefore it is suggested that *in vivo* community assessment (such as a work trial) is used to augment neuropsychological assessments and to 'test the limits' to evaluate at what point cognitive and behavioural problems interfere with job performance. Given the difficulty experienced by clients with cognitive deficits in generalizing learned skills to the workplace, the need to simulate the actual work situation as closely as possible is stressed. This is particularly important in the case of executive difficulties. However, the practical assessment of executive-based difficulties is complex (Crepeau *et al.* 1997; Bamdad *et al.* 2003).

Warren (2000) suggests a number of evaluative questions concerning executive function and the person's ability to:

- plan activities and decide which are important and which are not
- initiate activities and get going on a plan of action
- continue to prioritize activities
- problem-solve or resolve issues that do not have an obvious next step
- make appropriate decisions and/or learn from mistakes
- monitor/evaluate actions and make appropriate changes with environmental feedback
- adapt when plans need to change.

Uomoto (2000) discusses some of the specific vocational implications of executive dysfunction after ABI. These include the following.

1. The importance of work trials, 'job stations', or 'on-the-job' training to examine new learning, to help in assessing the person's ability to adjust to novel situations and perform multiple tasks simultaneously, and to observe how problem-solving deficits impede job performance.

2. The more familiar the tasks the better—relying on overly learned tasks and minimizing the need for new learning.

3. Training the client in a method of problem-solving that is job or task specific because of difficulty in transferring learned skills from one group of tasks or job setting to another.

4. The probable need for supervision by coworkers or other supervisors for clients with problem-solving deficits. It is suggested that job coaches or coworker trainers can provide feedback and cues to prevent the client from making too many errors.

Cicerone and Fraser (2000) discuss the importance of the therapeutic relationship, client–therapist expectancies and collaboration, goal-setting, self-monitoring, and the management of self-awareness. Several of the suggested counselling interventions within vocational rehabilitation are relevant to executive difficulties: teaching a self-checking routine to detect errors; manipulation of the environment to reduce distractors; use of a formal problem-solving framework; teaching self-management techniques and checklists to increase independence in the workplace; help with social judgement and communication. The authors note that a problem-solving framework (identification of the problem, review of alternative solutions, selection of a response, and verification of a solution) can be taught in a therapy context and then applied to counselling about job options, specific work behaviours, and interpersonal behaviours. Particular attention is given to identifying the costs and benefits of a specific solution. von Cramon and Matthes-von Cramon (1994) describe a case study of a medical doctor who completed extensive training in a problem-solving technique (2–3 hours/week for 12 months) in a work trial within a department of pathology. However, despite successfully learning the technique, the client was unable to apply this to novel or changing situations. This highlights the difficulty that people with executive difficulties have in generalizing taught coping strategies.

The suggested help with social judgement and communication includes feedback on difficulties, modelling of appropriate behaviour, and use of role-playing to develop a repertoire of well-practised and routine responses for different social situations (e.g. greeting/responding to supervisors/coworkers, waiting for appropriate moments to speak or make non-disruptive interruptions, responding to suggestions or criticisms). Cicerone and Fraser (2000) suggest that practised routines also reduce social anxiety and the emotional consequences of difficult social interactions, and that self-monitoring of inappropriate verbalizations and social behaviours can be conducted through diaries, notebooks, and checklists.

Cicerone and Fraser (2000) also stress the value of group work and group therapy as a means of clients experiencing the effects of ABI on their social behaviour and the effects of their social behaviour on others. It is suggested that the experience of turn-taking, compromise, personal risk-taking, self-disclosure, and other social skills is readily transferred to work situations, and that the use of structured exercises, homework assignments, and videotape feedback can be of assistance in developing awareness and in generalizing skills or behaviours. In addition to alleviating a sense of alienation and demoralization, clients benefit from peer feedback regarding their cognitive limitations, emotional reactions, and social behaviours. It is suggested that support groups may be structured around specific vocational issues such as job-seeking and job placement using a combination of psychoeducational, behaviour change, and support group emphases.

In summarizing the supported employment model after ABI, Wehman *et al.* (2000) outline the role of the job coach/trainer advocate/employment specialist. This typically involves the following steps: developing a customer profile, performing a career search, job-site training and support services, extended support services, and case management. Although the authors do not comment specifically on the needs of people with executive difficulties, many of the interventions outlined (e.g. instructional techniques, job accommodations, and compensatory strategies) are likely to be of benefit. Wehman *et al.* (1989) report an example of a person whose primary cognitive impairments included poor planning and organizational skills, distractibility, limited self-awareness, and inconsistent error recognition. Kreutzer *et al.* (1988) stress the importance of feedback regarding work performance because of reduced self-awareness and outline the benefits of the job coach in providing or facilitating employer feedback, drawing on neuropsychological expertise if the feedback is not accepted. The two examples described to illustrate compensatory strategies in improving work performance had difficulty with organizational and reasoning skills. Kreutzer *et al.* (1990) report on a more challenging example. In guidelines for supported employment, Yasuda *et al.* (2001) comment specifically on the need for the employment specialist to help the client to develop compensatory skills for executive difficulties.

The training of 'natural supports' in the workplace (i.e. employer/supervisor and/or coworkers) also offers considerable potential benefit because of the hidden but complex nature of executive difficulties and the need for external support (Curl *et al.* 1996; Fraser and Curl 2000). In outlining the use of assistive technology, Warren (2000) describes two case studies of people with executive difficulties: a person with a tendency to wander into dangerous areas assisted by a remote controlled flashing light to summon help, and a student having difficulties with self-regulation and time management provided with a palm top and desktop computer to create and respond to daily and weekly schedules.

A service example

Many of the specialist brain injury rehabilitation programme components of the Working Out programme (Tyerman *et al.* 2008) have been observed to be of assistance to people with executive difficulties.

Specialist vocational assessment typically combines vocational interviews, formal tests (i.e. neuropsychological and occupational therapy), group work, and observations/ratings of work attitude, performance, and behaviour on practical work activities in the community. When the person has recently been on placement or in work post-injury, feedback is sought from relevant supervisors. Work assessment projects are often set up and evaluated on site to look at specific work skills and performance. Other assessments (e.g. medical, physiotherapy, speech and language) are incorporated as required.

The neuropsychological assessment routinely includes tests of executive function (e.g. Trail Making Test and the Multiple Errands Test, Six Elements Test, or other tests from the Behavioural Assessment of the Dysexecutive Syndrome or Delis Kaplan Executive Function System) alongside tests of general intellectual ability, attention, memory, and information processing (plus other language, perceptual, and spatial skills as appropriate). The Chessington Occupational Therapy Neurological Assessment Battery commonly highlights executive difficulties in the ability to follow complex instructions (written, visual, and spoken), along with any difficulties in visual perception, constructional ability, and sensory–motor ability.

In parallel with formal testing, work attitude, performance, and behaviour are observed on practical work activities and rated on two vocational scales— the Functional Assessment Inventory (FAI) and the Work Personality Profile (WPP). The FAI (Crew and Athelstan 1981, 1984) comprises 30 items of vocational strengths/limitations across seven factors: adaptive behaviour, motor functioning, cognition, physical condition, communication, vocational qualifications, and vision. The WPP (Bolton and Roessler 1986a,b) has 58 items relating to work attitudes, values, habits and behaviours across five factors: task orientation, social skills, work motivation, work conformance, and personal presentation. The comparison of self-ratings with staff ratings often highlights reduced awareness, as well as the extent of vocational restrictions, as the WPP includes items sensitive to executive difficulties. However, it is also important to record qualitative observations of executive function in practical work activities. Executive difficulties are also often apparent in vocational guidance interviews (e.g. in evaluating vocational implications and realistic future options).

The weekly work preparation group helps people to re-evaluate strengths and weaknesses, discuss the implications of ABI for re-employment, explore suitable jobs, and manage issues related to ABI in job applications/interviews etc. through education, role plays, group discussions, peer group sharing/ support, and 'homework' exercises. On community-based vocational activities the feedback and advice from both programme staff and supervisors from the

relevant organizations helps clients to develop greater awareness of their difficulties and appropriate coping strategies. Individual projects within a specific
area of work help to identify potential difficulties, refine coping strategies, and
explore whether this might offer a realistic avenue of future work. Individual
vocational counselling helps clients to develop a clearer understanding of
vocational aptitudes and resources, limitations arising from ABI, and current
opportunities and prospects, before exploring a realistic future occupation
through job-matching etc. In parallel, many clients, particularly those with
executive difficulties, require individual psychological therapy to facilitate
vocational adjustment, as well as attending brain injury educational sessions
and other group programmes (e.g. cognitive rehabilitation group, personal
issues group).

When clients are considered ready for the workplace, the placement consultant
works with them to find and set up suitable individually tailored voluntary
work trials. These typically start with one or two half-days per week and gradually increase in line with progress. Work trials serve a number of vital
functions, most of which are likely to be of particular potential benefit for
people with executive difficulties: independent assessment of work potential;
identification of residual difficulties in the workplace; development, evaluation,
and refinement of coping strategies; and re-establishment of work routines
and behaviours.

In parallel with the work trial, clients typically progress from the work
preparation group to a fortnightly placement support group. This promotes
understanding of and adjustment to the world of work after ABI. One of the
functions of the group is to help clients form a balanced view of difficulties in
the workplace, as well as alerting programme staff early to emerging difficulties,
enabling a proactive response before the situation escalates. For those with
executive difficulties, this group provides an opportunity to consider how the
effects of ABI in general, and executive difficulties in particular, may (or may
not) be contributing to difficulties at work and to assist them with any
required action. This might include increased structure, mechanisms for
providing external feedback on work performance, refinement of coping
strategies, or broader problem-solving about other work adjustments. This
may be discussed initially in the group, and then addressed individually or
jointly with the workplace supervisor.

Long-term supported placements may include full- or part-time employment,
vocational training, supported employment, adult education, permitted work,
and voluntary work. Clients are assisted, as required, both individually and in
a 'job search club' in finding and applying for suitable positions. Whenever
possible the placement consultant assists in setting up, supporting, monitoring,

reviewing, and refining work placements. Once established, there is usually a phased reduction in support but attendance at the placement support group is open-ended. Whilst some clients, such as the example described by Tyerman *et al.* (2008), are able to absorb and apply independently the learning from the programme, people with executive difficulties often require ongoing access to advice/support because of reduced awareness and difficulties in monitoring and adjusting their work performance in the light of feedback. For this group in particular the open-door review policy is critical to respond to emerging difficulties.

As with the models of brain injury vocational rehabilitation reviewed above, many of the core components of the Working Out programme are of assistance in managing executive difficulties. However, people with executive difficulties commonly require considerable additional individual input throughout the rehabilitation process.

- In vocational assessment/work preparation:
  - ongoing education, feedback and support in recognizing the nature and extent of difficulties arising from ABI and their vocational implications
  - structured and explicit feedback from programme staff (from group rehabilitation activities and individual work) and from workplace supervisors/colleagues (from projects/trials) through feedback forms, rating scales, videotape feedback etc to assist the client in re-appraising vocational strengths and weaknesses
  - assisting clients in accepting identified work-related difficulties after ABI and in developing, testing and refining strategies to manage executive difficulties (eg planning, problem-solving, decision-making, time-management strategies)
  - providing extensive vocational counselling to assist in appropriate job selection.

- In voluntary work trials/supported placements:
  - assistance with job applications and interview preparation/behaviour
  - selecting work trials and long-term work placements with scope for a high degree of structure and clear expectations/boundaries
  - explicit explanation to the employer about the nature and potential impact of executive difficulties to reduce the risk of the client's difficulties being misconstrued (executive difficulties are often not readily apparent, especially during an induction period when jobs are often more tightly structured/supervised)
  - working closely with the person and supervisor (with short-term job coaching as necessary) to break down the specific requirement of the

job and to develop the work procedures, prompts, and compensation strategies necessary to meet these
- additional supervisory input to assist the client in organizing and prioritizing their work, boundary-setting, and managing time, fatigue, and work pressures.
♦ In ongoing placement monitoring/support:
  - setting up external mechanisms for monitoring and facilitating feedback of work performance and behaviour (including adherence to health and safety policies) in order to make necessary work adjustments and refine or develop new strategies
  - close liaison with close family or friends to obtain feedback of how the client is coping after work and in reaching a positive and sustainable work–life balance
  - ongoing availability of assistance in understanding and responding to difficulties that arise in relationships with colleagues and supervisors
  - proactive review and follow-up to assist the client and supervisor in recognizing and responding to any emerging difficulties and/or adjusting to change as the job role/requirements evolve over time and/or the client seeks career progression.

Through a combination of the core components of a specialist brain injury vocational rehabilitation programme and the provision of the above individual interventions, the Working Out programme has sought to manage the vocational needs of people with executive difficulties. The particular needs of people with executive difficulties has required close collaboration with Jobcentre Plus Disability Employment Advisors (DEAs)/Work Psychologists (and other vocational services) regarding the following: suitability and timing of individual referrals for specialist assessment, work preparation, and/or job retention; pooling of assessment results; joint goal-setting, monitoring, and progress review; joint consideration of ongoing support needs. Joint working across agencies is particularly important for people with executive difficulties as their difficulties are often not readily apparent or are misconstrued by those without brain injury training and experience. Joint working is also important for those with training and experience because of the challenging and ongoing nature of vocational needs and the need to pool brain injury and vocational expertise and resources.

Conclusions

Many people with ABI are unable to return to previous or alternative employment or other occupation. Executive difficulties are a key factor in limiting successful vocational outcome. In the UK people with ABI frequently do not receive the specialist support they require. This reflects a combination of under-developed brain injury services, shortage of both specialist ABI vocational rehabilitation and suitable alternative occupational provision, and a lack of joint working, both across statutory agencies and with independent vocational providers. However, there is consistent evidence worldwide of the value of specialist ABI vocational rehabilitation programmes.

It is hoped that the quality requirement on vocational rehabilitation in the National Service Framework for Long-term Conditions (Department of Health 2005) will provide impetus for services in developing their practice in assessing, preparing, and supporting people with ABI in their return to previous or alternative occupations. It is essential that the needs of people with executive difficulties are taken into account throughout the vocational rehabilitation process: in formal and practical assessments; in fostering awareness of vocational restrictions; in developing and evaluating coping strategies; in setting up and monitoring work trials; in job-matching and assisted job search/application; in placement set-up and support. It is vital both to build strategies for managing executive difficulties into the structure of the ABI vocational rehabilitation process and also to recognize the need for considerable individual input, close liaison with both supervisor and family, proactive review/follow-up and the availability of long-term specialist support to reduce the risk of avoidable breakdown in work placements.

Current statutory service provision and funding in the UK requires ABI rehabilitation services to work in partnership with Jobcentre Plus and vocational providers to address these needs through integrated brain injury and vocational rehabilitation expertise. There is an urgent need for research into the relative efficacy of models of brain injury vocational rehabilitation in general and of the management of executive difficulties in the workplace in particular.

References

Abrams, D., Barker, L.T., Haffey, W., and Nelson, H. (1993). The economics of return to work for survivors of traumatic brain injury: vocational services are worth the investment. *Journal of Head Trauma Rehabilitation*, **8**, 59–76.

Bach, L.J. and David, A.S. (2006). Self-awareness after acquired and traumatic brain injury. *Neuropsychological Rehabilitation*, **16**, 397–414.

Bamdad, M.J., Ryan, L.M., and Warden, D.L. (2003). Functional assessment of executive abilities following traumatic brain injury. *Brain Injury*, **17**, 1011–20.

Ben-Yishay, T., Silver, S.M., Piasetsky, E., and Rattok, J. (1987). Relationship between employability and vocational outcome after intensive holistic cognitive rehabilitation. *Journal of Head Trauma Rehabilitation*, **2**, 35–48.

Bolton, B. and Roessler, R. (1986a). *Manual for the Work Personality Profile*. Arkansas Research and Training Center in Vocational Rehabilitation, University of Arkansas, Fayetteville, AK.

Bolton, B. and Roessler, R. (1986b). The Work Personality Profile: factor scales, reliability, validity and norms. *Vocational Evaluation and Work Adjustment Bulletin*, **19**, 143–9.

Brooks, N., McKinlay, W., Symington, C., Beattie, A., and Campsie, L. (1987). Return to work within the first seven years of severe head injury. *Brain Injury*, **1**, 5–19.

BSRM/JCP/RCP (2004). *Vocational assessment and rehabilitation after acquired brain injury: Inter-Agency guidelines* (ed A. Tyerman and M.J. Meehan). Inter-Agency Advisory Group on Vocational Rehabilitation after Brain Injury, London.

Buffington, A.L.H. and Malec, J.F. (1997). The vocational rehabilitation continuum: maximising outcomes though bridging the gap from hospital to community based services. *Journal of Head Trauma Rehabilitation*, **12**, 1–13.

Burgess, P.W. and Alderman, N. (2004). Executive dysfunction. In: *Clinical neuropsychology: a practical guide to assessment and management for clinicians* (ed L.H. Goldstein and J. McNeil), pp. 185–209. Wiley, Chichester.

Callaghan, C.D. (2001). The assessment and rehabilitation of executive function disorders. In: *Rehabilitation of neuropsychologiocal disorders* (ed B. Johnstone and H.H. Stonnington), pp. 87–124. Psychology Press, Philadelphia, PA.

Cattelani, R., Tanzi, F., Lombardi, F., and Mazzucchi, A. (2002). Competitive re-employment after severe traumatic brain injury: clinical, cognitive and behavioural predictive variables. *Brain Injury*, **16**, 51–64.

Cicerone, K.D. and Fraser, R.T. (2000). Counseling interactions for clients with traumatic brain injury. In: *Traumatic brain injury: practical vocational,neuropsychological and psychotherapy interventions* (ed R.T. Fraser and D.C. Clemmons), pp. 95–127. CRC Press, Boca Raton, FL.

Crepeau, F. and Scherzer, P. (1993). Predictors and indicators of work status after traumatic brain injury: a meta-analysis. *Neuropsychological Rehabilitation*, **3**, 5–35.

Crepeau, F., Scherzer, B.P., Belleville, S., and Desmarais, A.G. (1997). A qualitative analysis of central executive disorders in a real-life work situation. *Neuropsychological Rehabilitation*, **7**, 147–65.

Crewe, N.M. and Athelstan, G.T. (1981). Functional assessment in vocational rehabilitation: a systematic approach to diagnosis and goal-setting. *Archives of Physical Medicine and Rehabilitation*, **62**, 299–305.

Crewe, N.M. and Athelstan, G.T. (1984). *Functional Assessment Inventory: manual*. University of Wisconsin-Stout, Menonomie, WI.

Curl, R.M., Fraser, R.T., Cook, R.G., and Clemmons, D. (1996). Traumatic brain injury vocational rehabilitation: preliminary findings for the co-worker as trainer project. *Journal of Head Trauma Rehabilitation*, **11**, 75–85.

Department of Health (2005). *The National Service Framework for Long-term Conditions*. Department of Health, London.

Deshpande, P. and Turner Stokes, L. (2004). Survey of vocational rehabilitation services available to people with acquired brain injury in the UK. In: *Vocational assessment and rehabilitation after acquired brain injury: Inter-Agency guidelines*. Inter-Agency Advisory Group on Vocational Rehabilitation after Brain Injury, BSRM/JCP/RCP London.

Evans, J.J. (2008). Executive and attentional problems. In A Tyerman and NS King. Psychological approaches to rehabilitation after traumatic brain injury. Oxford: BPS Blackwell.

Ezrachi, O., Ben-Yishay, Y., Kay, T., Diller, L., and Rattok, J. (1991). Predicting employment in traumatic brain injury following neuropsychological rehabilitation. *Journal of Head Trauma Rehabilitation*, **6**, 71–84.

Fleming, J.M. and Ownsworth, T. (2006). A review of awareness interventions in brain injury rehabilitation. *Neuropsychological Rehabilitation*, **16**, 474–500.

Fraser, R.T. and Curl, R. (2000). Choice of a placement model. In: T*raumatic brain injury rehabilitation: practical vocational, neuropsychological and psychotherapy interventions* (ed R.T. Fraser and D.C. Clemmons), pp. 185–99. Boca Raton, FL: CRC Press.

Fraser, R., Dikmen, S., McLean, A., Miller, B., and Temkin, N. (1988). Employability of head injury survivors: first year post-injury. *Rehabilitation Counselling Bulletin*, **31**, 276–88.

Girard, D., Brown, J., Burnett-Stolnack, M., *et al.* (1996). The relationship of neuropsychological status and productive outcomes following traumatic brain injury, *Brain Injury*, **10**, 663–76.

Gordon, W.A., Cantor, J., Ashman, T., and Brown, M. (2006). Treatment of post-TBI executive dysfunction: application of theory to clinical practice. *Journal of Head Trauma Rehabilitation*, **21**, 156–67.

Groswasser, Z., Melamed, S., Agranov, E., and Keren, O. (1999). Return to work as an integrative measure following traumatic brain injury. *Neuropsychological Rehabilitation*, **9**, 493–504.

Ip, R.Y., Dornan, J., and Schentag, C. (1995). Traumatic brain injury: factors predicting return to work or school. *Brain Injury*, **9**, 517–32.

Johnson, R. (1987). Return to work after severe head injury. *International Disability Studies*, **9**, 49–54.

Johnson, R. (1998). How do people get back to work after severe head injury? A 10 year follow-up study. *Neuropsychological Rehabilitation*, **8**, 61–79.

Johnstone, B., Schopp, L.H., Harper, J., and Koscuilek, J. (1999). Neuropsychological impairments, vocational outcomes, and financial costs for individuals with traumatic brain injury receiving state vocational rehabilitation services. *Journal of Head Trauma Rehabilitation*, **14**, 220–32.

Johnstone, B., Vessell, R., Bounds, T., Hoskins, S., and Sherman, A. (2003). Predictors of success for state vocational rehabilitation services with traumatic brain injury. *Archives of Physical Medicine and Rehabilitation*, **84**, 161–7.

Kregel, J., Parent, W., and West, M. (1994). The impact of behavioral deficits on employment retention: an illustration from supported employment. *Neurorehabilitation*, **4**, 1–14.

Kreutzer, J.S., Wehman, P., Morton, M.V., and Stonnington, H.H. (1988). Supported employment and compensatory strategies for enhancing vocational outcome following traumatic brain injury. *International Disability Studies*, **13**, 162–71.

Kreutzer, J.S., Leininger, B.E., Sherron, P.D., and Groah, C.H. (1990). Managing psychosocial dysfunction. In: *Vocational rehabilitation for persons with traumatic brain injury* (ed P. Wehman and J.S. Kreutzer), pp. 33–69. Aspen Publications, Rockville, MD.

Kreutzer, J.S., Marwitz, J.H., Walker, W., *et al.* (2003). Moderating factors in return to work and job stability after traumatic brain injury. *Journal of Head Trauma Rehabilitation*, **18**, 128–38.

Langer, K.G. and Padrone, F.J. (1992). Psychotherapeutic treatment of awareness in acute rehabilitation of traumatic brain injury. *Neuropsychological Rehabilitation*, **2**, 59–70.

McCrimmon, S. and Oddy, M. (2006). Return to work following moderate-to-severe traumatic brain injury. *Brain Injury*, **20**, 1037–46.

Malec, J.F. and Moessner, A.M. (2006). Replicated positive results for the VCC model of vocational intervention after ABI within the social model of disability. *Brain Injury*, **20**, 227–236.

Murphy, L., Chamberlain, E., Weir, J., Berry, A., Nathaniel-James, D., and Agnew, R. (2006). Effectiveness of vocational rehabilitation following acquired bran injury: preliminary evaluation of a UK specialist rehabilitation programme. *Brain Injury*, **20**, 1119–29.

Oddy, M., Coughlan, A., Tyerman, A., and Jenkins, D. (1985). Social adjustment after closed head injury: a further follow-up seven years after injury. *Journal of Neurology, Neurosurgery and Psychiatry*, **48**, 564–8.

Olver, J.H., Ponsford, J.L., and Curran, C.A. (1996). Outcome following traumatic brain injury: a comparison between 2 and 5 years after injury. *Brain Injury*, **10**, 841–8.

Ownsworth, T. and McKenna, K. (2004). Investigation of factors related to employment outcome following traumatic brain injury: a critical review and conceptual model. *Disability and Rehabilitation*, **26**, 765–84.

Ponsford, J.L., Olver, J.H., and Curran, C. (1995). A profile of outcome: 2 years after traumatic brain injury. *Brain Injury*, **9**, 1–10.

Price, P.L. and Baumann, W.L. (1990). Working: the key to normalisation after brain injury. In: *The neuropsychology of everyday issues: issues in development and rehabilitation* (ed D.E. Tupper and K.D. Cicerone). Kluwer Academic, Boston, MA.

Prigatano, G.P. (2005). Disturbances of self-awareness and rehabilitation of patients with traumatic brain injury: a 20-year perspective. *Journal of Head Trauma Rehabilitation*, **20**, 19–29.

Ryan, T.V., Sautter, S.W., Capps, C.F., Meneese, W., and Marth, J.T. (1992). Utilizing neuropsychological measures to predict vocational outcome in a head trauma population. *Brain Injury*, **6**, 175–82.

Sander, A.M., Kreutzer, J.S., Rosenthal, M., Delmonico, R., and Young, M.E. (1996). A multi-center longitudinal investigation of return to work community integration following traumatic brain injury. *Journal of Head Trauma Rehabilitation*, **11**, 70–84.

Sander, A.M., Kreutzer, J.S., and Fernandez, C.C. (1997). Neurobehavioral functioning, substance abuse, and employment after brain injury: implications for vocational rehabilitation. *Journal of Head Trauma Rehabilitation*, **12**, 28–41.

Scherer, M., Bergloff, P., Levin, E., High, W.M., Oden, K.E., and Nick, T.G. (1998). Impaired awareness and employment outcome after traumatic brain injury. *Journal of Head Trauma Rehabilitation*, **13**, 52–61.

Scherer, M., Hart, T., Nick, T.G., Whyte, J., Thompson, R.N., and Yablon, S.A. (2003). Early impaired self-awareness after traumatic brain injury. *Archives of Physical Medicine and Rehabilitation*, **84**, 168–76.

Simpson. A. and Schmitter-Edgecombe, M. (2002). Prediction of employment status following traumatic brain injury using a behavioural measure of frontal lobe functioning. *Brain Injury*, **16**, 1075–91.

Teasdale, T.W., Hansen, S., Gade, A., and Christensen, A.-L. (1997). Neuropsychological test scores before and after brain-injury rehabilitation in relation to return to employment. *Neuropsychological Rehabilitation*, **7**, 23–42.

Thornhill, A., Teasdale, G.M., Murray, G.D., McEwan, J., Roy, C.W., and Penny, H.I. (2000). Disability in young people and adults one year after head injury: a prospective cohort study. *British Medical Journal*, **320**, 1631–5.

Turner, G.R. and Levine, B. (2004). Disorders of executive functioning and self-awareness. In: *Cognitive and behavioral rehabilitation: from neurobiology to clinical practice* (ed J. Ponsford), pp. 224–68. Guilford Press, New York.

Tyerman, A. and Young, K. (1999). Vocational rehabilitation after severe traumatic brain injury: evaluation of a specialist assessment programme. *Journal of the Application of Occupational Psychology to Employment and Disability*, **2**, 31–41.

Tyerman, A. and Young, K. (2000). Vocational rehabilitation after severe traumatic brain injury. II: Specialist interventions and outcomes. *Journal of the Application of Occupational Psychology to Employment and Disability*, **2**, 13–20.

Tyerman, A., Tyerman, R., and Viney, P. (2008) Vocational rehabilitation programmes. In: *Psychological approaches to rehabilitation after traumatic brain injury* (ed A. Tyerman and N.S. King). Blackwell, Oxford.

Uomoto, J.M. (2000). Application of the neuropsychological evaluation in vocational planning after brain injury. In: *Traumatic brain injury: practical vocational, neuropsychological and psychotherapy interventions* (ed R.T. Fraser and D.C. Clemmons), pp. 1–94. CRC Press, Boca Raton, FL.

von Cramon and Matthes-von Cramon, G. (1994). Back to work with a chronic dysexecutive syndrome? (Case report). *Neuropsychological Rehabilitation*, **4**, 399–417.

Warren, C.G. (2000). Use of assistive technology in vocational rehabilitation of persons with traumatic brain injury. In: *Traumatic brain injury: practical vocational, neuropsychological and psychotherapy interventions* (ed R.T. Fraser and D.C. Clemmons), pp. 129–60. CRC Press, Boca Raton, FL.

Weddell, R., Oddy, M., and Jenkins, D. (1980). Social adjustment after rehabilitation: a two year follow-up of patients with severe head injury. *Psychological Medicine*, **10**, 257–63.

Wehman, P., Kreutzer, J., Wood, W., Morton, M.V., and Sherron, P. (1988). Supported work model for persons with traumatic brain injury: toward job placement and retention. *Rehabilitation Counselling Bulletin*, **31**, 298–312.

Wehman, P., Kreutzer, J., Sale, P., West, M., Morton, M.V., and Diambra, J. (1989). Cognitive impairment and remediation: implications for employment following traumatic brain injury. *Journal of Head Trauma Rehabilitation*, **4**, 66–75.

Wehman, P., Kregel, J., Sherron, P., *et al.* (1993). Critical factors associated with the successful employment placement of patients with severe traumatic brain injury. *Brain Injury*, **7**, 31–44.

Wehman, P., Bricourt, J., and Targett, P. (2000). Supported employment for persons with traumatic brain injury: a guide for implementation. In: *Traumatic brain injury: practical vocational, neuropsychological and psychotherapy interventions* (ed R.T. Fraser and D.C. Clemmons), pp. 201–40. CRC Press, Boca Raton, FL.

Wehman, P., Kregel, J., Keyser-Marcus, L., *et al.* (2003). Supported employment for person with traumatic brain injury: a preliminary investigation of long-term follow-up costs and program efficiency. *Archives of Physical Medicine and Rehabilitation*, **84**, 192–6.

Wise, K., Ownsworth, T., and Fleming, J. (2005). Convergent validity of self-awareness measures and their association with employment outcome in adults following acquired brain injury. *Brain Injury*, **19**, 765–75.

Yasuda, S., Wehman, P., Targett, P., Cifu, D., and West, M. (2001). Return to work for persons with traumatic brain injury. *American Journal of Physical Medicine and Rehabilitation*, **80**, 852–64.

13

The use of smart technology in the management and rehabilitation of executive disorders

Roger Orpwood

Bath Institute of Medical Engineering, University of Bath

Introduction

There has been a growing interest in the use of intelligent homes to support people with a variety of disabilities (Bjørneby 1997; Dewsbury *et al.* 2004; Orpwood 2006). Initial work has focused on supporting people with physical disabilities (Gann *et al.* 1999), and these studies clearly showed the potential of such approaches. Most work on intelligent homes has used the established devices that have been available for automatic environmental control for many years and applied them to supporting the new client group (Porteus and Brownsell 2000). For people with physical disabilities, this approach was sensible and provided many benefits. However, when attempts were made to apply the same approach to people with cognitive problems it was clear that some rethinking was necessary. For example, one very useful development concerned the operation of bathroom taps. Taps that can be linked to smart home environments and can be operated purely by moving your hands under the tap have been available for some time. An infrared beam is activated that initiates the flow of water. Such remote activation is really useful for someone with poor hand function from, say, arthritis. However, such operations can be very confusing for someone with an executive disorder leading to cognitive problems. Understanding that moving your hands under the tap is needed in order to make water come out is cognitively challenging, and not part of common experience.

Therefore a new approach is needed for people with cognitive problems. The work to support people with cognitive problems that is being explored at the Bath Institute of Medical Engineering (BIME) has taken a very needs-led approach. Most of the original work has been carried out with people with dementia, but the basic principles apply to anyone with executive control problems. Rather than simply matching people against the technology that was available, the approach was to explore the needs of the client group in the first instance to obtain an understanding of the key issues that needed to be addressed (Jepson and Orpwood 2000). This understanding was then used to define potentially useful technology. If established technology were available, clearly this could be used, but there were many situations where it was quite obvious there was nothing suitable available, and a programme of new design and development was initiated (Orpwood *et al.* 2005). Therefore the work was very much needs led rather than technology led.

In this chapter we explore the way that this technology has been developed to support people with cognitive problems, and in particular executive disorders. We examine the kind of technology that is needed, and look at the results of some initial work in applying it. We discuss how this potentially very beneficial technology can be tailored to suit the needs of this client group.

What is smart home technology?

The smart home descriptor is somewhat over-employed these days, with many technologies using the 'smart' label to imply something with a bit of intelligence. Of course, manufacturers have jumped on the bandwagon in the hope that the label imbues some added value to their products. This has happened, for example, with Telecare technology where the manufacturers have been using the 'smart house' label for the last few years, even though Telecare is far from having much intelligence. It is often no more than a basic community alarm system that involves a round-the-clock call centre able to respond in an emergency or provide regular contact by telephone. The work described in this chapter uses technology that does include a level of intelligence, and is able to provide autonomous assistance rather than simply detecting problems and calling for help via call centres or through nurse call systems.

The infrastructure for providing homes with autonomous capabilities requires three key components: behaviour monitoring sensors, assistive support technology, and a communication link between the two (Figure 13.1).

Sensors

Sensing technology is used to monitor the behaviour of people in the home, or the way they interact with their environment. Many sensors are already available for the mainstream application of the technology. Components such

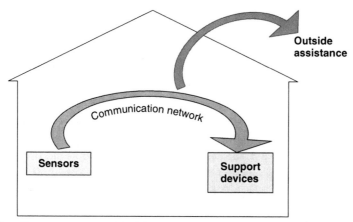

Fig.13.1 The components required for an autonomous smart home. Outside help is only required in the event of the home not being able to deal with problems itself.

as movement sensors using passive infra-red (PIR) units, similar to those used for burglar alarms, are well developed. For similar applications, sensors are available to monitor whether windows or doors are open. Further sensors have been developed as part of the current interest in Telecare technology, such as bed-occupancy sensors. However, there is an important need for further work to develop sensors that are specific to the needs of this client group. Some, such as toilet-usage monitors and fall detectors, are the subject of much current research (e.g. McKenna and Nait Charif 2005).

Support devices

Support technology is used to react to the information being provided by the sensors, and to try and assist the occupant to maintain independence and a good quality of life. It is in the area of support devices that most work is now needed. Again, some devices, such as automatic cooker shut-off valves (Gibbs *et al.* 2003), are fairly straightforward, but others, such as bath tap shut-off devices that do not take control away from the user, are still quite experimental. An important area of work, described in more detail below, is a means for providing prompts and reminders to occupants.

Communication bus

A key component of all autonomous installations is a means for all the sensors and the support devices to talk to each other. This communication is provided through what is known as a communication bus. This bus can simply be a set of extra wiring that links all the components together, but it can also be via a radio and, therefore, wireless link. The bus does rather more than just allow a sensor such as a bed-occupancy sensor to turn on a bedroom light. It has computing facilities embedded within it to enable judgements to be made about appropriate actions on the part of the support devices, depending on what the sensors are telling it. It also provides a means for coded messages to be sent from the sensors to the whole smart installation so that any component can know what has just happened. It also has facilities for checking that the message it has just sent out has been received, and will send the message repeatedly until this is assured. These systems were developed for providing automatic control in large public buildings such as airports, and needed to be extremely reliable and effective, and require minimal intervention. Therefore they are ideal for the kinds of application described here where someone's safety or security is at stake. The work undertaken in Bath has used a communication bus known as the European Installation Bus (EIB), which is now incorporated in the KNX system. It is the most popular system in Europe and many components are available, such as different sensors that can work with it. However, radio-based versions have only been made available recently, and the range is still rather limited. Other systems are in use, and one still evolving which looks to have much promise for these kinds of applications, particularly where radio communication is involved, is a system known as Ziggbee.

To recap, the sensors monitor the user's behaviour, and this monitoring provides the basis for judgements to be made about how the user can be helped. The communication bus is able to listen to all the sensors and to talk to appropriate support devices to initiate their action, depending on the judgements made by its embedded computer. In many ways the effective function of an autonomous smart installation is to emulate the behaviour of a good carer, but of course without getting tired or frustrated or emotionally involved in other ways. However, what the technology cannot do is to replace the love, affection, personal understanding, and social interaction that a carer can provide. Some have criticized the work for that reason. If service providers see the technology as a complete replacement of human carers, possibly with a view to saving money, then this criticism would be valid. However, most can see that there is a lot of potential for this kind of technology to augment personal human care, and in many ways it can be more effective in situations where constant close monitoring is needed. It can also provide the client with some dignity and self respect by giving them some independence and low-level back-up for daily activities, without having to rely on human carers or interventions from others to resolve their difficulties.

What kind of support can be provided?

Examples of technology

What sort of support can this technology provide? A few examples can illustrate its potential. Sensors can detect user's movements around their living space and use this information to provide support. This support could simply be turning off appliances that had been forgotten about, like the cooker or the bath taps. It could provide automatic lighting when someone gets out of bed at night to provide orientation and help prevent falls. However, such systems really come into their own when they are linked to voice prompting devices. For example, if someone was confused about time and tended to go out of the house at inappropriate times, it is quite easy to detect their movement near an external door and, knowing that it is an inappropriate time to go out, to prompt them with a message to that effect. Similarly, if someone was prone to getting up in the middle of the night and becoming a little disoriented, their movements and the fact that they were out of bed could be used to provide them with a prompt about the time and to suggest that they go back to bed. If a user had a habit of putting something on the cooker and wandering off, they could be prompted when they left the room. The house could intervene to turn the cooker off if smoke were detected or the kettle had boiled dry, or with appropriate sensors turn off a gas cooker if the gas had not been lit.

Voice prompts

When voice prompts were originally planned some concern was expressed about how people would react to them. It was felt that users with cognitive problems would become anxious and a little alarmed about voices coming out of nowhere. When the use of such prompts was originally explored, the voices came out of appliances that people expected voices to emanate from, such as the TV or the radio. This was quite difficult to configure but could be done. If the radio was off it would be automatically turned on to play a message. If it were on, and playing a broadcast, it would be overridden to play the message. However. some work was carried out using simple speaker boxes, and these were found to be just as effective (Orpwood *et al.* 2004). Users were not at all concerned about the disembodied voice. They could see that the voice was coming out of a box, and it was part of their common experience that voices come out of things like tape recorders and record players.

It was unclear as to what would be the best voice to use. Should it be a known voice or an anonymous one? Should it perhaps be the person's own voice? A concern was expressed that the voice ought not be recognizable as the user might think the speaker was in the home, and go looking for him/her.

For this reason, all the early voice prompts used a warm anonymous voice. However, it was found that people do not behave inappropriately if they hear a voice that they recognize. On the contrary, it appears that people respond better to a voice they trust, which inevitably means that it is recognized. Recent work with a client with quite severe dementia (MMSE score of 10) has found that he has no problem with his daughter's voice coming out of speaker boxes mounted in the rooms (Evans *et al.* 2007). He knows that she is not really there, but he also knows that she cares for him and would give him good advice. When the system was set up various messages were recorded for him to use. His daughter was asked to imagine she was standing next to her father when, for example, he was about to go outside in the middle of the night, and to talk to him in a way that she felt would prompt him to respond. Her messages were quite assertive and even a little angry, and there was a concern that they might just upset or alienate him. However, they have worked very well, and when asked about her tone of voice the daughter said that she knew that this was the kind of tone that her father would respond to if she had to advise him. Her father is quite accepting and pleased with the messages, and accepts that they help him. The messages would appear to have some emotional value because, despite his dementia, he can relate the content of the messages during subsequent interviews.

Some of this experience of using voice prompts has been applied to people with acquired brain injuries, and the indications are that they are well accepted and acted upon. They have much potential for providing prompts and reminders for people with memory problems.

Flexibility

One of the benefits of the kind of technology that has been discussed is the flexible way in which it can be applied. Of course, people are very different and their needs vary enormously. Their needs will also change with time. Such variability could be seen as a real problem, but the nature of autonomous smart environments is that it is fairly easy to adapt the technology to match the needs of the user. Some users may only need some lighting support at night. Others might benefit from simple prompts for things they tend to forget. Others might require something more substantial to deal with their problems of wandering or forgetful use of household appliances. All can benefit from the same installation, but it has to be configured by simple adjustments to suit their needs.

There are two issues which need to be dealt with to realize the inherent flexibility of these systems. It is fairly easy for an engineer to make the software adjustments once they have been identified, but it would be very confusing for a care professional without engineering skills. There is a real need for autonomous installations to be designed to allow easy changes to be made by intelligent but non-technical carers. The second important issue concerns the definition of the user's needs. Many aspects will be understood from prior assessments of the user carried out by occupational therapists and psychologists, but there are often issues which only come to light following the detailed monitoring that smart environments can provide. There is a need for careful procedures to be put in place to allow the tailoring of the environment for the individual to be an ongoing process, and for the system to provide care staff with constant reports of how the user is getting on.

Installations

To provide a home with the abilities described requires installation of the sensors, the support devices, and the communication bus. Of these, the one that can cause the most problems and most disruption is the communication linkage. If a new-build care home is being planned, it could make sense to install a hard-wired communication bus throughout new development, terminating the cabling in strategic positions within the rooms so that sensors and support devices can be connected at a later date according to the client's needs. However, it is extremely difficult to anticipate accurately where such wiring should terminate, and there always appears to be a need for a lot of extra wiring when it comes to subsequently installing the smart equipment. When such hard-wired systems are to be installed in people's homes the situation is far worse. The installer will probably have to bury wires in the plaster or take up floor boards, and the whole process would be extremely disruptive. This could be a very traumatic experience for clients with cognitive problems.

Radio-based systems have many advantages because of ease of installation and adaptability. Sensors and support devices can be placed where required for a particular client, and therefore retrospective installations in people's own homes are much less disruptive and far quicker. The downside for radio-based systems is that they require electrical power from somewhere, and this usually means battery power for most of the equipment. The installed devices will indicate when their batteries are getting flat, but the use of batteries means that a battery-checking and replacement policy is required to ensure that they are replaced before they go completely flat and lose their function, with potentially dangerous consequences. Fortunately, battery life is quite good with modern devices, and with the advent of communication protocols such as Ziggbee with excellent power management, the battery life for many appliances would be over a year. The other downside with radio-based systems is the existence of radio dead-spots where communication to a sensor or support device would not be possible. However, a good installer would check such things, and find alternative placements.

In recent developments, the power management issue has been addressed by the use of so-called power scavenging. The power levels needed for, say, signalling that a light switch has been turned on are very low. Power scavenging utilizes the user's own actions to generate some power. For example, the act of turning on a switch will generate some power, and this can be collected and used to augment the power being supplied from the battery. In this way such sensors could run almost indefinitely without any battery changing being needed. Such approaches will only work for very-low-power situations, such as switches or for movement sensors, and would not be appropriate where large amounts of power are needed, such as tap turning-off devices.

In conclusion, it is likely that the use of radio-based system will be the system of choice for many of these kinds of installations, even in the case of new buildings.

Application of the technology to people with acquired brain injuries

The basic work described above was mostly carried out with people with dementia, but the problems tackled were very similar to those experienced by people with ABIs. Some applications of the technology to this group are described below.

Needs surveys

Much technology has been developed that can potentially provide the basic structure for an intelligent smart home environment for people with ABIs. In order to assess its potential, and to highlight any further developments needed, it is important to try to obtain a better understanding of the needs of such clients, and to assess these needs in the light of the kind of interventions that can be provided. An initial study was carried out using paper records to identify when problems arose during the day for a group of people with brain injuries, and when interventions were necessary to provide support. Originally care staff were asked to keep notes of all the interventions they provided over a month-long period. However, it was found that the records were not comprehensive, and often missed crucial data that would be relevant to the provision of automatic support. The exercise was repeated using observations from psychology assistants over a shorter period. A large amount of data was collected, and was categorized according to the issues that arose. Table 13.1 categorizes the data into various difficulties such as sleeping problems, problems with toileting, etc. It shows that there are many issues that cause problems, and it also provides some quantitative information about their relative importance.

Automatic lifestyle monitoring

The data collected from these exercises was useful in that it identified issues to be tackled, but it did not provide very detailed information about their nature or about the user's behaviour in relation to them. Therefore a further exercise was carried out using automatic data collection via sensors. Such systems provide very good lifestyle-monitoring capabilities, and can show the way that the user is interacting with their environment in great detail. Several sensors have been developed for this work. These include movement monitors based on PIR sensors, bed-occupancy monitors, and monitors to detect door opening. Each sensor contains a small data logger that records all the events that triggered it, and when they occurred. The loggers can subsequently be attached to a computer to download the information stored. By using the data collected from all the sensors a picture can be generated of the user's behaviour during the monitoring period.

Figure 13.2 shows some typical data for a client in a sheltered environment who was having problems with sleeping. As can be seen he was out of bed frequently during the night. Some of these episodes were clearly to go to the toilet, but during many he just wandered about his apartment. A paper record would just have reported that he had had a disturbed night, but the lifestyle monitoring enabled a much clearer picture to be generated of how he had behaved during the night and gave much more insight into the problem he was experiencing. Such data can be very helpful for making judgements about what sort of interventions would be helpful for clients because it is very detailed, and by definition objective. Of course, it still requires judgements to be made about what kind of intervention might be supportive, but it enables those judgements to be based on a much clearer picture of what is going on. The other major advantage of using such lifestyle monitoring is that, once interventions have been provided, it can provide a great deal of data about how effective the interventions have been, and can be used to quantify their outcome.

Sensors can uncover unknown behaviours

Another client in a sheltered housing scheme had such an installation provided. His assessment prior to moving in showed that he had some continence

Table 13.1 Analysis of data from paper study of the difficulties faced in the home by people with acquired brain injury

No.	Sex	Age group	Calling for help in the night	Getting dressed approp.	Knowing right time to get up	Taking medication correct time	Remembering correct dosage	Understand reason for taking medicine
1	M	51–60	1	2	1	2	3	1
2	M	51–60	1	1	1	2	1	1
3	M	51–60		1	1			
4	M	41–50						
5	M	41–50	2	3	3			
6	F	41–50	1	1	1			1
7	M	21–30	1	1	1	1	1	1
8	M	21–30	1	1	1	3	3	1
9	F	<20						
10	M	?	3	3	3			
11	?	?						
12	F	31–40	2	1	2	3	4	4
13	M	21–30	1	2	2	4	3	4
14	M	41–50	1	3	3	1	1	2
15	M	31–40	4	4	4	4	4	4
16	M	31–40	1	1	1	1	1	1
17	M	41–50	1	2	1			2
18	M	51–60	2	2	1	2	2	2
19	M	41–50	1	1	2	2	4	2
20	M	21–30	1	2	3	1		2
21	M	21–30	1	2	2	1	1	1
22	F	41–50	1	1	1			
23	M	21–30	3		3			
24	F	31–40	1	2	2	4	4	4
1	NOT A PROBLEM		14	9	10	5	5	7
2	OCCASIONAL PROBLEM		3	7	5	4	1	5
3	REGULAR PROBLEM		2	3	5	2	3	0
4	VERY SERIOUS		1	1	1	3	4	4
TOTAL SCORE			30	36	39	31	32	33
NUMBER OF PEOPLE			20	20	21	14	13	16
AVERAGE			1.50	1.80	1.86	2.21	2.46	2.06

Using appliances safely	Choosing approp. food to eat	Keeping home clean	Dealing with laundry	Regulating heating in the home	Handling money	Shopping	Forgetting time/date/ year etc	Using the telephone
2	2	2	2	3	2	2	2	1
1	1	2	2	2	1	1	1	1
2	2	2	3	4	1	2	3	3
4	1						4	3
2	1	1	2		2	2	2	2
2	1	2	1	2	2	1	1	1
2	2	2	2	4	2	2	1	1
	3	1	1	1	3	4	3	2
3	3	3	2	2	4	3	2	2
4	4	4	3		4	4	4	2
1	1	1	1	1	1	1	3	4
4	4	4	4	4	4	4	2	4
1	1	2	1	1	1	1	1	
	1	2			3	2	3	2
2	2				2	2	2	1
2	2	3	3	3	2	2	2	2
	1		1	1	4		3	1
	2	2	1	1	1		3	1
2	1	1	2		1	2	2	1
	1						3	4
3	4	4	4	4	3	3	3	1
3	10	4	6	5	6	4	4	9
8	6	8	6	3	6	8	7	6
2	2	2	3	2	3	2	8	2
3	3	3	2	4	4	3	2	3
37	40	38	35	33	43	38	50	39
16	21	17	17	14	19	17	21	20
2.31	1.90	2.24	2.06	2.36	2.26	2.24	2.38	1.95

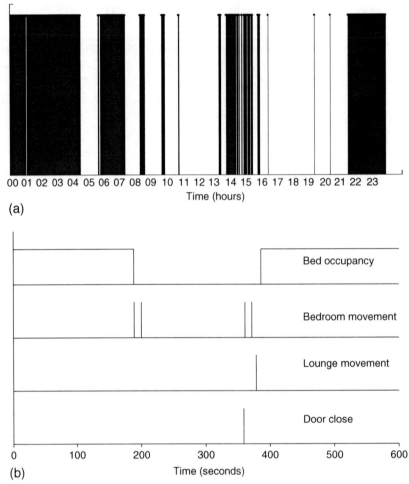

Fig.13.2 (a) Bed occupancy shown for a 24-hour period starting from midnight. (b). Details of bed occupancy and movements within an apartment for a 10-minute period during the night.

problems and a tendency to wander at night, but was mostly quite inactive. A standard set of smart technology had been installed in his apartment, and prior to any of the support devices being activated the sensors were used to record his behaviour in a similar manner to that described above. In this case the house had been fitted with a compete smart home infrastructure, and so the computer embedded within in it could directly log all the information provided by the sensors, as well as its own support activities. The initial recording period showed that his behaviour was much more complex than had previously been understood (Evans *et al.* 2007). For example, he did interact with the cooker,although his family and care-staff were quite adamant that he never did any cooking. His night-time wandering was also quite severe, and his behaviour when he got out of bed also showed signs of confusion, particularly about the location of the toilet. He seemed to follow a very complicated path through the apartment before he went to the toilet (Figure 13.3(a)). These data were invaluable in providing an understanding of his difficulties and for planning appropriate interventions. What came as a complete surprise was that he was getting very little sleep at night (average of 3.53 hours per night). With automatic lighting at night, including toilet guidance and messages from his carer to encourage him to go back to bed rather than wander about the apartment or to go outside, his sleep increased to an average of 5.39 hours per night (Figure 13.3(b)) and his wandering out of the flat markedly reduced. He also had far fewer toileting accidents.

The sensors and the data-logging used for the work described above were purpose designed for the project. However, a number of other groups are exploring this kind of lifestyle monitoring and ways in which the data can be presented to give care-staff a clear view of what has been going on (e.g. Perry *et al.* 2004), although there are clearly problems in interpreting such complex behavioural data (Hanson *et al.* 2007). Some of this work has translated into commercial products. A system known as JustChecking has been quite successful. It uses a small series of sensors that can be simply mounted on the wall using self-adhesive Velcro. The sensors have a radio link to a centralized data logger which sends the information to a secure web-site. The data can then be downloaded onto a PC for display. This kind of technology is clearly going to be a very useful tool for care staff to ascertain in more detail how their clients are getting on, and to assess the outcome of interventions. A major issue with this technology is how the data is presented. For research purposes it is important to obtain quite detailed indications of how someone is behaving on a second-by-second basis. However, for use in a care setting it would be more important to provide automatic interpretation of the data that would be meaningful to care staff and the kind of understanding they require. For example, some processing of the data that would indicate that the client was feeling anxious or restless, or flagged up how long the client had been sleeping, would be much more useful. Some work on manipulating such data for these purposes has been completed (Evans *et al.* 2007), but much more needs to be done in this area in collaboration with care staff. A large amount of useful data can be collected, but it will all go to waste unless some kind of intelligent automatic interpretation is possible.

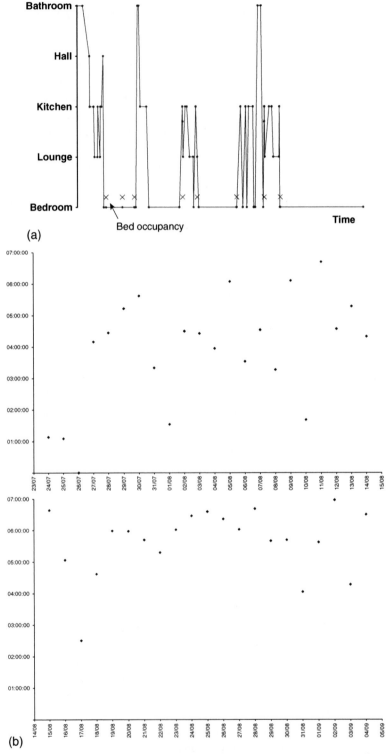

Fig.13.3 (a). Complex movements around an apartment, and bed occupancy, from midnight to 2 a.m. for a client showing signs of confusion, before support equipment was turned on. (b). Bed occupancy before and after turning on support equipment.

The need for close involvement of users

It would be useful to relate a case study that illustrates very well the importance of close user involvement to enable appropriate support to be provided. A client reported being restless at night, and staff complained that he would often wander out of his room. A wander reminder was tried with him. These devices just detect movement near a door during the night and replay a message to discourage the client from going out. He was happy to have one installed but it did not really make much difference. He would still go looking for staff in the night. Discussions with him indicated that his sleeping was severely affected by night-time anxieties. He reported that he would often wake up with some deep concern that he wished to talk about, and could not get back to sleep. He said that he knew his memory was poor, and that if he had waited until the morning he would have forgotten all about the issue that was bothering him. Consequently, he would try to find a staff member to relay his anxious thoughts. Given this understanding, a piece of technology was developed for him. He was asked how he would feel if he were provided with a voice recorder that would enable him to record his concerns during the night rather than go and search for a staff member. He could then replay it to the staff in the morning. He seemed quite happy with this proposal as it meant that the issue would still be dealt with in the morning even though he knew he would have forgotten about it. Care staff felt that normal recorders would be too difficult for him to operate, and after discussion with him a design was constructed that just used one large 'record' button on the top. He found this very easy to operate, as he just had to reach over to his bedside cabinet, press the button, and say what was bothering him. Several messages could be recorded.

The device was partially successful. He was able to use it, and was happy that it was an effective substitute for finding care staff to talk to in the night. Unfortunately, the messages that he recorded were not very coherent, and it was difficult for care staff to understand what was bothering him. Although he could not remember what the issue was by the morning, he realized that care staff were not clear about what was bothering him, and this decreased his satisfaction with this method of reporting his concerns. Therefore the device was not completely successful, but the experience is included to give an insight into both the potential of simple technological interventions once a clear understanding of the problem is known, and the need for close and careful involvement of the user in any design solutions.

Interactions between technology and people

Behaviour monitoring

A key aim of the use of sensors is to enable the house to make judgements about the behaviour of the occupants. These behavioural judgements can in turn be used to initiate the action of a support device, or to call for assistance. For example, the bed-occupancy sensors can be used to make a judgement about whether someone is in bed or not, and then turn on lights accordingly. Movement sensors can be used to make a judgement about whether the occupant is showing signs of restlessness, and then initiate a voice prompt to encourage the occupant to go back to bed. Such judgements are relatively easy for human carers to make. For personal carers there is an understanding of the person's behaviour from a history of living with the person. The carer would know the particular circumstances occurring at any given time that might be affecting behaviour, and, of course, carers have that crucial human capability of empathy, of being able to intimately relate to how the person is feeling at any given moment. Consequently, the judgement of human carers about when to provide assistance, and what kind of help to give, are based on a very sophisticated understanding of the user's requirements. (Of course, it is common experience that some people are far more skilful in this area than others.) Trying to emulate such approaches through the use of technology is bound to be very difficult, and quite crude in its application. The technology can mostly only respond according to the algorithms, or programme plans, built into it. These, in turn, have been designed according to very simple cause-and-effect rules that reflect the designer's general understanding of the significance of the information that has been obtained. This information is primarily the sensor data, although it is possible for the system to take past behaviour of the user into account.

Therefore the technology is quite primitive in its ability to make accurate judgements about user's behaviour, and it is often likely to be inaccurate. Therefore the kind of support that it can initiate is often going to be far from ideal. This is an important issue because so much exploratory work in this field is technology led, and assumes that these judgements are much easier to make and much more accurate than they often are. If judgements are being made about whether someone is in bed or not, these errors would be annoying, and possible confusing, but are not likely to affect the user's safety. However, if judgements are made about the occupant's use of a cooker, there is a real risk that the user's safety could be compromised.

An illustration of the difficulty of making such judgements with cookers concerns a system used to assess whether someone had left a pan or kettle on too long, and it had boiled dry. The technology was based around simple infra-red sensors. These sensors looked at the side of the pan, and could provide information about the temperature of the pan from the infra-red light that is emitted. The pan temperatures monitored can determine within a few seconds if a pan has boiled dry. Based on these observations a simple sensor system was developed that was mounted at the side of a cooker and looked at one spot on the side of the pan on a cooker ring (Figure 13.4). Figure 13.5 shows the kind of data that such a sensor collected. As can be seen the signal increased as the pan was being heated to boiling, then stayed the same during boiling, and then rapidly increased when the pan boiled dry. It was hoped that the rapid increase when the pan boiled dry could be detected, and used to turn off the ring.

Unfortunately, the behaviour of people is more complicated than this simple model assumes. When cooking, people will often turn the heat up and down. They will move pans around between rings. These and other behaviours make it very difficult to use the raw sensor data to make a judgement about what is going on. In order to develop appropriate control algorithms it is important in these situations to collect a lot of data from real-life usage of cookers to see how people react, and to try and design the algorithm to accommodate the variabilities that occur. Having followed this procedure, it was anticipated that the algorithm could make a correct judgement about 80 per cent of the time. This was a high rate, but still meant that in 20 per cent of the cases it was making wrong judgements. The next step was to allow false-positive decisions, where the cooker turned itself off even though there was no danger, but this proved to be very irritating to users. In such a situation it might be possible to improve the success rate by incorporating learning capabilities in the control software so that the cooker adapted to the kind of behaviour displayed by a particular user, but even then the success rate would not be 100%. It has to be accepted that the judgements being made when human behaviour is involved are probabilistic and that there will be errors. Consequently, it is very important that some form of back-up is provided to deal with these errors. In the case of the cooker it was decided that if any of the sensors continued to indicate danger for more than a short time after the cooker had acted to prevent it, the house would turn the whole cooker off, or shut off the gas if it was a gas cooker, and then call for some assistance. The helper would then have to check that everything was in order before turning the cooker on again. Such back-up facilities are very important when dealing with the variability of human behaviour, and safety critical judgements are being made.

User interactions

Most of the technology discussed does not require much in the way of direct user interaction. It has a monitoring role, and it is linked to simple support devices that are brought into play in an autonomous fashion. This is the beauty of smart home technology. Its operation is not dependent on the executive

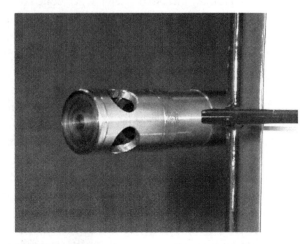

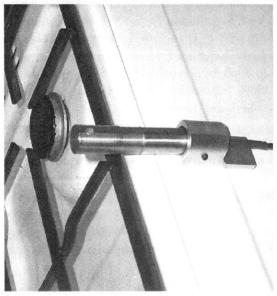

Fig.13.4 Pan-boiling-dry sensor mounted on the side of a cooker.

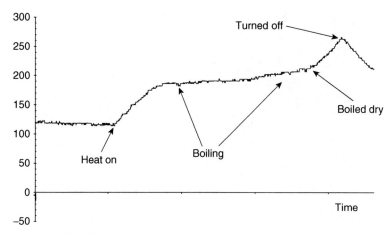

Fig.13.5 Raw data from a sensor showing the time course of pan temperature as the pan boiled dry.

skills of the user. However, there is still a need for some interaction and choice on the part of the user. Interactions can be quite simple. If a cooker monitor detects that excessive smoke is being generated by hot fat and turns the cooker off, it needs to provide the user with some feedback and the opportunity to resolve the situation. The feedback can probably best be done using voice information, but if the user is given the opportunity to turn the system back on there will inevitable be some interaction and control that the user has to follow. The same requirement can arise from specialist devices such as the night-time message system described above. The user had to initiate the recording facility. If such interactions are going to be done confidently, and effectively, by the user, some thought has to be given to the nature of such controls. A useful rule of thumb for users with executive problems is to make controls look and feel familiar to ones experienced before. Therefore no learning is involved.

The approach of maintaining familiarity works quite well, but this is not always possible. However, evidence is emerging that for all such users it is possible to develop controls that are very intuitive to use. For example, a simple music player was developed that enabled someone with cognitive problems to turn it both on and off and to select the kind of recorded music they wished to listen to (Figure 13.6) (Orpwood *et al.* 2007; Sixsmith *et al.* 2007). The controls typically fitted to recorded music players, with their multitude of small buttons and little lights, would be quite inappropriate for these users. The simple music player stored many recordings, like an MP3 player. It was turned on and off by lifting and shutting its lid, like an old

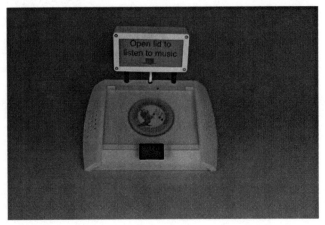

Fig.13.6 Music player designed to be very intuitive to operate by someone with cognitive problems.

musical box. Inside was a large illuminated and raised button decorated with icons that communicated 'music'. When the user pressed the button the player changed the kind of music it was playing, like changing a CD. Users just pressed the button until something arose that they wanted to listen to at that time. These simple controls worked well, but they were far more than just a good idea on the part of the designer. A lot of time was spent with potential users exploring in an iterative manner how they reacted to different kinds of controls, and evolving systems that were intuitive. The design of such controls requires a lot of work with users, and certainly is not something that can be done successfully from a third-party understanding of the issues.

Future

The technology used for autonomous homes is developing all the time, and this development is being directed by the accumulating experience of what works and what still causes problems. It is clear that wireless-based sensors and support devices will continue to evolve further until a truly comprehensive range of equipment is available. The power management of these devices is also likely to improve with time. It is also likely that adaptive control systems will be used more. Such systems learn from their experiences, and so adapt themselves more closely to the behaviour and the needs of the individual (e.g. Mozer 2004). A number of such systems are being investigated, and these are likely to become more mainstream. The link between technology and service provision reqires much research, and this area will surely see many improvements.

It is important to ensure that care plans can easily be adapted to incorporate the facilities the technology can provide, and for the technology to link into the kind of clinical information required for revision of care plans. There is a need for the information collected from the sensors to be made available in an easily understandable form to give care-providers more insight into how the user is getting on. But, most importantly for the future of this technology, there is a real need to gain far more experience of how users react to these systems. What are the main benefits? What are the problems? Confident adoption of the technology will only take place once this evidence is available and confirmed by different evaluation programmes.

Conclusions

The use of autonomous smart environments for people with executive problems is still in its infancy and many issues need exploring. However, there is no doubt that the potential of the technology has been demonstrated. It can provide support alongside human care and augment the assistance that support staff can provide. Its future development and the work needed to realize its potential depends very much on ensuring such developments are user led. Its development has to reflect a growing understanding of how people can interact with the technology, and how its support can be applied most effectively. Given these important provisos, the use of smart technology has an important future in the care of people with executive disorders.

References

Bjørneby, S. (1997). *The BESTA flats in Tonsberg. Using technology for people with dementia.* Human Factors Solutions, Oslo.

Dewsbury, G., Clarke, K., Rouncefield, M., Sommerville, I., Taylor, B., and Edge, M. (2004). Designing acceptable 'smart' home technology to support people in the home. *Technology and Disability*, **15**, 191–201.

Evans, N., Orpwood, R., Adlam, T., Chadd, J., and Self, D. (2007). Evaluation of an enabling smart flat for people with dementia. *Journal of Dementia Care*, **15**, 33–6.

Gann, D., Barlow, J., and Venables, T. (1999). *Digital futures: making homes smarter.* Chartered Institute of Housing, Coventry.

Gibbs, C., Adlam, T., Faulkner, R., and Orpwood, R. (2003). Development of a cooker monitor for people with dementia. In *Assistive technology: shaping the future* (ed G.M. Craddock, L.P. McCormack, R.B. Reilly, and H.T.P. Knops), pp. 771–5. IOS Press, Amsterdam.

Hanson, J., Osipovic, D., Hine, N., Amaral, T., Curry, R., and Barlow, J. (2007). Lifestyle monitoring as a predictive tool in telecare. *Journal of Telemedicine and Telecare*, **13** (Suppl 1), 26–8.

Jepson, J. and Orpwood, R. (2000). The use of SMART home technology in dementia care. *Proceedings of the Annual Conference of the College of Occupational Therapy.*

McKenna, S.J. and Nait Charif, H. (2005). Summarising contextual activity and detecting unusual inactivity in a supportive home environment. *Pattern Analysis and Applications*, **7**, 386–401.

Mozer, M.C. (2004). Lessons from an adaptive house. In: *Smart environments: technology, protocols, and applications* (ed D. Cook and S. Sas), pp. 273–94. John Wiley, Hoboken, NJ.

Orpwood, R. (2006). Smart homes. In: *Principles and practice of geriatric medicine* (4th edn) (ed M. Pathy, J. Morley, and A.Sinclair), pp 189–198. John Wiley: Chichester.

Orpwood, R., Gibbs, C., Adlam, T., Faulkner, R., and Meegahawatte, D. (2004). The Gloucester Smart House for people with dementia: user-interface aspects. In: *Designing a more inclusive world* (ed S. Keates, J. Clarkson, P. Langdon, and P. Robinson), pp. 237–245. Springer-Verlag, London.

Orpwood, R., Gibbs, C., Adlam, T., Faulkner, R., and Meegahawatte, D. (2005). The design of smart homes for people with dementia: user-interface aspects. *Universal Access in the Information Society*, **4**, 156–64.

Orpwood, R., Sixsmith, A., Torrington, J., Chadd, J., Gibson, G., and Chalfont, G. (2007). Designing technology to support quality of life of people with dementia. *Technology and Disability*, **19**, 103–13.

Perry, M., Dowdall, A., Lines, L., and Hone, K. (2004). Multimodal and ubiquitous computing systems: supporting independent-living older users. *IEEE Transactions on Information Technology in Biomedicine*, **8**, 258–70.

Porteus, J. and Brownsell, S.J. (2000). *Using Telecare: exploring technologies for independent living for older people*. Anchor Trust, Oxford.

Sixsmith, A., Orpwood, R., and Torrington, J. (2007). Quality of life technologies for people with dementia. *Topics in Geriatric Rehabilitation*, **23**, 85–93.

14

The use of virtual reality in the assessment and rehabilitation of executive dysfunction

Paul Penn*, David Rose*, and
David Johnson†

*School of Psychology, The University of East London
†Child Life and Health, University of Edinburgh

Virtual reality: definition and brief overview

Virtual reality (VR), familiar to the layperson as the technology underpinning computer games, has been more usefully defined by Schultheis and Rizzo (2001) as 'an advanced form of human–computer interface that allows the user to interact with and become immersed in a computer-generated environment in a naturalistic fashion'. Whilst VR can take many forms (Isdale 1998), the form of most relevance to the present chapter is known as Window on World or Desktop VR. Here, a conventional computer monitor is used to present a virtual environment (VE) and users control their movement within, and interaction with, the VE by means of a joystick and/or keyboard.

The last decade has been a hugely exciting time for researchers interested in VR. This period has witnessed a truly remarkable growth in the power and, most importantly, the affordability of computer hardware and software which has taken VR, 'out of the realm of expensive toy and into that of functional technology' (Schultheis et al. 2002, p. 3). Indeed, the range of areas in which VR has been applied, for example engineering, defence, medicine, entertainment, art, education, design, and visualization (Stone 2002), is truly impressive.

The emergence of VR in neuropsychological rehabilitation

One application of VR that was identified over 10 years ago (Rose et al. 1996), but which has attracted increasing interest in recent times, is neuropsychological assessment and rehabilitation (Rizzo *et al.* 2004a). Empirical investigations in this area are looking very promising (Heyn *et al.* 2004). VR has been applied to a number of domains of cognitive assessment and rehabilitation, such as attention (Rizzo *et al.* 2004a), memory (Brooks *et al.* 2004), and spatial transformation (Rizzo *et al.* 1998).

VR and executive functioning

Lezak *et al.* (2004) proposed that executive functioning has four basic components: (1) volition, (2) planning, (3) purposive action, and (4) effective performance. Each of these components has associated behaviours. Volition involves determining what an individual needs or wants, i.e. a goal. Planning entails identifying and organizing what is required to achieve a desired goal. Purposive action relates to bringing a planned goal to fruition by initiating and regulating the orderly execution of appropriate sequences of action in order to achieve the desired goal. Finally, effective performance concerns an individual's ability to monitor their purposive actions and correct for mistakes/ineffective performance.

Deficits in executive function are usually, although not exclusively, the result of damage to the frontal lobes (Lo Priore *et al.* 2003) and can involve problems with one or more of the above components of executive functioning. Alderman and Burgess (2003) list 20 common deficits including problems with abstract thinking, temporal sequencing, apathy and lack of drive, lack of insight and social awareness, and loss of decision-making ability. The term 'dysexecutive syndrome' is often used to encompass such deficits. Deficits in executive functioning cause highly pervasive problems in daily life (Nies 1999).

The advantages of VR in the assessment and rehabilitation of executive dysfunction

The characteristics of VR that are of potential value in neuropsychological assessment and rehabilitation have been rehearsed comprehensively on several occasions (Rose *et al.* 1996, 2005; Rizzo *et al.* 2004). Several have particular relevance in the context of executive dysfunction. In the following sections some of these characteristics are outlined and are illustrated with reference to existing research on VR and executive dysfunction. Although the characteristics of VR discussed below are beneficial to both the assessment and rehabilitation of executive dysfunction, the research cited deals exclusively with assessment. This is simply a reflection of the research available at the time of the publication of this book.

Ecological validity

Elkind *et al.* (2001) argue that: 'The artificiality of executive functioning assessments limits their capacity to predict real-life functioning'. VR has the potential to address this problem of ecological validity. It has the capacity to simulate almost any real-world environment, from entire cities (e.g. Shopland *et al.* 2004) right down to a home environment (e.g. Brooks *et al.* 2004). VR can also be used to simulate situations and tasks that people experience in their daily lives, such as food preparation (Rose and Brooks 2004), shopping (Lo Priore *et al.* 2003), banking (Wallergård *et al.* 2002), office skills (Brooks *et al.* 2004), use of public transport (Brown *et al.* 1998), and driving (Liu *et al.* 1999, Lengenfelder *et al.* 2002, Rose *et al.* 2004).

Much of the work on executive functioning and VR to date has used analogues of existing assessments, presented in VR in order to address issues of ecological validity. For example, some of the earliest research into the application of VR to executive dysfunction used an immersive VR system, in which the VE is presented to the user via a head-mounted display (HMD), to replicate the features of the Wisconsin Card Sorting Task (WCST) (Pugnetti *et al.* 1995). This VE involved participants using visual cues (colour and shape) located on doors as matching criteria to use in navigating between a series of rooms and connecting corridors, whilst avoiding dead ends. The matching criteria were changed after every seven consecutive correct selections, so that the participants needed to evaluate and amend the effectiveness of their matching strategies to be successful. Pugnetti *et al.* (1998) compared the performance of patients with neurological impairments and non-impaired control participants on the WCST and their VR test and found that the controls performed better than patients in both tests, and that there was a modest correlation between the WCST and the VR test. Hit rates for the WCST and VR tests were 60.3 per cent and 71.4 per cent, respectively. Of particular note was that more patients were correctly classified by the VR test than by the WCST (68 per cent vs. 41 per cent). Interestingly, a clearly significant difference between patients and controls only emerged after the fourth category in the WCST, whereas this difference was apparent in the first category in the VR test. The authors suggested that: '...this finding depends on the more complex (and complete) cognitive demands of the VE setting at the beginning of the test when perceptuomotor, visuospatial (orientation), memory, and conceptual aspects of the task need to be fully integrated into an efficient routine' (Pugnetti *et al.* 1998, p.160). A test's sensitivity to 'integrative' difficulties is likely to be particularly relevant for the task of predicting real world capabilities.

The VR 'doors and rooms' task received additional support from Mendozzi *et al.* (1998) who conducted a detailed case study of a highly educated patient 2 years after sustaining a stroke. The results indicated that this VR test was successful in detecting deficits that adversely affected the patient's everyday life, yet were missed using traditional neuropsychological tests.

Another example of a VR analogue of an existing test of executive function, the Multiple Errands Test (Shallice and Burgess 1991), was developed by McGeorge *et al.* (2001). In this study, participants with traumatic brain injury (TBI), whose family members had indicated suffered with planning deficits, and healthy control participants were asked to complete both real-world and VR-based vocationally oriented planning tasks administered within a simulated work setting (an office). The tasks included collecting office equipment and preparing refreshments. Despite the patients not differing from normative values on the Behavioural Assessment of the Dysexecutive Syndrome (BADS) battery (Wilson *et al.* 1996), they were impaired relative to controls on the real and virtual versions of the Multiple Errands Task. Additionally, there was a significant correlation between performance in the real and virtual tasks. The authors concluded that VEs provide a more discriminating method of assessing planning impairments than currently available standardized tests. They also indicated that the concordance between real and virtual task performance (together with the difference in performance between the TBI and control participants) suggests that the VR method has a significant pragmatic advantage over real-world-based testing, as it is much easier to administer while offering more systematic stimulus control and accurate response measurement.

Titov and Knight (2005) reached similar conclusions after conducting pilot tests involving three neurological patients with functional impairments on a virtual street environment that they had developed, also based on the Multiple Errands Test. Once again, the patients' performances on the VR-based tests were consistent with their reported difficulties in everyday life and clinical accounts of their deficits. Jansari *et al.* (personal communication) have developed a VE based around the kind of office tasks used by McGeorge *et al.* (2001), but featuring additional tasks that assess a broader array of components of executive functioning, such as planning, selection, prioritizing, creative thinking, adaptive thinking, and multi-tasking. The aim was to create an assessment tool that could reliably be used to predict the type of problems that an individual was likely to experience upon returning to work after a brain injury (Jansari *et al.* 2004).

The concept of ecological validity encompasses many different strands. Some which have particular relevance to VR are considered further below.

The provision of real world distractions and stressors

Elkind *et al.* (2001) note that conventional tests of executive functioning are usually devoid of the stressors, distractions, and complexities that one might find in everyday life. However, action slips, or 'errors at the level of intentional action production resulting from the execution of an action that was not intended' (Zalla *et al.* 2001, p. 760), which are frequently observed in patients with deficits in executive functioning, are primarily attributed to an inability to inhibit external distractions (Norman, 1981). Extraneous distractions can easily be controlled in VR, and their presence or absence can be manipulated such that the conditions of testing are more representative of real life. Distractions can be removed to facilitate the initial stages of rehabilitation (Brooks *et al.* 1999) and then systematically re-introduced in accordance with the patient's progress.

A number of VR assessments of executive functioning have incorporated distractions. For example, the Virtual Store (V-STORE) (Lo Priore *et al.* 2003), which can be considered a hybrid of the Tower of London Task and the WCST, consisted of a virtual fruit shop in which a representation of the user was depicted in front of a conveyor belt on which a number of baskets (from one to three) traversed the room. The participants' task was to fill up the baskets with pieces of fruit that could be found on four shelves in the VE according to verbal instructions. The clinician could introduce distractions, such as the room light switching off or progressively dimming, the telephone ringing, or the belt speed changing. These distractions were designed to increase task difficulty and generate time pressure. When the distractions occurred, the focus was on how participants adapted their strategy to compensate. Comprehensive data about the participants' performance, in addition to the way that they adapted to distractions, was recorded for each trial. Morganti (2004) referred to a pilot study involving V-STORE and frontal lobe patients; unfortunately, the present authors could find no further details on this study.

Interactivity and immersion

On another issue that may be seen as a particular aspect of ecological validity, Elkind *et al.* (2001, p. 491) pointed out that conventional neuropsychological assessments of executive dysfunction have 'difficulty in creating the type of interactivity and immersion that occurs in day-to-day life, which limits their usefulness and application to real life'. This comment seems to correspond to Damasio's (1994) observations that situations devised to assess executive functioning by conventional means are not so much presented, as they are described, and that they often lack the chain of events (actions and reactions) that occur in real life. VR environments consist of rich three-dimensional depictions of real-world locations and scenarios, and induce in the user a clear feeling of immersion and interaction with appropriate auditory stimuli. A good example of this was provided by Josman *et al.* (2006), who conducted a study to determine the feasibility of using a virtual supermarket to assess executive function deficits in individuals following a stroke. The VR supermarket task involved selecting and paying for a pre-defined list of products. Users were assessed relative to eight measures, including the total distance (in metres) traversed by the patient, the total time in seconds taken to complete the task, the number of correct actions (e.g. selecting the correct product), the number of incorrect actions (e.g. exiting the supermarket without paying), and the number of pauses. In this study, 26 participants who had previously sustained a stroke interacted with the virtual supermarket and also completed the BADS. Significant correlations were found between performance in the virtual super-market and on the key search subtest of the BADS (which is designed to assess planning ability).

A significant addition featured in the work of Josman and colleagues was the incorporation of virtual representations of humans, commonly referred to as 'avatars' (Rizzo *et al.* 2004a), in the VE. In real life, other shoppers provide perhaps the greatest single source of distractions from the primary task. The use of such avatars is becoming more frequent in neuropsychological applica-tions of VR (e.g. Rose and Brooks 2004; Rizzo *et al.* 2002b). Potentially, this could be a critical feature in VR assessment and rehabilitation of executive dysfunction, as it is disturbances in social skills such as impulsivity, lack of social awareness, and lack of concern for social rules that present some of the most significant challenges for social reintegration (Mazaux and Richer 1998). Incorporating convincing artificial intelligence in VEs is no small undertaking. Avatars can often look relatively simplistic and have a limited repertoire of behaviours. However, research has indicated that even basic avatars are often entirely suitable for introducing a social dimension into the test situation (e.g. Blascovich *et al.* 2002; Pertaub *et al.* 2002).

Flexibility and the provision of the capacity for self-initiation and structuring of behaviour

Lezak *et al.* (2004. p. 611) eloquently describe a further fundamental issue with conventional assessment and rehabilitation of executive dysfunction as 'the paradoxical need to structure a situation in which patients can show whether and how well they can make structure for themselves'. This problem is, at least to some extent, a consequence of the need to ensure that clinicians have sufficient opportunity for comprehensive observations and accurate recordings of patients' performance. However, this is not an issue in VR, as the limitations of monitoring and recording of behaviour and performance are removed. It is possible to monitor and record every movement an individual makes in a VE and, where applicable, automatically score any interactions/activities according to pre-determined performance criteria. This enables the creation of much less rigid assessments that take place in a more natural environment and allow patients to exercise discretion in how they go about a task. For example, Morris *et al.* (2002) used a virtual bungalow originally designed to assess prospective memory (Brooks *et al.* 2002b) to examine strategy formation, rule-breaking (a common feature of executive dysfunction), and prospective memory in 35 patients who had undergone prefrontal lobe surgery and 35 age- and IQ-matched controls. The virtual bungalow consisted of four rooms, and the participants' task was to help the owner of the virtual bungalow move to a larger house comprising eight rooms. Participants had to search all the rooms of the bungalow and collect items for the rooms in the new house (e.g. items for the new lounge first, followed by the other rooms of the new house in a specified order). Participants were also given prospective memory tasks such as remembering to put 'Fragile' notices on five glass items. The VE allowed Morris and colleagues to monitor the strategy or pattern used in searching the rooms of the bungalow for items for the designated room in the new house (i.e. whether they were being searched in a systematic order or in a more haphazard fashion), instances of rule-breaking (i.e. when a participant selected a category of furniture inappropriate for the designated room of the new house), and instances where the participants failed to complete a prospective memory task. Both patients and controls were able to navigate around the virtual bungalow and perform the task. However, the patients showed significantly less efficient strategies for exploring the virtual bungalow and exhibited significantly more rule breaks compared with the controls. They also exhibited impairments in selected prospective memory tasks.

Reliability and control

Rigorous control over the test situation and ecological validity are often seen as being mutually exclusive (e.g. Banaji and Crowder 1989). Perhaps the most impressive benefit of using VR is that increases in ecological validity do not come at the expense of control over the VE. The use of VR ensures test and rehabilitation materials of consistent quality, can significantly reduce the chances of errors and inconsistencies by the clinician in administering the assessment or rehabilitation strategy, and avoids unwanted variations in the environment in which the assessment or rehabilitation is being conducted. As noted above, in a VE the user's performance can also be documented in great detail. This is nicely reflected in a study by Zalla *et al.* (2001) who argued that although there was an extensive literature documenting problems with everyday activity after frontal lobe damage, there was a paucity of studies providing quantitative evidence of the behavioural impairments of these patients in ecologically valid situations. Zalla and colleagues used a VR apartment consisting of a bedroom, bathroom, kitchen, and living room in an attempt to determine whether patients' impairments reflected reduced supervisory attention capacity or deficits in the ability to take context into account when executing and monitoring tasks. The participants' task was to verbally formulate a plan of action for getting ready for work in the morning (e.g. preparing breakfast, getting washed, dressed, etc.), which they would then use to execute the actions in the VR apartment. The participants consisted of seven patients with prefrontal cortex damage and 16 control participants. The results indicated that the presence of the realistic context (i.e. the virtual apartment) benefited patients' performance in terms of constraining some types of errors, such as those relating to the sequencing of actions. However, patients did exhibit specific impairments in the execution condition, namely action slips, omissions, and failure to initiate actions. Control participants took significantly less time to verbally generate the action sequence than to actually execute the actions, whereas the patients took similar times to plan and then execute the actions. Zalla and colleagues suggested that control participants were taking longer to execute than to plan the actions as they were actively adapting the plan to the context for optimal execution, whereas the patients were not evaluating the effect of the context on their plan during its execution.

The degree of control afforded by VR generates exciting opportunities to combine the technology with brain-scanning technology such as functional magnetic resonance imaging (fMRI). This provides researchers with precise insights into the neurological correlates of executive functioning in everyday activities, which would not be possible in the real world. Baumann (2005) developed a VR apartment consisting of seven rooms and, with VR apparatus that could be used by the subject whilst inside the fMRI equipment, sought to establish if performance on a simple test of executive function, such as task loading, would produce a detectable response in fMRI in healthy controls. The task-loading paradigm entailed participants being given 2 minutes to complete a contiguous set of five runs through the apartment, each run featuring tasks of increasing difficulty. For example, the first run featured the instruction to examine the apartment, but not to interact with any of the objects within. In the third run, participants were asked to change the state of all the lights in the apartment, and in the final run, their task was to open all of the four closets in the apartment and to mentally count and categorize all the clothing within. At the conclusion of the runs, participants were asked to subjectively rate the difficulty of each run. Baumann found a statistically significant correlation between subjective rating of task difficulty and pixel intensity in the anterior frontal lobes compatible with highly significant bilateral activation when the more difficult tasks were compared with the less difficult tasks.

Patient compliance and motivation

Patients with cognitive deficits often exhibit low motivation and compliance in assessment and rehabilitation tasks that are repetitive and not stimulating (Castelnuovo *et al.* 2003). Again, VR has potential in this regard. The peak age range for traumatic brain injury is 15–24 years, and it is precisely this age range that constitutes the largest proportion of commercial video games users. Thus an age group well represented in brain injury statistics may be particularly receptive to assessment and rehabilitation strategies that feature gaming elements.

Increasing the perceived challenge and enjoyment of VEs has been of concern to some researchers involved with the application of VR to the assessment of executive dysfunction. For example, Elkind *et al.* (2001) developed an analogue of the WCST featuring a virtual beach, a matching task that involved delivering frisbees, sodas, ice lollies, and beach balls to bathers sitting under umbrellas, each featuring a depiction of one of the above four objects, differing in colour and number. In all other respects the test procedure matched that of the WCST. Non-impaired participants performed both a WCST (presented on a PC) and the VR-based test (counterbalanced across participants). Participants' subjective ratings of the tests indicated that the majority found the VR test more difficult, interesting, and enjoyable than the WCST.

Practical considerations

Rose *et al.* (1998) have explained in some detail a fundamental neuroscience justification for using VR in rehabilitation. They argued that the reduction in individuals' ability to interact with their environment that often follows a significant brain injury leads to a form of 'environmental impoverishment'. This situation is compounded by staffing and budget constraints that mean, for example, that stroke patients in the UK spend, on average, just 1 hour a day in formal therapy (DeWit *et al.* 2005). Clinicians would agree that this is not conducive to optimal rehabilitation outcomes. There is extensive animal research, a full review of which is beyond the scope of this chapter, indicating that if this reduction in interaction can be reversed via 'environmental enrichment', i.e. enforced interaction with the brain-damaged animal's physical environment, the functional consequences of the brain damage are often ameliorated (e.g. Rose *et al.* 1998; Johansson 2003). Unfortunately, providing enriched environments for patients, given practical constraints such as clinician time, budget, and safety concerns, is highly problematical. This is where VR could be of very significant benefit (Rose *et al.* 1998). If one cannot take the patient to real enriched environments, VR affords clinicians with the opportunity to take virtual enriched environments to the patient, thus negating the practical constraints identified above. This application of VR becomes all the more compelling now that researchers have started to develop ways of measuring brain activity during interaction with VEs, affording the exciting opportunity to study the impact of exposure to VEs on the damaged brain (e.g. Parslow *et al.* 2004; Baumann 2005).

Summary of progress and future directions

Research incorporating VR into the assessment and rehabilitation of executive dysfunction has been, at best, sporadic over the last decade. Moreover, it has often been preliminary in nature and consequently open to criticisms such as small number of participants (Baumann 2005), use of purely normal populations (Elkind *et al.* 2001), lack of information regarding the nature of brain injuries and patients' prior functioning (Josman *et al.* 2006), and lack of follow-ups to initial investigations (Lo Priore *et al.* 2003).

However, the available literature has demonstrated that presenting conventional tests of executive function in a VR format can make them more efficient in identifying deficits (e.g. Pugnetti *et al.* 1998). In some instances, the VR assessments have identified errors that have been missed by conventional tests (e.g. Mendozzi *et al.* 1998) and identified deficits that occur in everyday scenarios that would have been difficult to detect using conventional testing (McGeorge *et al.* 2001). The potential of VR in the rehabilitation, as opposed to assessment, of executive dysfunction has yet to be realized. This is the most obvious and fundamentally important suggestion for further research.

The full potential of VR in the field of the assessment and rehabilitation of executive dysfunction is still to be harnessed. Ten years ago, the technology was playing catch up with the aspirations of the researchers. Now it is the researchers' turn to catch up with the potential of the technology.

References

Alderman, N. and Burgess, P.W. (2003). Assessment and rehabilitation of the dysexecutive syndrome. In: *Handbook of neurological rehabilitation* (2nd edn) (ed R.J. Greenwood, M.P. Barnes, T.M. McMillan, and C.D. Ward), pp. 387–402. Psychology Press, Hove.

Banaji, M.R. and Crowder, R.G. (1989). The bankruptcy of everyday memory. *American Psychologist*, **44**, 1185–93.

Baumann, S.A. (2005). Neuroimaging pilot study of task loading and executive function using a virtual apartment. *Presence: Teleoperators and Virtual Environments*, **14**, 183–90.

Blascovich, J., Loomis, J., Beall, A.C., Swinth, K.R., Hoyt, C.L., and Bailenson, J.N. (2002). Immersive virtual environment technology as a methodological tool for social psychology. *Psychological Inquiry*, **13**, 103–24.

Brooks, B.M., McNeil, J.E., Rose, F.D., Greenwood, R.J., Attree, E.A., and Leadbetter, A.G. (1999). Route learning in a case of amnesia: a preliminary investigation into the efficacy of training in a virtual environment. *Neuropsychological Rehabilitation*, **9**, 63–76.

Brooks, B.M., Rose, F.D., Attree, E.A., and Elliot-Square, A. (2002a). An evaluation of the efficacy of training people with learning disabilities in a virtual environment. *Disability and Rehabilitation*, **24**, 622–6.

Brooks, B.M., Rose, F.D., Potter, J., Attree, E.A., Jayawardena, S., and Morling, A. (2002b). Assessing stroke patients' ability to remember to perform actions in the future using virtual reality. In: *Proceedings of the 4th International Conference on Disability, Virtual Reality and Associated Technologies* (ed P. Sharkey, C.S. Lányi, and P. Standen) pp. 239–45. Reading University Press.

Brooks, B.M., Rose, F.D., Potter, J., Jawawardena, S., and Morling, A. (2004). Assessing stroke patients' prospective memory using virtual reality. *Brain Injury*, **18**, 391–401.

Brown, D.J., Kerr, S.J., and Bayon, V. (1998). The development of the Virtual City: a user centred approach. In: *Proceedings of the 2nd European Conference on Disability, Virtual Reality and Associated Techniques* (ed P. Sharkey, D. Rose, and J. Lindstrom), pp. 11–16. Reading University Press.

Castelnuovo, G., Lo Priore, C., Liccione, D., and Ciuffi G. (2003). Virtual reality based tools for the rehabilitation of cognitive and executive functions: the V-STORE. *Psychology Journal*, **1**, 310–25

Damasio, A.R. (1994). *Descartes' error: emotion, reason, and the human brain*. Putnam, New York.

DeWit, L., Putman, K., Dejaeger, E., *et al.* (2005). Use of time by stroke patients: a comparison of four european rehabilitation centers. *Journal of the American Heart Association*. Available on-line at: http://stroke.ahajournals.org/cgi/content/full/36/9/1977

Elkind, J.S., Rubin, E., Rosenthal, S., Skoff, B., and Prather, P. (2001). A simulated reality scenario compared with the computerized Winconsin Card Sorting test: an analysis of preliminary results. *CyberPsychology and Behaviour*, **4**, 489–96.

Heyn, P., Abreu, B.C., and Ottenbacher, K. (2004). A systematic review of the effectiveness of virtual-reality intervention on physical, mental, and behavioral rehabilitation outcomes. *Neurorehabilitation and Neural Repair*, **17**, 227–44.

Isdale (1998). What is VR? A web based introduction. Available on-line at: http://vr.isdale.com/WhatIsVR/frames/WhatIsVR4.1.html

Jansari, A., Agnew, R., Akesson, K., and Murphy, L. (2004). The use of virtual reality to assess and predict real-world executive dysfunction: can VR help for work-placement rehabilitation? In: *Abstracts of the Symposium on Neuropsychological Rehabilitation*, Uluru, Australia, 12–13 July 2004.

Johansson, B.B. (2003). Environmental influence on recovery after brain lesions: experimental and clinical data. *Journal of Rehabilitation Medicine*, **41**, 11–16.

Josman, N., Hof, E., Klinger, E., *et al.* (2006). Performance within a virtual supermarket and its relationship to executive functions in post-stroke patients. In: *Proceedings of the 5th International Workshop on Virtual Reality Rehabilitation (IWVR)*, pp 106–9.

Lengenfelder, J., Schultheis, M.T., Ali-Shihabi, T., DeLuca, J., and Mourant, R. (2002). Divided attention and driving: a pilot study using virtual reality technology. *Journal of Head Trauma Rehabilitation*, **17**, 26–37.

Lezak, M., Howieson, D., and Loring, D. (2004). *Neuropsychological assessment*. Oxford University Press.

Liu, L., Miyazaki, M., and Watson, B. (1999). Norms and validity of the 'DriVR'—a virtual reality driving assessment for persons with head injury. *CyberPsychology and Behavior*, **2**, 53–67.

Lo Priore, C., Castelnuovo, G., Liccione, D., and Liccione, D. (2003). Experience with V-STORE: considerations on presence in virtual environments for effective neuropsychological rehabilitation of executive functions. *Cyberpsychology and Behaviour*, **6**, 281–7.

McGeorge, P., Phillips, L.H., and Crawford, J.R. (2001). Using virtual environments in the assessment of executive dysfunction. *Presence: Teleoperators and Virtual Environments* **10**, 375–83.

Mazaux, J.M. and Richer, E. (1998). Rehabilitation after traumatic brain injury in adults. *Disability and Rehabilitation*, **20**, 435–47.

Mendozzi, L., Motta, A., Barbieri, E., Alpini, D., and Pugnetti, L. (1998). The application of virtual reality to document coping deficits after a stroke: report of a case. *CyberPsychology and Behavior*, **1**, 79–91.

Morganti, F. (2004). Virtual interaction in cognitive neuropsychology. *Studies in Health Technology and Informatics*, **99**, 55–70.

Morris, R.G., Kotitsa, M., Bramham, J., *et al.* (2002). Virtual reality investigation of strategy formation, rule breaking and prospective memory in patients with focal prefrontal neurosurgical lesions. In: *Proceedings of the 4th International Conference on Disability, Virtual Reality and Associated Technologies* (ed P. Sharkey, C.S. Lányi, and P. Standen). Reading University Press.

Nies, K.J. (1999). Cognitive and social–emotional changes associated with mesial orbitofrontal damage:assessment and implications for treatment. *Neurocase*, **5**, 313–24.

Norman, D.A. (1981). Categorization of action slips. *Psychological Review*, **88**, 1–15.

Parslow, D.M., Rose, F.D., Brooks, B.M., *et al.* (2004). Allocentric spatial memory activation of the hippocampal formation measured using MRI. *Neuropsychology*, **18**, 450–61.

Pertaub, D., Slater, M., and Barker, C. (2002). An experiment on fear of public speaking anxiety in response to three different types of virtual audience. *Presence: Teleoperators and Virtual Environments*, **11**, 68–78.

Pugnetti, L., Mendozzi, L., Motta, A., *et al.* (1995). Evaluation and retraining of adults' cognitive impairments: which role for virtual reality technology? *Computers in Biology and Medicine*, **25**, 213–227

Pugnetti, L., Mendozzi, L., Attree, E., *et al.* (1998). Probing memory and executive functions with virtual reality: past and present studies. *CyberPsychology and Behavior*, **1**, 151–62

Rizzo, A.A., Buckwalter, J.G., Neumann, U., *et al.* (1998). The virtual reality mental rotation/spatial skills project: preliminary findings. *CyberPsychology and Behavior*, **1**, 107–13.

Rizzo, A., Buckwalter, J.G., and van der Zaag, C. (2002a). Virtual environment applications in clinical neuropsychology. In: *Handbook of virtual environments* (ed K. Stanney), pp. 1027–64. Lawrence Erlbaum, Mahwah, NJ.

Rizzo, A.A., Bowerly, T., Buckwalter, J.G., *et al.* (2002b). Virtual environments for the assessment of attention and memory processes: the virtual classroom and office. In: *Proceedings of the 4th International Conference on Disability, Virtual Reality and Associated Technologies* (ed P. Sharkey, C.S. Lányi, and P. Standen), pp. 3–12. Reading University Press.

Rizzo, A.A., Schultheis, M.T., Kerns K., and Mateer C. (2004a). Analysis of assets for virtual reality applications in neuropsychology. *Neuropsychological Rehabilitation*, **14**, 207–39.

Rizzo, A., Pryor, L., Matheis, R., Schultheis, M., Ghahremani, K., and Sey, A. (2004b). Memory assessment using graphics-based and panoramic video virtual environments. In: *Proceedings of the 5th International Conference on Disability, Virtual Reality and Associated Technologies* (ed P. Sharkey *et al.*), pp. 331–8. Reading University Press.

Rose, F.D. and Brooks, B.M. (2004). The virtual office trainer: a teaching tool for people with learning disabilities. *International Journal of Therapy and Rehabilitation*, **11**, 96.

Rose, F.D., Attree, E.A., and Johnson, D.A. (1996). Virtual reality: an assistive technology in neurological rehabilitation. *Current Opinion in Neurology*, **9**, 461–7.

Rose, F.D., Attree, E.A., Brooks, B.M., and Johnson, D.H. (1998). Virtual environments in brain damage rehabilitation: a rationale from basic neuroscience. In: *Virtual environments in clinical psychology and neuroscience: methods and techniques in advanced patient–therapist interaction* (ed G. Riva, B.K. Wiederhold, and E. Molinan), pp. 233–42. IOS Press, Amsterdam.

Rose, F.D., Brooks, B.M., and Leadbetter, A.G. (2004). Preliminary evaluation of a virtual reality-based driving assessment test. In: *Proceedings of the 5th International Conference on Disability, Virtual Reality and Associated Technologies* (ed P. Sharkey *et al.*). Reading University Press.

Rose, F.D., Brooks, B.M., and Rizzo, A. (2005). Virtual reality in brain damage rehabilitation. *CyberPsychology and Behaviour*, **8**, 241–62.

Schultheis, M.T. and Rizzo, A.A. (2001), The application of virtual reality technology in rehabilitation. *Rehabilitation Psychology*, **46**, 296–311.

Schultheis, M.T., Himelstein, J., and Rizzo, A.A. (2002). Virtual reality and neuropsychology: upgrading the current tools. *Journal of Head Trauma Rehabilitation*, **17**, 379–94.

Shallice, T., and Burgess, P.W. (1991). Deficits in strategy application following frontal lobe damage in man. *Brain*, **114**, 727–41.

Shopland, N., Lewis, J., Brown, D.J., and Dattani-Pitt, K. (2004). Design and evaluation of a flexible travel training environment for use in a supported employment setting. In: *Proceedings of the 5th International Conference on Disability, Virtual Reality and Associated Technologies* (ed P. Sharkey *et al.*), pp 69–76. Reading University Press.

Stone, R.J. (2002). Applications of virtual environments: an overview. In: *Handbook of virtual environments* (ed K.M. Stanney) pp. 827–56. Lawrence Erlbaum, Mahwah, NJ.

Titov, N. and Knight, R.G. (2005). A computer-based procedure for assessing functional cognitive skills in patients with neurological injuries: the virtual street. *Brain Injury*, **19**, 315–22.

Wallergård, M., Cepciansky, M., Lindén, A., *et al.* (2002), Developing virtual vending and automatic service machines for brain injury rehabilitation, In: *Proceedings of the 4th International Conference on Disability, Virtual Reality and Associated Technologies* (ed P. Sharkey, C.S. Lányi, and P. Standen), pp. 109–15. Reading University Press.

Wilson, B.A., Alderman, N., Burgess, P.W., *et al.* (1996). *Behavioural Assessment of the Dysexecutive Syndrome Test (BADS)*. Thames Valley Test, Bury St. Edmunds.

Worthington, A. (2005). rehabilitation of executive deficits: effective treatment of related disabilities. In: *The effectiveness of rehabilitation for cognitive deficits* (ed P.W. Halligan and D.T. Wade). Oxford University Press.

Zalla, T., Plassiart, C., Pillon, B., Grafman, J., and Sirigu, A. (2001). Action planning in a virtual context after prefrontal cortex damage. *Neuropsychologia*, **39**, 759–70.

Part 3

Professional issues

Michael Oddy and Andrew Worthington

Part 3 considers some key aspects of professional practice that are important in working with people with executive disorders. In Chapter 15, Rickards picks up on the theme raised by Stuss: the importance of identifying particular aspects of executive disorder that can then be targeted by specific intervention, in this case pharmacological. Once again there is a lack of research evidence and Rickards calls for larger trials employing standardized outcome measures. Rickards also notes the problem of obtaining consent to treatment from people with executive deficits who may have little insight into their vulnerabilities or need for treatment. He discusses the implications of the legislative framework of the Mental Health Act in England and Wales in such cases.

Decision making is often compromised by executive disorders with potentially serious consequences for individuals and their families. This can also be a difficult management issue for practitioners who have a duty of care to maintain and an obligation to promote personal choices in rehabilitation. This topic provides the focus of the next two chapters. Writing at the time of the implementation of a new Mental Capacity Act in England and Wales, Herbert considers the particular difficulties involved in assessing the capacity of those with executive disorders. This is a complex issue, not least because capacity in law is seen as specific to the issue in question. Once again the difficulty of explaining executive disorders to the uninitiated raises its head.

The balancing act between managing risk and the dangers of constraining autonomy is explored in the chapter by Worthington and Archer. They point out that not only is risk increased by the presence of executive disorder (impulsivity, poor monitoring etc.) but, at least those with traumatic brain injuries tend to be a group with a high level of pre-morbid risk-taking.

Nevertheless, drawing on a range of sources from healthcare and beyond they suggest a number of ways in which risk can be assessed and managed.

The family plays a crucial role in the rehabilitation and long-term support of those who acquire a brain injury. In Chapter 18 Oddy and Herbert explore the particular problems experienced by families when faced with executive disorder and the ways in which these can be ameliorated by professional intervention and support. Yet again the theme of the difficulty of explaining executive disorder to those who are unfamiliar comes through as does both the nebulous and all-pervasive nature of the effects of executive disorder.

After the family, those having the most contact with (and arguably influence upon) those with executive disorders are often the least experienced and trained staff such as rehabilitation assistants and support workers. McCrea and Sharma discuss their years of experience of training this group of staff to work with those with executive disorders. They emphasise the importance of educating such staff to understand the nature of executive disorder and helping them to avoid making erroneous attributions and interpretations of client behaviour. In particular they emphasise the value of training staff in a neurobehavioural approach which focuses upon experiential learning when working with this client group.

15

Psychopharmacological treatment of executive disorders following brain injury

Hugh Rickards

Birmingham and Solihull Mental Health Trust, and
University of Birmingham

Introduction

The term 'executive function' covers a range of brain activities which are essential to modern human existence. The 'dysexecutive syndrome' is a constellation of symptoms which can significantly impair function and quality of life and lead to significant carer distress. There is no specific pharmacological treatment for the dysexecutive syndrome. This is partly because this is a heterogeneous group of conditions presenting differently in different people and is caused by pathology in different areas of the brain (around a third of brain substance may be involved in executive tasks). However, some pharmacological treatments can target specific areas of function and lead to improvements.

Broadly speaking, there are three areas of executive function that may be targeted by pharmacological agents:

- problems with inhibition, including irritability, sexual and social disinhibition, and aggressive behaviour
- problems with drive and initiation
- problems with organization, concentration, and mental focus.

There are differing rationales for the choice of treatments in these three areas. Some treatments are tried because they have been successfully used to manage similar problems in other disorders. An example of this is the use of stimulant medications to improve concentration and mental focus. This beneficial effect is seen in children and adults with attention deficit–hyperactivity disorder and in normal adolescents. Other treatments are tried because there is a rationale in terms of the underlying pathology. An example of this is the use of dopamine receptor agonists such as bromocriptine in drive disorders said to be caused by damage to dopamine pathways between the midbrain and the orbitofrontal cortex. On occasion, there may be conflicts in rationale— a drug which may help with one area of executive function may lead to problems in another. For instance, some drugs which reduce irritability and aggression may directly reduce drive and initiation (examples of this include dopamine blocking agents). Conversely, medicines which increase drive and initiation may lead to problems with disinhibition and disorganized behaviours (an example of this is bromocriptine).

There are a number of methodological problems in the study of pharmacological treatments of dysexecutive syndrome. Brain injuries are a highly heterogeneous group of conditions, varying in type and location. This makes patient selection difficult in trials and can limit generalization of results. Executive dysfunction is broadly defined and exists on a spectrum with normal function. This again creates difficulties in defining the boundaries of the syndrome for the purposes of research. Numbers are relatively small and so the majority of studies are underpowered. Some of the rating scales used may not have been defined specifically for people with brain injury, and this may affect reliability and validity. Finally, communication problems in relation to brain injury can affect consent and data gathering in research.

Treating irritability and disinhibition after brain injury

Irritability is relatively common after brain injury, occurring in around 35 per cent of brain-injured individuals in the first year (Deb *et al.* 1999). Irritability may occur as a direct consequence of brain injury or may arise from secondary causes, which need to be fully explored before direct pharmacological treatments for irritability are tried. Irritability may be secondary to a variety of primary psychiatric disorders, including depression, anxiety disorders, and psychosis, which require assessment and treatment in their own right. The frustrations of physical and specific cognitive impairments may be a direct cause of irritable behaviour. Systemic illnesses, particularly infections, can lead to irritable behaviour, and pain is a strong trigger for irritability. Misunderstandings caused by cognitive problems can lead to aggressive behaviour. Examples of this include patients with receptive aprosodias who may perceive a friendly verbal approach as threatening and react accordingly. Irritability may also be a long-standing trait not related to the brain injury at all.

Why might executive function problems lead to irritability?

There is no clear explanation for the genesis of irritability. One possible explanation takes in two aspects of executive dysfunction—multi-tasking problems and disinhibition. An individual with a brain injury is faced with an everyday situation which requires multi-tasking that they had previously found easy to perform (e.g. making a cup of tea or organizing a visit to a friend). Realization that this task is now extremely difficult leads to an increase in anxiety and arousal. A disinhibited individual may then express this increased arousal as paroxysmal verbal or physical aggression.

What treatments work for irritability or temper control after brain injury?

If underlying causes for irritability have been identified and treated as far as possible, primary irritability may still remain and often requires treatment. A wide variety of treatments have been tried in the treatment of irritability; however, trials have been on relatively small numbers of patients and randomized controlled trials (RCTs) are sparse. A recent Cochrane review (Fleminger *et al.* 2003) identified only six RCTs on the treatment of aggressive behaviour. Four of these studies looked at the effectiveness of beta-blockers (two studies examined propranolol and two examined pindolol) in a total of 43 patients (Greendyke and Kanter 1986; Greendyke *et al.* 1986, 1989; Brooke *et al.* 1992). The doses used were very high (520 mg of propranolol daily in one study and up to 420 mg daily in another) and a number of the patients had been non-responsive to other treatments. In all the studies, beta-blockers produced a reduction in frequency of outbursts. In at least one of the studies (Greendyke *et al.* 1986) marked adverse effects were reported.

One trial of the stimulant methylphenidate (MPH) examined its effect on anger or temper in 38 people using a randomized placebo-controlled single-blind design over 6 weeks (Mooney and Haas 1993). The treatment led to a decrease in anger-type symptoms with no measurable effect upon cognitive function. The final RCT reported in the Cochrane review was a trial of amantadine (Schneider *et al.* 1999). This was a crossover trial in 10 brain-injured individuals and showed no differences between the treatment and placebo arms.

The conclusion of the Cochrane review was that there was some evidence for the efficacy of beta-blockers in the treatment of agitation after brain injury and that the drug effects are seen early (within 2–6 weeks of starting medication). The authors also recommend that 'if no benefit (is) observed by the end of six weeks, then the drug should be tailed off and another one tried after a suitable interval'.

Apart from the RCTs, a range of smaller and less robust trials of the treatment of irritability/aggression have been reported. These are described in the Cochrane review (Fleminger *et al.* 2003) and summarized by Deb and Crownshaw (2004). There are six case reports of the use of buspirone, a partial agonist at 5-HT2A receptors and an anxiolytic, in a total of 38 patients with a mixed response. Even allowing for publication bias, only 16 patients were said to respond to treatment, with 22 either not responding or getting worse. In one study (Gualtieri 1991) five of the drop-outs were in relation to adverse effects. In the largest case series relating to buspirone, Stanislav *et al.* (1994) reported 14 brain-injured patients of whom only four or five responded to treatment within the first month. They required relatively high doses to have an effect (30–60 mg daily).

Neuroleptic medications have commonly been used to control irritable behaviour following brain injury, but evidence for their effectiveness is lacking. In the largest of the existing trials, Maryniak *et al.* (2001) examined the effect of methotrimeprazine in the first 3 months following brain injury and found that most of the patients improved in the domain of agitation. This trial was severely limited in that there was no control group, the data were retrospective, and the outcome measures used were not validated. Other small trials indicated that neuroleptics may worsen cognitive function after acquired brain injury (ABI) and, especially in the instance of clozapine, may lower the seizure threshold (Michals *et al.* 1993).

Reports on lithium in agitated behaviour are largely from case reports or small case series, the largest of which (Glenn *et al.* 1989) involved 10 cases of brain injury with very mixed results, including three patients who deteriorated (one of whom had an epileptic seizure).

Two case series using selective serotonin-reuptake inhibitor (SSRI) in agitated brain-injured patients have been reported. Kant *et al.* (1998) used therapeutic doses of sertraline in 13 cases and found reductions in aggression and independent improvement in mood. Fann *et al.* (2000) found similar results from a similar methodology, but used the Brief Anger and Aggression Questionnaire as an outcome measure. There are also two case series of tricyclic antidepressant usage. Jackson *et al.* (1985) reported 35 cases, two-thirds of whom had reduced agitation with either amitriptyline or desipramine. However, those people with previous psychiatric diagnosis were excluded, leading to a significant bias in the study. Mysiw *et al.* (1988) described 20 cases of agitated TBI patients treated with therapeutic doses of amitriptyline, 13 of whom responded within a week of treatment.

There is surprisingly little published data on the use of anticonvulsant drugs in the management of agitated, aggressive, or irritable brain-injured patients, even though this group of drugs is probably still the most widely prescribed group in agitated brain-injured patients. Azouvi *et al.* (1999) reported an 8-week open trial of carbamazepine in agitated patients using a variety of outcome scales (Neurobehavioural Rating Scale–Revised, the Katz Adjustment Scale and the Mini Mental State Examination). Out of a total of 10 cases, five improved on treatment, a 'moderate effect' was seen in three further cases, and a 'negligible' effect in two cases. Four of the the cases reported drowsiness during the treatment on doses of up to 800 mg daily. Chatham-Showalter (1996) used larger doses of carbamazepine (up to 1600 mg daily) in a case series of seven patients and found a decrease in 'combative behaviour' as measured by the Rancho Los Amigos scale. This allowed for the reduction in other medications such as neuroleptics or benzodiazepines.

There are two reported studies of valproate in agitated brain injury patients (Chatham-Showalter and Kimmel 2000; Kim and Humaran 2002). Both are limited by the fact that they are retrospective studies with no control groups. The two studies had a total of 40 patients, the vast majority of whom showed improvement in agitation and impulsiveness following treatment.

Managing hypersexuality and disinhibition

No good epidemiological studies exist to inform us of the prevalence of hypersexuality following traumatic brain injury. Case reports suggest that in fact hyposexuality is the most common form of sexual problem after brain injury (probably in relation to abulia). However, hypersexual behaviour and altered sexual preference have been clearly described and, at times, this can lead to significant risk.

There are only 10 cases in the literature reporting the use of hormone treatments to reduce sexual behaviour (Arnold 1993; Emory *et al.* 1995; Britton 1998). In the first of these (Emory *et al.* 1995), the cases of eight men who had developed hypersexual behaviours following brain injury were reviewed. They were treated with medroxyprogesterone acetate (Depo-Provera) at a dose of 400 mg weekly for 6 months. Testosterone levels were also measured and dropped very significantly during treatment. None of the patients exhibited significant inappropriate behaviour during the study, and increases in attention span were noted as well as reduction in impulsivity and emotional lability. This study is compromised by the lack of a control group and of standardized measures.

Summary of treatments for aggressive, irritable, and disinhibited behaviours

There is very little high-quality evidence to support the use of any pharmacological treatments in this area. Almost all the studies have at least one major methodological flaw. However, the absence of good-quality evidence does not mean that these treatments are necessarily ineffective. Indeed, most of the available evidence points towards the effectiveness of beta-blockers, antidepressants, and anticonvulsants as well as the effectiveness of hormonal treatments on sexually aggressive behaviour. Further randomized studies are needed in this area.

Problems with drive, initiation and focus

Problems with initiating and maintaining goal-directed behaviours are common following brain injury. Two main classes of drugs, stimulants and dopamine agonists, are used in the management of this group of problems.

Stimulants

Stimulants have a reasonable adverse effect profile in the area of brain injury. Alban *et al.* (2004) studied tolerability and vital signs in 35 adults with TBI as part of another trial. They found that reduction in appetite was the only adverse effect that was significantly higher in the treated group. They also found a small rise in heart rate (+7 beats/minute) and blood pressure (+2.5 mmHg) in the treated patients. There are four published RCTs on the effects of stimulants on attention and drive following brain injury. Whyte *et al.* (1997) reported on 19 patients who participated in an RCT of MPH. They used cognitive tests to assess sustained arousal, phasic arousal, distraction, choice reaction time, and behavioural inattention. They found that MPH increased the speed of mental processing, but motor speed and most aspects of sustained attention were unaffected. Speech *et al.* (1993) used a crossover design in 12 chronically head-injured patients and found that MPH had no significant effect on a variety of tests of attention and processing speed, including digit span, Stroop Interference Test, Complex Reaction Time Test, and others. In contrast, Gualtieri and Evans (1988) found significant improvements in cognition in 14 of 15 patients using a similar methodology and similar dosages (0.15–0.3 mg/kg) but different outcome measures. The measures in this study included the Selective Attention Test, the Verbal Fluency Test, the Non-verbal Fluency Test, the Selective Reminding Test, the Continuous Performance Test, and the Benton Visual Retention Test. Finally, Plenger *et al.* (1996) randomized 23 patients to MPH (0.3mg/kg) or placebo in the post-acute phase. This trial was underpowered because of patient dropout. However, at 30 days into treatment, the MPH group performed significantly better on tests of attention and motor performance. These differences disappeared at 90 days, but this may have been due to the low power of the study to detect a difference between groups. Thus the existing trials provide a 'mixed bag' of results clouded by a relative underpowering of studies.

Dopamine agonists

Decelerating injuries to the brain commonly affect areas rich in dopaminergic neurons including the basal forebrain and pathways to this area from the midbrain (Gennarelli *et al.* 1982). These pathways have also been associated with executive function problems, especially initiation of new behaviours and changing the cognitive or behavioural set. There is a little evidence from rodent models that dopaminergic drugs could prevent brain damage and enhance recovery. Kline *et al.* (2004) showed how the oxidative stress induced by brain injury could be attenuated by bromocriptine. A similar pattern was found using cognitive outcome measures in rats who had sustained ischaemic brain damage (Micale *et al.* 2006). O'Neill *et al.* (1998) showed how a variety of dopamine 2 agonists (including bromocriptine and pergolide) could protect against ischaemia-induced hippocampal damage.

There are a number of potential problems in the usage of dopaminergic medications in patients who lack drive and focus following brain injury. One practical problem, mentioned earlier, is that an increase in drive and focus could lead to a higher level of inappropriate and aggressive behaviours which may actually diminish the rehabilitation potential of the individual. Dopamine agonists as a group have been associated with exacerbation of psychotic symptoms. In addition, abrupt withdrawal of dopamine agonists can trigger a neuroleptic malignant syndrome.

There are two RCTs of dopamine agonists looking specifically at cognitive outcomes. Meythaler *et al.* (2002) studied 35 subjects using a randomized crossover design. One of their outcome measures, the FIM-Cog score, was a measure of cognition in relation to function (Heinemann *et al.* 1991). Other scales used in this study included MMSE, the Disability Rating Scale, and the Glasgow Outcome Scale. Although trends in favour of amantadine were reported, the comparisons did not reveal significant differences between the groups (amantadine 200 mg vs. placebo).

McDowell *et al.* (1998) looked at a range of cognitive tasks in a double-blind crossover trial of low-dose bromocriptine after TBI. Their results were particularly interesting as they showed a preferential effect of bromocriptine on cognitive functions served by the prefrontal cortex in 24 patients. Tasks which were significantly better on bromocriptine included Trail Making, Stroop, the FAS Test, and the Wisconsin Card Sorting Test. However, tests of working memory and non-executive tasks were no different between the treatment and the placebo group. The authors concluded that bromocriptine had a specific effect on some types of cognitive function and did not exert its effect through a non-specific increase in arousal, attention, or response speed. A smaller less robust trial looked specifically at the use of dopaminergic medications for motivational problems. Powell *et al.* (1996) studied 11 patients in an open-label trial and gave bromocriptine in gradually escalating doses; they reported increases in motivation by their own rating scale which was separate from any effect upon mood.

Ethical and legal considerations of the use of pharmacological treatments in brain-injured people

In most cases pharmacological treatments require consent from the patient. However, there are a number of scenarios where this is problematic. These include the following:

- the patient is unconscious or semi-conscious
- the patient is not able to understand the nature or effects of the proposed treatment because of receptive language problems
- the patient has difficulty communicating their consent
- the patient is actively refusing treatment which the clinicians and/or carers feel is in their best interests.

In the case of the unconscious or semi conscious patient, decisions about treatment should be made collaboratively within the clinical team, informed by significant carers or relatives and mindful of any previous wishes expressed by the patient prior to the injury. In this case, treatment would probably be parenteral (intramuscular, intravenous, subcutaneous, or through gastrostomy). The Mental Capacity Act now provides a statutory framework for decision-making in these cases. This Act now puts the onus on clinicians to have tried all reasonable methods for eliciting capacity. In cases where the patient does not have the capacity to make or communicate decisions, these decisions have to be made in the 'best interests' of the patient, in consultation with significant relatives or carers, the multidisciplinary team and, where appropriate, an independent mental capacity advocate (IMCA).

In cases where consent is hampered by communication problems, every effort should be made to secure informed consent to treatment. A full assessment of language function is needed and augmentative methods of communication investigated. Non-verbal behaviour, especially in relation to oral medication, can provide information about non-consent in particular, but the problem of patients passively receiving mediation without full consent may remain.

At times patients can actively refuse treatment which the clinicians and carers feel is in their best interests. This is particularly true for patients with irritable or disinhibited behaviours for which they have no insight. In the acute phase, if there is a clear threat to the patient, carer, or health professional, medication may be given under common law to prevent or manage a crisis situation. In this situation, medication is often given via the intramuscular route.

If medication needs to be given over a period of time against the wishes of the patient, then the Mental Health Act 1983 should be used. This legislation applies predominantly to England and Wales. For the most part, it does not apply to Scotland and Northern Ireland. Section 3 of the Mental Health Act allows the treatment of in-patients against their wishes with the following provisos:

(1) that they are suffering from a mental illness of a 'nature or degree' which makes it appropriate for them to be treated in a hospital (or registered unit)

(2) that it is necessary for the patient's health or safety or the protection of others that he receives treatment

(3) that the treatment cannot be provided in any other way.

Are problems with executive function treatable as 'mental illness' under the Mental Health Act?

It is very clear that people with dysexecutive syndrome can in many cases be deemed to be mentally ill from a legal standpoint. The Mental Health Act takes the international classifications of disease as a yardstick to decide whether someone has mental illness. The most pertinent category in the ICD-10 Classification of Mental Disorders (World Health Organization 1992) is F07.0: Organic personality disorder. The diagnostic guidelines for this category include 'consistently reduced ability to persevere with goal-directed activities', 'emotional lability', 'expression of needs and impulses without consideration of consequences or social convention', and 'altered sexual behaviour'.

It is also worth noting that a patient does not have to be deemed 'dangerous' in order to be subject to detention under the Mental Health Act. As long as admission for treatment is justifiable in the 'interests of the patient's health', this is sufficient, provided that the other criteria are met. Finally, section 3 (the main treatment section) only allows for treatment in a hospital or registered setting, which includes some specialist residential and nursing facilities.

Advantages and disadvantages of treatment under the Mental Health Act 1983

The Mental Health Act can be used in the setting of executive dysfunction in two main situations. First, it can be used if a patient requires treatment of any kind, including care intervention to which they are clearly not consenting or are resisting. In this situation, detention under the Act can protect the rights of staff who might otherwise be open to charges of assault. The second situation is one where the patient has clearly expressed a wish to leave an inpatient setting but, because of their executive dysfunction, they are unable to see or deal with risk outside an inpatient setting. In this situation, the Act can provide a frame of reference for detention against the patient's wishes. The Act specifies time periods for detention and includes rights for legal representation of the patient and independent tribunals to verify the legality of detention. Finally, some sections of the Act put a duty upon local health and social services providers to fund appropriate care over the long term.

Section 117 specificies that 'It shall be the duty of the District Health Authority and of the local social services authority to provide…after-care services for any person to whom this section applies until such time…the person concerned is no longer in need of them'.

This section of the Act empowers the judge of a Mental Health Review tribunal to subpoena the directors of primary care trusts or social services to appear and explain why funding for further placement is not forthcoming. In an era where people with brain injury are often excluded from the mainstream debate about health funding, this can often provide leverage to fund appropriate longer-term placements.

However, patients who have been subject to detention under the Mental Health Act can have difficulties in obtaining visas for travel to some countries and may experience discrimination in employment if they declare it.

Summary

In this chapter it has been shown that when executive function following brain injury is broken down into separate groups of symptoms, each group can be managed by different classes of drug treatment. This field is still in its infancy. Functional neuroimaging after brain injury may help us to narrow down further those pathways responsible for the different elements of executive function. From this information, more specific treatments could be developed to improve outcome. As in many fields, larger trials with standardized outcome measures are the priority for further research in this promising area.

References

Alban, J.P., Hopson, M.M., Ly, V., and Whyte, J. (2004). Effect of methylphenidate on vital signs and adverse effects in adults with traumatic brain injury. *American Journal of Physical Medicine and Rehabilitation*, **83**, 131–7.

Arnold, S.E. (1993). Estrogen for refractory aggression after traumatic brain injury. *American Journal of Psychiatry*, **150**, 1564–5.

Azouvi, P., Jokic, C., Attal, N., Denys, P., Markabi, S., and Bussel, B. (1999). Carbamazepine in agitation and aggressive behaviour following severe closed head injury. *Brain Injury* 13(10): 797–804.

Britton, K.R. (1998). Medroxyprogesterone in the treatment of aggressive hypersexual behaviour in traumatic brain injury. *Brain Injury*, **12**, 702–7.

Brooke, M.M., Patterson, D.R., Questad, K.A., Cardenas, D., and Farrel-Roberts, L. (1992). The treatment of agitation during initial hospitalization after traumatic brain injury. *Archives of Physical Medicine and Rehabilitation*, **73**, 917–21.

Chatham-Showalter, P.E. (1996). Carbamazepine for combativeness in acute traumatic brain injury. *Journal of Neuropsychiatry and Clinical Neurosciences*, **8**, 96–9.

Chatham-Showalter, P.E. and Kimmel, D.N. (2000). Agitated symptom response to divalproex following acute brain injury. *Journal of Neuropsychiatry and Clinical Neurosciences*, **12**, 395–7.

Deb, S. and Crownshaw, T. (2004). The role of pharmacotherapy in the management of behaviour disorders in traumatic brain injury patients. *Brain Injury*, **18**, 1–31.

Deb, S., Lyons, I., and Koutzoukis, C. (1999). Neurobehavioural symptoms one year after a head injury. *British Journal of Psychiatry*, **174**, 360–5.

Mental Health Act 1983, Chapter 20, p. 3. Stationery Office, London.

Emory, L.E., Cole, C.M., and Meyer, W.J. (1995). Use of Depo-Provera to control sexual aggression in persons with traumatic brain injury. *Journal of Head Trauma Rehabilitation*, **10**, 47–58.

Fann, J.R., Uomoto, J.M., and Katon, W.J. (2000). Sertraline in the treatment of major depression following mild traumatic brain injury. *Journal of Neuropsychiatry and Clinical Neurosciences*, **12**, 226–32.

Fleminger, S., Greenwood, R.J., and Oliver, D.L. (2003). Pharmacological management for agitation and aggression in people with acquired brain injury. *Cochrane Database of Systematic Reviews*, Issue 1, Art No. CD003299.

Gennarelli, T.A., Thibault, L.E., Adams, J.H., Graham, D.I., Thompson, C.J., and Marcincin, R.P. (1982). Diffuse axonal injury and traumatic coma in the primate. *Annals of Neurology*, **12**, 564–74.

Glenn, M.B., Wroblewski, B., Parziale, J., Levine, L., Whyte, J., and Rosenthal, M. (1989). Lithium carbonate for aggressive behaviour or affective instability in ten brain-injured patients. *American Journal of Physical Medicine and Rehabilitation*, **68**, 221–6.

Greendyke, R.M. and Kanter, D.R. (1986). Thereapeutic effects of pindolol on behavioural disturbances associated with organic brain disease: a double-blind study. *Journal of Clinical Psychiatry*, **47**, 423–6.

Greendyke, R.M., Kanter, D.R., Schuster, D.B., Verstreate, S., and Wootton, J. (1986). Propranolol treatment of assaultative patients with organic brain disease: a double-blind crossover, placebo controlled study. *Journal of Nervous and Mental Disease*, **174**, 290–4.

Greendyke, R.M., Berkner, J.P., Webster, J.C., and Gulya, A. (1989). Treatment of behavioural problems with pindolol. *Psychosomatics*, **30**, 161–5.

Gualtieri, C.T. (1991). Buspirone for the behaviour problems of patients with organic brain disorders. *Journal of Clinical Psychopharmacology*, **6**, 90–2.

Gualtieri, C.T. and Evans, R.W. (1988). Stimulant treatment for the neurobehavioural sequelae of traumatic brain injury. *Brain Injury*, **2**, 273–290.

Heinemann, A.W., Hamilton, B.B., Granger CV, *et al.* (1991). *Rating scale analysis of functional assessment measures (final report)*. Rehabilitation Institute of Chicago.

Jackson, R.D., Corrigan, J.D., and Arnett, J.A. (1985). Amitryptiline for agitation in head injury. *Archives of Physical Medicine and Rehabilitation*, **66**, 180–1.

Kant, R., Snith-Seemiller, L., and Zeiler, D. (1998). Treatment of aggression and irritability after head injury. *Brain Injury*, **12**, 661–6.

Kim, E. and Humaran, T.J. (2002). Divalproax in the management of neuropsychiatric complications of remote acquired brain injury. *Journal of Neuropsychiatry and Clinical Neurosciences*, **14**, 202–5.

Kline, A.E., Massucci, J.L., Ma, X., Zafonte, R.D., and Dixon, C.E. (2004). Bromocriptine reduces lipid peroxidation and enhances spatial learning and hippocampal neuron survival in a rodent model of focal brain trauma. *Journal of Neurotrauma*, **21**, 1712–22.

McDowell, S., Whyte, J., and D'Esposito, M. (1998). Differential effect of dopaminergic agonist on prefrontal function in traumatic brain injury patients. *Brain*, **121**, 1155–64.

Maryniak, O., Manchandra, R., and Velani, A. (2001). Methotrimeprazine in the treatment of agitation in acquired brain injury patients. *Brain Injury*, **15**, 321–31.

Mental Health Act 1983, Chapter 20, p. 3. Stationery Office, London.

Meythaler, J.M., Brunner, R.C., Johnson, A., and Novack, T.A. (2002). Amantadine to improve neurorecovery in traumatic brain injury-associated diffuse axonal injury: a pilot double-blind randomized trial. *Journal of Head Trauma Rehabilitation*, **17**, 300–13.

Micale, V., Incognito, T., Rampello, L., Rampello, L., Spartà, M., Drago, F. (2006). Dopaminergic drugs may counteract behavioural and biochemical changes induced by models of brain injury. *European Neuropsychopharmacology*, **16**, 195–203.

Michals, M.L., Crismon, M.L., and Childs, A. (1993). Clozapine response and adverse effects in nine brain-injured patients. *Journal of Clinical Psychopharmacology*, **13**, 198–203.

Mooney, G.F and Haas, L.J.(1993). Effect of methylphenidate on brain injury related anger. *Archives of Physical Medicine and Rehabilitation*, **74**, 153–60.

Mysiw, W.J., Jackson, R.D., and Corrigan, J.D. (1988). Amitryptiline for post-traumatic agitation. *American Journal of Physical Medicine and Rehabilitation*, **67**, 29–33.

O'Neill, M.J., Hicks, C.A., Ward, M.A., *et al.* (1998). Dopamine D2 receptor agonists protect against ischaemia-induced hippocampal neurodegeneration in global cerebral ischaemia. *European Journal of Pharmacology*, **352**, 37–46.

Plenger, P.M., Dixon, C.E., Castillo, R.M., Frankowski, R.F., Yablon, S.A., and Levin, H.S. (1996). Subacute methylphenidate treatment for moderate to severe traumatic brain injury: a preliminary double-blind placebo-controlled study. *Archives of Physical Medicine and Rehabilitation*, **77**, 536–40.

Powell, J.H., Al-Adawi, S., Morgan, J., and Greenwood, R.J. (1996). Motivational deficits after brain injury: effects of bromocriptine in 11 patients. *Journal of Neurology, Neurosurgery, and Psychiatry*, **60**, 416–42.

Schneider, W.N., Drew-Cates, J., Wong, T.M., and Dombovy, M.L. (1999). Cognitive and behavioural efficacy of amantadine in acute traumatic brain injury: an initial double-blind placebo controlled study. *Brain Injury* 13(11):863–872.

Speech, T.J., Rao, S.M., Osmon, D.C., and Sperry, L.T. (1993). A double-blind controlled study of methylphenidate in closed head injury. *Brain Injury*, **7**, 333–8.

Stanislav, S.W., Fabre, T., Crismon, M.L., and Childs, A. (1994). Buspirone's efficacy in organic-induced aggression. *Journal of Clinical Psychopharmacology*, **14**, 126–30.

Whyte, J., Hart, T., Schuster, K., Fleming, M., Polansky, M., and Coslett, H.B. (1997). Effects of methylphenidate on atentional function after traumatic brain injury. *American Journal of Physical Medicine and Rehabilitation*, **76**, 440–50.

World Health Organization (1992). *The ICD-10 Classification of Mental and Behavioural Disorders: clinical descriptions and diagnostic guidelines*, pp. 66–7. World Health Organization, Geneva.

16

Assessment of capacity in clients with executive dysfunction

Camilla Herbert
Brain Injury Rehabilitation Trust, Horsham, West Sussex

Introduction

Assessment of capacity has always been a relevant question in relation to people with neurological disorders, but it has become increasingly prominent in the UK following the legislative changes agreed by the Parliaments for Scotland (Adults with Incapacity Act (Scotland) 2000) and for England and Wales (Mental Capacity Act (England and Wales) 2005). Other jurisdictions (e.g. Australia, Canada, and the USA) have already established legislation and codes of practice.

Capacity (or 'competence' in the USA) is a legal question, and therefore reference must be made to the law and relevant codes of practice. The law uses a **functional** approach, i.e. one that is based on each individual decision at each particular point in time. This is distinguishable from an **outcome** approach, in which making an unwise decision is taken as evidence of incapacity, and from a **diagnostic** approach, in which a person is deemed to lack capacity purely because of their status or diagnosis. However, the assessment of capacity is often a clinical process, and there are clearly examples where the diagnosis of acquired brain injury or progressive dementia will raise questions about decision-making capacity. Questions may arise in relation to individuals with post-traumatic amnesia, those who lack insight, those who have significant cognitive difficulties or severe challenging behaviour, or clients with impulsive and disinhibited behaviours. Other dilemmas may arise around treatment approaches such as behavioural programmes, use of time out, restraint, or the more general issue of 'engagement' in rehabilitation. Multidisciplinary treatment programmes often work around clients' lack of awareness of their problems, which may manifest itself in the form of 'refusal to participate', by engaging clients in activities that they will participate in but at the same time using these activities to achieve other therapeutic goals, which might include raising levels of awareness.

Central to many of these capacity questions are impairments of executive functioning, and these provide some of the greatest challenges to the assessment process. Based on case law, and now enshrined in the Mental Capacity Act itself, there are four areas of functioning deemed to be required for the capacity to make decisions. These are the abilities to (a) understand the information relevant to the decision, (b) retain that information, (c) use or weigh that information as part of the process of making the decision, and (d) communicate that decision (whether by talking, sign language, or other means). Executive dysfunction can affect the cognitive skills relevant to each of these processes, and in turn affect an individual's ability to carry out actions and behaviours.

Some of the key points from the Act and Code of Practice (published in 2007) in relation to the assessment of capacity to make decisions are presented in this chapter. These issues are explored further through the use of case vignettes, focusing particularly on the impact of executive dysfunction.

The Mental Capacity Act (England and Wales) 2005

The Mental Capacity Act 2005 (MCA 2005), implemented in full from October 2007, provides a legal framework for decision-making on behalf of adults who lack capacity. The Scottish Parliament passed similar legislation in 2000 (Incapacity Act (Scotland) 2000) and there are some differences in terminology and procedures. In this chapter we focus on the legislation for England and Wales, but many of the questions and issues raised will be familiar to clinicians working within the Scottish legislation and in other jurisdictions.

MCA 2005 clarifies the legal position in relation to the definition of capacity, but there will inevitably be ongoing discussion and case law to establish how the new legislation applies in practice. In addition, there are some areas of legal decision-making not covered by the Act where existing legal tests will continue to apply. For example, the Act does not cover areas of family relationships including consenting to marriage/civil partnerships, divorce, issues around adoption, or consenting to have sexual relations (see section 27). Consent to Sexual Relationships is covered under the Sexual Offences Act 2003. MCA 2005 also excludes treatment under the Mental Health Act (see section 28) and Voting Rights (see section 29).

MCA 2005 includes a set of guiding principles and definitions of capacity which are summarized below.

The principles

1. A person must be assumed to have capacity unless it is established that he/she lacks capacity.
2. A person is not to be treated as unable to make a decision unless all practicable steps to help him/her to do so have been taken without success
3. A person is not to be treated as unable to make a decision merely because he/she makes an unwise decision.
4. An act done, or decisions made, under this Act or on behalf of someone who lacks capacity must be done, or made, in his/her best interests.
5. Before the act is done, or the decision is made, regard must be had to whether the purpose for which it is needed can be as effectively achieved in a way that is less restrictive of the person's rights and freedom of action

How the Act defines capacity

For the purposes of this Act, a person lacks capacity in relation to a matter if at the material time he/she is unable to make a decision for him/herself in relation to the matter because of an impairment of, or a disturbance in the functioning of, the mind or brain (whether permanent or temporary) *and* if he/she is unable to make any of the following steps in decision-making:

- understand the information relevant to the decision
- retain that information
- use or weigh that information as part of the process of making the decision
- communicate his/her decision (whether by talking, sign language, or other means).

The information relevant to a decision includes information about the reasonably foreseeable consequences of (a) deciding one way or another or (b) failing to make the decision. The fact that a person is able to retain information relevant to a decision for a short period only does not prevent him/her from being regarded as able to make the decision.

Assessment of capacity

Assessment of capacity to make a specific decision where a concern has been raised about cognitive functioning will inevitably include a more general understanding of the client's neuropsychological status than purely executive skills. Some areas of cognitive skills are easier to assess than others, and it is particularly difficult to evaluate more covert processes such as the ability to sequence thoughts or to exercise judgement about relative risks and benefits of various options (Reid-Proctor *et al.* 2001). This chapter will focus as far as is practicable on the issues arising from executive disorders or frontal lobe damage.

Understanding information relevant to the decision

Before assessing a person's understanding of information relevant to the decision, efforts must be made to provide the information and explain it in a way that is most appropriate for that individual (section 3(2) of the Act). The emphasis is on information being presented in a *simple* form. Relevant information includes:

- the particular nature of the decision in question
- the purpose for which the decision is needed
- the likely effects of making or not making the decision.

The onus is on the assessor to use the appropriate form of communication (simple language, signing, visual aids, Makaton, etc.).

Providing information in simple language, using visual aids etc., is important but does not in itself guarantee comprehension of information when other cognitive limitations are present. It is likely that longer interviews, or several interviews focused on the key decision topic and which explore the pros and cons in a number of different ways, will be most useful in clarifying the extent to which the individual has genuinely understood and followed the relevant information.

More difficult to assess are the effects of executive functioning on understanding and decision-making. Using a framework such as that presented by Powell (2004) is one approach to explore the relevant executive skills and their potential impact. Powell's framework is based on the theory of reasoned action and planned behaviour (Ajzen and Fishbein 1980) and examines the impact of neuropsychological (in particular executive) functioning on an individual's ability to form reasoned actions. These include (modified from Powell 2004):

- reduced ability to conceptualize future events, which affects one's beliefs about possible consequences
- reduced ability to weigh up consequences, and hence the impact that these consequences may have on one's behaviour
- altered motivation to comply because of one's beliefs about others and their motives
- reduced ability to identify social prohibitions, which in turn affects the individual's view of what is normal behaviour

- reduced time devoted to decision-making, reflected in impulsive behaviour or reduced ability to form an intent
- reduced ability to plan, including the ability to make a plan as to how to behave.

Retaining the information long enough to use it

Section 3(3) of the Act stipulates that the ability to retain information for a short period only should not automatically disqualify the person from making a decision. The use of aids such as notebooks, photographs, videos, and voice recorders is encouraged. Where there are concerns about retention of information, it is good practice to repeat the discussion on several occasions. If there is consistency in the individual's responses on different occasions, given the same information, then one can be more confident than if their response is highly variable. However, the fact that someone has retained the information is not in itself a guarantee that they will/can use it in their decision-making, particularly where individuals are prone to impulsive behaviour.

Using and weighing information as part of the process of making the decision

The courts have described the ability to weigh all relevant information in the balance as part of the process of making a decision and then using that information to arrive at a choice. It is recognized that there are cases where the effects of mental impairment or disturbance prevent an individual using the information or taking it into account, or cause a person to make decisions that are inevitable, regardless of the information and his/her understanding of it. Here one may also need to recognize the impact of other psychological factors, such as mood, suggestibility, external influences, and previous life experiences, since these are all known to affect decision-making ability. One may also need to take into account the role of individual beliefs (including religious beliefs), as these can have an impact on individual judgements. Finally, one has to ensure that evidence of logical processes and reasoning ability is not given such weight as to exclude 'irrational' decisions (thereby introducing a covert 'outcome' approach).

Communication of the decision

In most cases this is the easiest aspect to assess. The requirement is merely to produce a response (not necessarily verbal) that indicates choice. However, being able to communicate a decision does not necessarily mean that a person meets the other criteria of being able to understand the information, retain it, and weigh it in the balance.

Whilst individuals who are unconscious would clearly fail to meet the criterion for 'communicating a decision', there is more scope for ambiguity for individuals who are mute and unresponsive, or where there is evidence of repetitive utterances without evidence of engagement in the decision-making process. Where the underlying condition is treatable and the decision is not critical, the principles of the Act would support delaying the decision until the individual is able to participate with the decision-making process.

Assessment tools

There are a number of standardized assessments of capacity, which may be of assistance in some circumstances (Grisso and Appelbaum 1998). However, the emphasis on a particular decision at a particular time means that individualized assessments will often be required. Information from notes/clinical history plus interview with the individual and significant others will be more relevant in most cases. Unfortunately, the ability of many people with executive impairments following brain injuries to present a competent verbal description when they are actually unable to put into practice what they can recount is common, and can be misleading for the naive questioner. Therefore it is crucial that the interviewer has training in and understanding of the nature of brain injury, in particular the role of executive dysfunction. The focus of the assessment does need to be on the specifics of the topic under discussion but carried out in such a way that issues of awareness, impulsivity, and other executive skills are explored and checked. This might take the form of a detailed interview not only with the individual but also with other relevant people.

There may be a role for psychometric assessment both to gauge the level of questioning/interview that is appropriate for that individual and to highlight more subtle deficits. However, the choice of assessment tools and their interpretation remains very important. Whyte *et al.* (2003) compared the results of 'capacity assessments' carried out by a medical practitioner and a neuropsychologist, and found that those patients with executive functioning problems who presented well at interview were most likely to be judged as capable by the assessing doctor but as lacking capacity by the neuropsychologist. There was a particular problem with the use of the Mini Mental State Examination (MMSE) (Folstein *et al.* 1975) within the medical assessment in this study as this test is insensitive to executive functioning difficulties.

Reid-Proctor *et al.* (2001) make the point that 'neuropsychological assessment alone cannot be used to make competency decision, since the patient's executive dysfunction may not be obvious in the structured testing session' or if inappropriate measures such as the MMSE are used. In general one needs to consider how well standardized assessments relate to everyday functioning. There are numerous examples where individuals, particularly those with more subtle frontal deficits, can achieve a normal, and in some cases excellent, cognitive profile on tests such as the Wechsler scales or on tests often associated with frontal brain dysfunction such as the verbal fluency or subtests from the Behavioural Assessment of Dysexecutive Syndrome (BADS) (Wilson *et al.* 1996), but are unable to function in everyday life without high levels of support. The converse is also true in that individuals with significant cognitive deficits can cope well within their normal environment and be capable of making decisions relevant to their everyday functioning. Therefore emphasis has to be on interpreting the test results and all other sources of information in terms of their relevance to the specific decision under consideration.

There will be cases where neither standardized assessment nor interview will be sufficient, and specific and individualized assessments will need to be designed to identify the means by which an individual can best communicate their thoughts and wishes (e.g. McMillan 1997; McMillan and Herbert 2000). In these single-case studies of a young woman with severe physical, cognitive, and communication deficits, a series of questions requiring yes/no responses were repeated in a predetermined sequence over a period of weeks to ascertain the consistency of her responses. In the first study it was clear that simple autobiographical questions were consistently responded to but that her responses to more complex or abstract questions were less consistent or even at chance level. The follow-up study 5 years later showed progress in terms of both her ability to respond (now verbal rather than by pressing a buzzer) and the level of questions to which she could consistently respond.

Case vignettes

Case 1

Brief summary

Sheila was a 37-year-old female in an acute hospital ward 5 weeks after sustaining a severe traumatic brain injury in a road traffic accident. Although she was medically stable, she remained confused and agitated. She was assessed on the ward for suitability for transfer to a rehabilitation unit. The neuropsychologist interviewed her, the staff working with her, and a close relative. At this stage Sheila was too disoriented and distractible to focus on any systematic questions or to engage in discussions about her condition and treatment options. The view was taken that Sheila could benefit from transfer for rehabilitation, and the question of consent to treatment (rehabilitation) was discussed (see below). The decision to transfer Sheila to the rehabilitation unit was taken following consultation with staff and family, and over the next few weeks she gradually became more oriented and her capacity to consent to the admission was reviewed on a regular basis. After 4 weeks Sheila stated that she did not wish to remain on the unit and that she wanted to return home. Therefore further discussions were held as to whether Sheila was now capable of consenting to treatment (rehabilitation) and what the various options were at this stage.

Capable to consent to or refuse rehabilitation

When Sheila was first assessed on the medical ward she was unable to engage in conversation, being highly distractible and disoriented. At this stage she was not capable of consenting to treatment on the grounds of lack of understanding, appreciation, and reasoning. It was clear that Sheila's condition was likely to improve, and therefore there was a valid question as to whether treatment decisions should be postponed until she was able to make her own decisions. However, consideration of her best interests at this stage was that management on an acute medical ward was not conducive to optimal recovery, and the time-scales of such recovery are highly variable. Therefore it was agreed, on the grounds of her best interests and in accordance with Acts in Connection with Care and Treatment (MCA 2005), to support her transfer to a rehabilitation facility despite her inability to consent. The additional stipulation was made that that Sheila's capacity to consent should be reviewed regularly, in accordance with good practice and knowledge of recovery rates from traumatic brain injury.

During her initial period of admission to the rehabilitation facility Sheila underwent more extensive assessment including:

- neuropsychology testing
- occupational therapy assessment, including functional assessments including in the kitchen
- road safety assessment
- staff observations and feedback with her.

Her progress was monitored at weekly review meetings where her orientation and engagement with the programme was discussed. The question as to her capacity to consent to treatment was reviewed, but initially she remained very confused and unable to understand or appreciate the nature of her condition or appropriate treatment options. During the first 3 weeks Sheila was compliant with requests from staff and did not express any concerns about her presence on the unit. During the fourth week Sheila became more consistently oriented to time and place, and she began asking questions about her accident and why she was on the unit. These questions were repetitive and at this stage there was little evidence that Sheila was absorbing the information being given to her. However, she began to express repeatedly a wish to leave the facility, stating that she was capable of returning to her own home and managing independently. The question of capacity to consent to treatment was reviewed again.

On the basis of the neuropsychological testing, functional assessments, and observations on the unit, it was the view of the team that Sheila's extensive executive impairments continued to affect her appreciation of her situation and her understanding of the consequences of her decision. She was not able to weigh and use this information as part of her decision-making, and so it was the opinion of the team that she remained unable to consent to (or refuse) treatment. Discussion with her family highlighted the pressure they felt under to respond to her telephone calls in which she would cry and ask to be taken home, but also that there were differing views as to what would be in her best interests, with some family members supporting the need for continuing with the rehabilitation programme and others agreeing with Sheila in believing that she would be better when she came home.

Following further discussion with her family, Sheila herself, and her care manager, it was identified that the risks at home, whilst real, could be managed by an extensive package of support, and her rehabilitation needs could be reviewed with her at a subsequent date. The balance between respecting her wishes (even though at this stage she had been assessed as lacking capacity to make this decision herself) and prevention of harm is sometimes a pragmatic, not an ethical or legal, issue.

The other problem, not addressed in this case because of the decision to support Sheila at home, was the clinical problem of how best to support and work with someone like Sheila if she refused to engage in any aspect of the programme. Even if the decision had been taken that it was in her best interests to remain at the rehabilitation unit, the staff would still have had to find a way of working with someone who does not either see the problem or want to be there. These are very real practical issues but they are not necessarily 'capacity' questions.

Case 2

Brief summary

Sally was a 24-year-old female with severe cognitive problems following an assault five years previously. Sally had made a good physical recovery but had both executive deficits and memory problems. She had developed post-traumatic epilepsy and required daily anticonvulsant medication. Her combination of memory deficits and poor organizational skills meant that she required supervision and prompting to ensure that she took her medication regularly. At times Sally was aggressive and non-cooperative with professionals, and she would disappear from contact for days or weeks at a time

Concerns had arisen because Sally's behaviour had been observed to be impulsive and disinhibited, and she was known to be sexually active and at risk from unplanned pregnancy. In addition to the concerns about Sally's vulnerability and behaviours that put her 'at risk' of assault and/or unwanted sexual activity, there were also questions around the management of her epilepsy if she became pregnant and ensuring that there was adequate support and information available for her. Therefore there was an option of using long-term contraceptive medication (Depo-Provera injections) in order to reduce the risks of unplanned pregnancy.

What are relevant capacity questions?

The MCA 2005 specifically excludes considerations of personal relationships. It does not address the question of capacity to consent to sexual relationships. These issues are dealt with under the Sexual Offences Act 2003. Under Section 7 of this Act consent is defined thus: 'a person consents if he/she agrees by choice and has the freedom and capacity to make that choice'. In this case it was acknowledged that Sally was capable of consenting to sexual relationships, although there were concerns that her impulsive behaviour might place her in situations that she found difficult to manage and which might put her at risk in other ways.

The specific 'capacity' question raised was in relation to Sally's ability to consent to take medication, and in particular her understanding of contraception and her ability to choose to use contraception on an ad hoc basis or to remember to take a daily contraceptive pill consistently.

The guidance on assessment of capacity requires that Sally can do the following.

- ◆ **Communicate her decision** Sally had no problem providing a verbal response at the end of a discussion. This response was relevant to the content of the discussion, i.e. it was not a random response or one that showed no evidence of decision-making. However, the response could vary according to the way the evidence was presented to her, and the same person could present different arguments persuasively and Sally would agree. She was clearly suggestible, although this was not formally tested. Thus the ability to communicate her decision was a necessary but not sufficient criterion in terms of assessing her capacity in relation to the decision in question.

- **Understand the risks/benefits** Sally could follow an argument and discuss the pros and cons of Depo-Provera injections vs. daily contraceptive vs. 'spur of the moment' decisions. She could also recognize that there could be risks attached to any pregnancy given her epilepsy and medication.

- **Retain the information long enough to use it** What was less certain was whether Sally could retain this information for very long, and subsequent discussions on the same topic always required a repetition of the information at some length. Although presenting the information with a different emphasis could alter her response, if the same information was presented she did come up with the same response, i.e. there was a level of consistency in her respones even if she remained vulnerable to suggestion.

- **Use and weigh the information as part of the process of making the decision** It was also uncertain, and there was evidence to suggest the contrary, that she could or would act on the information outside the discussion. Her impulsive behaviour strongly suggested that she would react to situations as they appeared to her at the time, without pausing to reflect on the implications. In addition, Sally's insight into her condition and her needs was variable, depending on her mood and what else was happening in her life at that time. During the discussions she could sometimes, but not always, recognize how these issues applied to her, and there was evidence from previous incidents that her ability to apply this information was weakest when she was in the most vulnerable positions.

Capacity to consent to long-term contraceptive medication

Capacity in the legal sense is about a specific decision at a specific time. The issues around Sally's decision-making ability are more subtle and provide a good example of why clinicians are often troubled by 'capacity' questions, particularly those involving impaired executive functioning. Sally clearly had the relevant skills to communicate her decision, to problem-solve and reason (with some support), and to weigh up information. What she also had was the tendency to be easily swayed by different points of view, which made her suggestible and possibly called into question the extent to which any decision she made was 'free from coercion'. Secondly, she had an impulsive pattern of behaving which affected her ability to put her decisions into practice.

The specific question was whether or not Sally could consent to a particular treatment option. At one level the answer to this question was 'yes', in which case the injection could go ahead if she chose to proceed. However, if one took the view that her suggestibility meant that she was not 'free from coercion', then on this basis it could be argued that she was not capable of consenting to treatment. The option of longer-term contraceptive could still be considered to be in her best interests, and at this stage in her life it could be argued that it reduced the risks of unwanted pregnancy whilst not restricting her lifestyle excessively or being unduly invasive. In this particular case it was felt that without Sally's consent the issue of longer-term contraceptive injections would not be pursued as it was considered to be only one element, albeit a useful one, in a more general management strategy to support her.

There were more general questions around her impulsive behaviour of which her sexual relationships were just one manifestation. There was a requirement for a more general programme of intervention to guide her impulsive responding, which in itself raised questions about her consent to this. The capacity questions raised by her behaviour were many and frequent, but each had to be treated as a specific issue (e.g. consent to medication, consent to a placement). Her status as a vulnerable adult was a general and lifelong issue and provided the overarching framework for the attempts to support her that persisted over many years.

In the event Sally did agree that the use of longer-term contraception was a reasonable suggestion and with staff support made and attended an initial appointment with her GP. Here she still had the option of refusing the injection but chose to go ahead. On subsequent occasions Sally had the opportunity to change her mind, and over a period of more than 12 months she continued to consent to the injections. Subsequently she entered into a stable relationship and chose to discontinue the injections and did become pregnant. This in turn raised further questions of capacity in terms of managing her pregnancy, childbirth, and child rearing, which are beyond the scope of this chapter.

Summary

The Mental Capacity Act 2005 provides a framework within which to assess capacity to make a particular decision at a particular time. The legislation reflects existing case law and practice in that there is a presumption of capacity. The Act emphasizes the need to maximize an individual's engagement in decision-making and for consultation with relevant others. In clinical practice with people with executive disorders, the complexity and subtlety of the cognitive and psychological processes involved in decision-making are inevitably going to provide examples where there is a range of opinion concerning a particular case. Over time case law will provide further guidance for clinicians. In the mean time, clinicians should ensure that they are aware of the principles underlying the Act and the key areas that should be considered when they are asked to assess capacity to make a decision, and that they have consulted appropriately. Clinicians should be able to demonstrate that in providing an opinion they have acted 'reasonably', but capacity is a legal concept and where there is dispute it is ultimately up to the court to make a decision.

References

Adults with Incapacity Act (Scotland) 2000. Stationery Office, London.

Ajzen, I. and Fishbein, M. (1980). *Understanding attitudes and predicting social behaviour.* Prentice Hall, Englewood Cliffs, NJ.

British Psychological Society (2006). *Assessment of capacity in adults: interim guidance for psychologists.* Professional Practice Board, British Psychological Society, Leicester

Folstein, M.F., Folstein, S.E., and McHugh, P.R. (1975). Mini-Mental State: a practical method for grading the cognitive state of patients for the clinician. *Journal of Psychiatric Research,* **12,** *189–198*

Grisso, T. and Appelbaum, P. (1998). *Assessing competence to consent to treatment: a guide for physicians and other health professionals.* Oxford University Press, New York.

McMillan, T.M. (1997). Neuropsychological assessment after severe head injury in a case of life or death. *Brain Injury,* **11,** 481–90.

McMillan, T.M. and Herbert, C.M. (2000). Neuropsychological assessment of a potential 'euthanasia' case: a five-year follow up. *Brain Injury,* **14,** 197–203.

Mental Capacity (England & Wales) Act 2005. Stationery Office, London.

Mental Capacity Act 2005 Code of Practice. Stationery Office, London.

Powell, G.E. (2004). Capacity to manage financial affairs—the legal perspective. Presented at: Division of Neuropsychology Study Day, London, 17 September 2004.

Reid-Proctor, G.M., Galen, K., and Cummings, M.A. (2001). *Brain Injury,* **15,** 377–86.

Sexual Offences Act 2003. Stationery Office, London.

Whyte, M., Wilson, M., Hamilton, J., Primrose, W., and Summers, F. (2003). Adults with Incapacity (Scotland) Act 2000: implications for clinical psychology. *Clinical Psychology,* **31,** 5–8.

Wilson, B.A., Alderman, N., Burgess, P.W., Emslie, H., and Evans, J.J. (1996). *Behavioural Assessment of the Dysexecutive Syndrome.* Harcourt Assessment, London.

17

Assessment and management of risk associated with executive dysfunction

Andrew Worthington and Nicola Archer

Brain Injury Rehabilitation Trust, Birmingham

Introduction

All activity where the outcome is unknown beforehand involves an element of risk, and in daily life we rely on our executive functions to act as a personal 'risk manager'. Anticipation of potential problems is crucial to effective planning; reasoning and judgment are involved in assessing the likelihood that a particular course of action will achieve a specific objective; and when the unexpected happens we may need to adapt accordingly. When the executive risk manager fails to function, as it can do in all of us from time to time, for example under the influence of alcohol or sleep deprivation, the result is poor decision-making and ineffective action. After brain injury such difficulties may become chronic problems, undermining engagement in rehabilitation and promising a lifetime of supervision. Consequently, one of the greatest (though largely unspoken) challenges in the rehabilitation of executive disorders is the management of risk associated with such diverse behaviours as leaving the gas on, forgetting to take medication, accruing debt, and making personally offensive remarks, all signs often associated with executive dysfunction.

Therefore this chapter is about risk-taking by adults with brain injury and how so-called 'risky behaviour' can be understood and managed by health care professionals. Executive dysfunction can set particular constraints on individual autonomy, and otherwise intelligent adults can feel aggrieved that their independence is undermined by what appear to be the paternalistic attitudes of others. Mindful of this experience, the authors' perspective is one of education and empowerment for brain-injured adults. This can be difficult to achieve, as risk assessment in a clinical context often highlights the very different views about risky actions that may exist between organizations, professionals, their clients, and the public at large. The process of managing risk is not simply a matter of evaluating 'the risk' and acting accordingly—there may be divergent opinions at each step. Therefore, in a departure from the more traditional approach to clinical risk assessment, this chapter will consider what all parties bring to the risk assessment process at an individual, organization, and societal level. It is intended to provide practitioners with conceptual and pragmatic tools to apply in the workplace while encouraging the reader to consider how their own implicit views about risk might influence this process.

Risk in contemporary life

The acrobat Karl Wallenda (1905–1978) once said: 'Being on a tightrope is living, everything else is just waiting'. Not everyone would embrace danger in such a manner, but interviews with the general public reveal a consensus that risk-taking is essential to everyday living. Tulloch and Lupton's case Isobel is typical:

> I think risk and pain and misery are all parts of existence, and they are part of what makes us impelled to success. If we lived in a garden of paradise we would still be there munching on food and saying oh, this is quite nice, we really don't need any more.

> (Tulloch and Lupton 2003, p. 72).

Except Isobel is wrong about Paradise; even the Garden of Eden was not immune. In taking the forbidden fruit, Eve's 'rash hand in evil hour' immortalized by Milton is perhaps the first example of risk-taking in human history.

Modern life seems to have more than its fair share of risks. In the UK in 2005–2006, six million working days were lost through workplace injury alone (Health and Safety Commission 2006). According to the Royal Society for the Prevention of Accidents there were over 328 000 injuries at work, more than 290 000 road accident casualties, and over 5.5 million accidents in the home or at recreation. Yet the notion that 'accidents will happen' is increasingly deemed unacceptable, as 'most injuries and their precipitating events are predictable and preventable' (Davis and Pless 2001). Such statements contribute to growing concern that clinicians are deemed to be at fault when adverse events occur (McCulloch *et al.* 2005). Sometimes even to speak of taking a risk is to invite social disapproval and professional criticism.

To some this betrays an insidious shift in attitudes to risk, from attributing adverse outcomes to bad luck or fate to assuming culpable negligence. Captain Scott's fateful Antarctic diary belies a stoicism rarely encountered today: 'We took risks, we knew we took them; things have come out against us, and therefore we have no cause for complaint'. In place of acceptance is an increasing public concern about risk. The 'nothing ventured, nothing gained' ethos has been replaced by a safety-first mantra. Suspicious of new technologies, wary of official reassurances, and anxious about their own well-being, lobby groups form to demand increasing government regulation (Furedi 2002; Poortinga and Pidgeon 2003). Thus the National Patient Safety Agency was created in 2001 in the wake of public concern after a series of health care crises. In a fast-moving world people are now more conscious of risk, even if their behaviour is less risky than that of previous generations. Journalists acknowledge that these perceptions may be fuelled by news media that are ill equipped to educate a largely risk-illiterate public with complex information (Oakley 2001; Marr 2004). Amongst the most contentious areas of risk management in the public mind, and consequently among the most likely to arouse media and political interest, are the risk of violence (Corbett and Westwood 2005) and the risk of abuse (Guldberg 2000), both of which are critical in the care of persons with executive disorder who may be both vulnerable and disposed to aggression.

May contain nuts ...

Popular news media carry daily examples of what some perceive as an increasing health and safety intrusion in daily life. Headlines such as 'Snowballs are banned unless you're 64 feet apart' (*Daily Mail*, 25 February 2005), 'Council spends £18,000 to find if donkey rides are dangerous' (*Daily Express*, 14 July 2006) and 'Outrage as council moves to ban tenants' homely doormats' (*The Guardian*, 14 September 2006) are not hard to find. The oft-cited explanation for the growth of health and safety legislation is a fear of litigation. The same media that revel in highlighting examples of excessive caution are quick to demand a scapegoat when a tragedy occurs ('How did boy die on school trip to "low risk" cave?' Daily Mail, 16 November 2005). Daytime television advertisements also seem to reinforce in the public mind that 'Where there's blame, there's a claim'. Not surprisingly perhaps, the Association of British Insurers (ABI) is worried that a perceived compensation culture damages the industry's reputation (ABI 2005), and yet the notion that our increasingly safety-conscious lifestyle reflects a more litigious society is not entirely supported by the evidence. Investigations by the House of Lords Select Committee on Economic Affairs revealed that legal compensation claims have actually been falling in recent years (House of Lords 2006).

Indeed, there are sound economic and scientific reasons for challenging the received wisdom that adverse events can simply be averted by greater caution. The financial costs of extreme caution following a safety incident may be considerable. Moreover, risk may be redistributed or even elevated by excessive safety measures by driving people into other more risky endeavours. Significantly, given the current climate of increased safety legislation, there are signs of a counter-response ('Chief nanny confesses: 'Health and safety is out of hand. We need to take risks', *Daily Mail*, 22 August 2006), and in 2005 the Health and Safety Executive convened a web forum to ascertain public perceptions of risk, and promised further research to examine factors behind the perception of excessive risk aversion in society. In a far-reaching consultation document the UK government has recently been challenged by the Better Regulation Commission (BRC) to redefine the nation's approach to risk, 'leaving the responsibility for managing risk with those best placed to manage it' and to do so in recognition of 'resilience, self-reliance, freedom, innovation and a spirit of adventure in today's society' (BRC 2006). Subsequently the Department of Health (2007) launched its best-practice guide *Independence, choice and risk: a guide to supported decision-making*, which was underpinned by a positive approach to risk management (see Appendix 1). This debate provides the contemporary backdrop for the operation of health and social services. The Commission for Social Care Inspection (CSCI), which regulates residential facilities in England and Wales, recently launched a discussion paper entitled *Making choices: taking risks* (CSCI 2006), in recognition that people 'want a life, not just services'. Similarly, the National Minimum Standards for Care Homes for adults (Department of Health 2003) specify that 'staff enable service users to take responsible risks' as part of an independent lifestyle. But what constitutes a responsible risk, and who should be the judge? There are no ready solutions to these challenges, as the factors affecting risk perception are many. Individuals vary in the degree to which they are risk averse, professional opinion may also differ according to one's role, parental and spousal attitudes may diverge, and finally a number of people suffer brain injury as a result of their predilection for relatively high-risk activities—to what extent should their premorbid attributes be respected in rehabilitation? In considering how to respond to these challenges it is important to review some key theoretical approaches to risk in relation to best practice in assessment and management of clinical risk.

Theoretical approaches to risk

The statistical (actuarial) approach

This approach, also known as probabilistic risk assessment, characterizes much of the health and safety industry (see Table 17.1) and is exemplified in public policy by the notion that government should make 'the environment safe, to remove all risk or as much of it as is reasonably possible' (Royal Society 1983).

Table 17.1 Stages of probabilistic risk assessment

Identify sources of potential hazard
Identify antecedent events that could precipitate hazard
Establish possible event sequences that could follow
Quantify likelihood of each event sequence
Determine overall risk

After Reason (1990)

Therefore actuarial risk management employs data on the occurrence of particular events to quantify risk (e.g. high, medium, or low risk). This has a superficial resonance: we can accept that our chance of being run over is greater than the likelihood of being hit by a meteorite or bumping into Elvis. It is also common in health care (Wreathall and Nemeth 2004) where individual judgements are considered readily biased and unreliable. Despite attracting criticism for promoting a risk averse approach to political and social concerns (Prins 2005), considerable effort has gone into the development of actuarial predictors of risks for certain categories of behaviour that society deems unacceptable (e.g. violence, re-offending). Such research requires a large representative sample, a lengthy time horizon, and sensitive measures to build up good base-rate information to avoid the problem of making false-positive predictive errors. This enterprise is hampered in brain injury by the absence of a coordinated database and communication network for the necessary collaboration between services. Moreover, if the objective is to individualize risk assessments, the probabilistic approach alone will fall short. Even advocates of this method acknowledge that it is at best an adjunct to clinical assessment (Craig *et al.* 2004).

The clinical approach

Clinical risk assessment has borrowed its approach from high-tech industries such as aviation (e.g. Wilf-Miron *et al.* 2003) and typically involves analysing incident data to inform decisions about how to reduce risk. It is a cornerstone of clinical governance (Scally and Donaldson 1998), and rehabilitation cannot be practised without an appreciation of its importance. For example, useful guidance is available on assessing and managing the risk of harm to others (Royal College of Psychiatrists 1996; Institute of Psychiatry 2002) and self-harm (British Psychological Society 1998; see also Appendix 2 for a practical tool developed by Worthington). Often, however, the aim is to reduce clinical errors and thereby the risk of harm to patients by professionals (e.g. Cavell 2004), but it may be driven by disproportionate anxiety about clinical negligence (Oyebode 2006). This chapter is essentially about clinical risk assessment and the balance between protection and empowerment for individuals with brain injury. It involves individual clinicians and others making judgements about health and social care interventions. However, frequently the process consists of little more than running through a list of 'risk factors' with little guidance as to how the data should be interpreted (e.g. Newell 2001). Such lists, if soundly based, can at least highlight risks that need further investigation or remedial action. Conversely, one can equate personal history with levels of impairment or disability in an attempt to identify persons most at risk. Thus Medley *et al.* (2006) tried to predict risk of falling in brain-injured adults by relating scores on various clinical measures with a personal history of falls.

The rise of evidence-based medicine offers a more empirical basis to the exercise (Walshe and Sheldon 1998), but strict selection criteria underpinning published data render clinical judgements preferable to actuarial tables in many circumstances (Norko and Baranoski 2005; Rakow *et al.* 2005). Readers will doubtless recall many high-profile cases of serious assault or death at the hands of persons judged by 'the authorities' to be safe to be in the community. The furore that accompanies such apparently ill-judged risk assessment makes clinicians understandably wary, and a safety-first approach can be the response. Yet practitioners may find that a precautionary principle conflicts with the present legislative promotion of individual autonomy through the Human Rights Act 1988, the NHS and Community Care Act 1990, and the recent Mental Capacity Act 2005. Furthermore, an overly restrictive stance on risk-taking can undermine the rehabilitation process and may lead to abuse (Murphy 2002). As a starting point, Greaves and Harris (2006) provide a useful summary of many of the factors that may need to be incorporated into a risk assessment for brain-injured persons living in the community. They also provide practical advice about how to draw up and communicate a risk management strategy.

Trait theories

Economists have long pondered why supposedly rational persons do not always act, as economic theory says they should, to maximize their expected utility (Coyle 2002). People generally prefer smaller immediate gains to larger longer-term benefits, but some people are naturally more inclined to take risks. There are strong links with age and sex, but also with personality (Nicholson *et al.* 2005). The literature is complex and fraught with methodological and interpretative qualifications, of which lack of space precludes further discussion. However, it is important to recognize that people can differ widely in their approach to risk and their attitudes may vary depending on the nature of the risk. While environmental factors influence risk-taking, genetic factors also appear to be important, with greater risk-taking characterizing the more extrovert personality (Zuckerman and Kuhlman 2000; Rowe *et al.* 2007), suggesting an interaction between disposition and opportunity. Brain injury often occurs in the context of a history of risky actions (e.g. taking drugs, not wearing a seatbelt, having unprotected sexual encounters), and this kind of pre-injury activity is likely to be very relevant when considering the likelihood of a particular risk being taken. Therefore it is important to obtain as full an account as possible of premorbid habits and propensities, as well as post-injury behaviour.

Sociocultural theories

There is an extensive literature concerning the cultural and social construction of risk. Influential research into public attitudes suggests that there are at least two kinds of belief about behaviour in society that are relevant to risk: an individualized–collectivized dimension, whereby risk-taking is more or less a responsibility of the individual, and an equality–inequality dimension, along which risky behaviour is more or less a matter of choice within parameters constrained by society (Thompson *et al.* 1990). These orthogonal dimensions yield four attitudes or 'types' of risk-taker variously characterized by their beliefs about the appropriate balance between autonomy and regulation (Adams 1995). This type of model extends the trait theories by setting personal propensities to take risks in the context of societal constraints. To the extent that therapists share similar societal values, we tend to treat professional risk assessment as if it were a more objective process. Consequently, differences of opinion in assessing risk are treated as matters of professional expertise when often they merely reflect personal preferences. Failure to recognize one's own inherent bias where clinical risk is concerned regularly leads to protracted dispute and poorer outcomes. Similarly, we fail to appreciate the impact of brain injury if we expect our patients to share the same societal constraints on behaviour.

Behavioural (risk compensation) theory

Under normal circumstances people react to reduce a risk when given information about possible hazards. Adams (1995) considers the example of an accident blackspot: when the road is marked with appropriate warnings, drivers change their behaviour and casualties reduce, which makes the area safer and no longer a site of accidents worthy of special attention. As well as reducing risky actions in response to a change in the world, it is equally possible that people may increase risk-taking behaviour under certain conditions. In this way, critics argue, many road safety measures merely redistribute the risks. If drivers feel safer, they may take more risks and thereby increase danger to other road users such as pedestrians and cyclists. While casualty rates for drivers have been falling, hospital admissions for road accidents (which include pedestrians and cyclists) have not reduced (Audit Commission 2007). Thus, the argument goes, when steps are taken to minimize a risk, behaviour changes in response.

Risk compensation theory embodies the notion that risk-taking can be predicted by knowing the individual values that people place on certain behavioural outcomes (Adams 1988). According to this approach, introducing a risk management intervention may lead to the emergence of new behaviours as the overall balance of costs and benefits is maintained. Hence, while the propensity to take risks can be seen as an inherent disposition, risk-taking itself is a function of costs and benefits associated with partaking in or abstaining from certain activities (Table 17.2). Risk compensation theory is controversial and empirical support is patchy (Hagel *et al.* 2006; Robinson 2006). Although the conditions under which risk compensation operates are poorly understood, clinicians should pay heed in their assessments to the possible value being attached to risk-taking. The authors have experience of substitute behaviours emerging in response to risk management interventions. For example, a 53-year-old woman with hemiplegia and a tendency to thrash out at care staff helping her to get dressed started attempting to bite carers for the first time when an intervention was introduced to prevent her using her arm to hit them. In another case, a 25-year-old man tried repeatedly to abscond from the rehabilitation unit through his bedroom window when a key-code was changed to prevent him leaving unnoticed through the main door at night. Risk compensation alerts clinicians to the possibility of new, possibly more dangerous, actions being substituted for other risky behaviours. The theory predicts that risk-taking should be reduced by interventions that target the underlying cost–benefit trade-off (Table 17.3). An example of how this might work in practice is shown in Appendix 3.

Table 17.2 Factors affecting risk-taking behaviour

Expected benefits of risky behaviour
Expected costs of cautious behaviour
Expected benefits of cautious behaviour
Expected costs of risky behaviour

Table 17.3 Interventions which should reduce risk-taking behaviour

Reduce the expected benefits of risky behaviour
Increase the expected costs of risky behaviour
Increase the expected benefits of less risky behaviour
Reduce the expected costs of safe behaviour

Cognitive and social cognition models

The idea that one can separate objective risk from perceived risk is 'no longer a mainstream position' (Royal Society 1992). All risk is based on subjective appraisal to some extent. Thus cognitive models have two uses in risk management: they can help in the analysis of adverse events to improve practice, and they can promote a more comprehensive understanding of risk-taking as a social and not just an individual phenomenon. In the first case, sound risk assessment requires analysis of previous behaviour relevant to the risk under consideration. In the clinical setting a failure to achieve an intended outcome, such as failure to prevent an injury or a criminal act, throws a spotlight on the risk assessment process. Reason's (2001) cognitive analysis of error is helpful here in distinguishing between (1) an inadequacy in the risk assessment process, such as insufficient prior knowledge or lack of training, and (2) a problem in the implementation of a risk management strategy, for example due to attentional lapses. Investigating incidents within this conceptual framework can ensure that lessons are learnt quickly and that the remedial steps taken are appropriate, not a knee-jerk reaction, so that the client does not suffer an unnecessary restriction of liberty.

Secondly, social cognition models (like sociocultural models) take the behavioural approach to risk-taking one step further by assimilating the role of social norms and values. If one accepts that people function as their own risk managers and act accordingly, it is possible to explore how they access information about risk. Sources include **primary agencies**, such as public health campaigns, government advice, and official reports, and **transmitters** of information such as the populist media and informal agencies, including anecdotes from friends and family and unsolicited information from the Internet. This fragmentary information, much of it contradictory, is filtered through a web of personal, political, and religious views, resulting in a highly idiosyncratic set of beliefs about a particular risk. The term 'mental model' has been adopted to describe this kind of thinking (Morgan *et al.* 2002), although there is nothing particularly formal about the result, which is often a tenuous mishmash of rumour, bias, and inconsistency. The complexity of these personal models is often revealed only after detailed interviews and sophisticated analysis. In a rehabilitation setting the unimpeded sharing of such loosely connected ideas underlies many misunderstandings about risk-taking—a process known as **social amplification** (Pidgeon *et al.* 1999). In the authors' experience professional staff may be overly restrictive with clients based on anecdotal evidence of an event long since lost amongst the client's extensive records. Similarly we recall a client from a small-town community who was unwilling to move to a new inner-city residence based on media-fuelled perceptions of a criminal populace. Acknowledging and challenging these lay beliefs can be very useful in changing behaviour.

There are many other theoretical perspectives of this kind that can be useful in considering risky activity, such as the health belief model, protection motivation theory, and theory of planned behaviour, all of which are reviewed by Conner and Norman (2005). The theory of planned behaviour, for example, has been reported to be useful in predicting self-harm and suicidal behaviour (O'Connor *et al.* 2006) and speed limit violations (Elliot *et al.* 2007). The importance of this framework in the context of executive dysfunction is that most adults will obtain their information about risk through informal sources that are difficult for their carers or therapists to control. Hence, where high-risk behaviour is repeatedly occurring, one should consider the value of an extended interview with clients to map out the factors influencing their behaviour (Morgan *et al.* 2002). Additional problems of concrete thinking, slow mental processing, and memory deficits might also be evident, but it may be possible to begin challenging the underlying beliefs with core cognitive-behavioural techniques such as presenting new information, encouraging alternative interpretations, and setting up behavioural experiments.

Human factors approach

Most clinical approaches to risk reduction focus on the individual decision-maker. However, outside the health care setting the contribution of environmental factors in risk reduction has long been recognized (Reason 1990), and the importance of safe design in health care facilities is belatedly being addressed (Reiling 2006). Practitioners will acknowledge that errors of judgement are more likely to be made (by clinicians and their clients) when the working environment (such as an office) and the tools of the job (such as a cognitive screening measure) are poorly designed for the task in hand. Hence ill-judged evaluations of risk are made by staff who have inadequate access to information and are working under excessive pressure in a noisy environment. This is not just a matter of aesthetics; the ability to respond to increased risk can be undermined by a working environment unsuited to managing vulnerable people. Individuals with executive deficits who have both poor self-awareness and poor self-monitoring skills can easily be placed at unnecessarily greater risk as a result of inadequate design of their living environment. Some risk-related environmental factors that should be considered by architects, designers, and therapists alike are summarized in Table 17.4.

Systems approach

The systems approach seeks to identify aspects of an organizational culture that perpetuate risky decision-making (Reason 1990). Relevant factors operating in health services include professional defensiveness, protectionism, deference to authority, secrecy, and perceived blame culture (Walshe and Shortell 2004). Other concerns reported by health workers include poor communication, inadequate resources, procedural loopholes, workload, and shift patterns (Dandurand 2004). Much of the challenge in improving risk assessment is trying to identify the chain of events that led to an adverse outcome. Based on techniques from the transport and power industries, the National Patient Safety Agency now promotes root cause analysis (RCA) as the method of choice in risk analysis in health care settings (Williams and Osborn 2004).

However, recognizing problems does not lead to safer practice if the shortcomings of the system are perceived to be unalterable (Waring 2007). Where adverse events occur, it is important for clinicians and managers to differentiate shortcomings within the system from any weaknesses in individual decision-making—a distinction between latent conditions for error, which includes poor design, and active failings (Reason 2000). In response to an adverse event, organizations need to look beyond the immediate antecedent actions of individuals to the basic assumptions and conditions that brought them about (Reason *et al.* 2001). For instance, having to report to an extended chain of command can impede local decision-making in response to a crisis. Bogner (2004)

Table 17.4 Elements of safe design in health care facilities

Effective use of space (e.g. busy thoroughfares, smoking areas)

Noise reduction (e.g. insulation, machinery, workstations)

Good visibility (e.g. sight-lines, lighting, use of colour-coding)

Mobility (e.g. flooring, type and location of furniture, use of space)

Communication (e.g. clearly marked areas for people with sensory/communication impairment)

Bedroom design (e.g. accessibility, hazards, privacy vs. visibility)

Access in emergencies (e.g. fire, personal injury, critical illness)

provides many examples of this and other failings operating in health care settings. It follows that effective risk management procedures require local accountability to enable decisions to be made quickly in response to changing conditions. Consideration should be given not simply to the most likely scenario, but also to the most difficult to manage, in order to ensure that risk management procedures are not encumbered by inefficient protocols. Consider a man with a tendency to impulsive spending. A risk assessment may reveal that he should not have more than £5 per day as he has spent excessively on alcohol in the past, with a consequent risk of falls and aggression, but this may be difficult to adhere to if he is angrily demanding his weekly allowance from an intimidated support worker. The risk assessment may state that no procedural change should be introduced until it has been discussed with his case manager and approved by his receiver, but to follow this course of action may aggravate the client and place the carer at greater risk of harm. It may be safer to keep a 'float' of additional monies available as an interim measure to pacify the client and buy time to discuss a more effective risk management strategy.

Risk-taking and executive dysfunction

Having examined a number of relevant approaches to risk, we turn now to the particular difficulties associated with brain injury, and especially executive function. Brain injury predisposes individuals towards greater risk-taking in three ways:

(1) cognitive limitations increase susceptibility to common information processing biases to which we are all prone;

(2) dysfunction of frontally mediated regulatory mechanisms can cause a general weakening of inhibitory control, increasing sensation-seeking behaviour and a shift towards extroversion on the normal introvert–extrovert personality dimension;

(3) damage to selective prefrontal regions disrupts the neural substrate for decision-making, causing poor decision-making and social judgement.

Taking each of these points in turn, first there is a range of information processing biases that can undermine efficient decision-making under uncertainty (Plous 1993). These include a tendency to make judgements based on appearance (halo effect), to overestimate positive outcomes for ourselves and negative outcomes for others, and to attribute one's own actions to situational influences but the actions of others to personal dispositions. Clinicians should take note of the possibility of their risk evaluations being influenced in this manner. Secondly, a general tendency towards impulsive or disinhibited behaviour after brain injury should be recognized as potentially having relevance for evaluation of risk, regardless of whether there is a history of a specific risk. There is evidence from healthy individuals that sensation-seeking is a stable trait across time (Zuckerman and Kuhlman 2000; Nicholson *et al.* 2005), but taking health risks (as opposed to risks associated with extreme sports for example) tends to be associated with other antisocial conduct. It follows that the emergence or exacerbation of asocial behaviour after brain injury will raise the likelihood of risks to the self.

We will focus particularly on the third point because this is unique to a subtype of executive dysfunction involving the orbitofrontal cortex and the ventromedial prefrontal areas, which are crucially implicated in decision-making (Walter *et al.* 2005). Neurons in these areas have been shown to respond to such diverse rewards as food and money, and are intimately involved in associative learning (Rolls 1999). People with known orbitofrontal damage often behave in a manner that suggests they are driven by their own impulses, showing a consequent disregard for social conventions (Eslinger and Damasio 1985; Varney and Menefee 1993). Such individuals may acquire a criminal or psychiatric history in the light of their antisocial behaviour (Pincus 1999; Brower and Price 2001). Investigations into this 'acquired sociopathy' have revealed underlying impairments in decision-making, especially in the social realm (see Table 17.5). For example, Dimitrov *et al.* (1999) described a Vietnam veteran with an exemplary military record who sustained a right ventromedial lesion in combat at 20 years of age. Despite average intelligence and retention of many executive skills, the following 30 years were a testimony to his poor judgement, social ineptitude, and diminished sense of responsibility, including three failed marriages, financial exploitation, and convictions for shoplifting and sexual offences. Importantly, this profile seems to be absent in persons with orbitofrontal damage sparing the ventral medial prefrontal (VMPF) structures (Satish *et al.* 1999).

Based on performance on what has become known as the Iowa Gambling Task (IGT) Bechara *et al.* (1997) developed a complex model of decision-making

Table 17.5 Characteristics of acquired sociopathy

Blunting of emotional experience
Inadequate control of emotional responses
Deficient goal-directed behaviour
Poor decision-making
Disturbances in social behaviour
Impoverished awareness of changes in personality

After Tranel 2002

incorporating both cognitive and emotional processes. This includes access to previous positive and negative outcomes, maintenance in working memory of information relevant to a current decision, and an action plan for achieving a specified goal. A deficit in any of these processes can result in impaired decision-making in the form of 'cognitive impulsivity'. In the IGT, decisions by patients with VMPF damage were weighted in favour of higher immediate gains, even where longer-term gains were reduced (Bechara *et al.* 1994). This bias was not evident for healthy controls or in a non-VMPF brain-injured group (see also Bechara *et al.* 2000).

Risk is involved whenever the outcome of a decision is uncertain, and it is generally assumed that risk-taking is guided by the perceived benefit of a favourable outcome (ie. the expected utility) for the risk-taker. This is traditionally conceived as a product of the value and the estimated probability of a particular outcome. It would be helpful for clinicians undertaking a risk assessment to know whether persons with executive disorder are willing to accept greater degrees of uncertainty or if they underestimate the likelihood of certain (negative) events. In other words, are their probability estimates awry or do they place disproportionate value on specific outcomes? Some evidence suggests the former. Using a computerized betting task, Salmond *et al.* (2005) reported that head-injured people were less likely than non-head-injured controls to change their betting preferences in response to a reduction in favourable odds. However, the compensation theory of risk tells us that the likelihood of risk-taking may also be influenced by the perceived benefits of an anticipated outcome, and so both possibilities need to be considered.

It has been argued that decision-making is normally influenced by the emotional feelings associated with the outcomes of previous decisions. For example, lower skin conductance responses, suggestive of lower arousal, are linked to greater risk-taking on the IGT (Suzuki *et al.* 2003). Decision-making may be compromised with damage to dorsolateral prefrontal areas (Fellows and Farah 2005), the amygdala (Bechara *et al.* 1999), and the hippocampus (Gutbrod *et al.* 2006), for different reasons in each case. However, according to one influential theory, the so-called somatic marker hypothesis (Damasio *et al.* 1991), it is structures in the ventromedial prefrontal region which provide the potential for learning an association between an event and the corresponding emotional state. The brain lays down a marker for future reference—the somatic marker. Thus negative outcomes can be anticipated and avoided. Tranel has described the process in the following manner:

> Somatic markers allow certain option–outcome pairs to be rapidly endorsed or rejected, making the decision-making space manageable for a logic-based cost-benefit analysis. In situations in which there is a lot of uncertainty regarding which course

of action is optimal, the constraints imposed by somatic markers would allow the individual to decide efficiently within reasonable time intervals, and to decide in a manner that is consistent with applicable social norms and with the best interests of the principal parties to the situation.

(Tranel 2000, p. 412.)

However, patients with VMPC lesions do not show this anticipatory response, making them more likely to repeat their mistakes, exhibiting a 'myopia for the future' (Bechara *et al.* 2002). Persons with orbitofrontal dysfunction (including the ventromedial region) tend to have particular problems with the neural processes that regulate feelings and emotions (intuitions) critical to decision-making (Bechara 2004). This may be related to underlying cognitive deficits. For example, ventromedial patients appear to adopt different strategies for decision-making than patients with dorsolateral damage (Fellows 2006). Moreover, Hinson *et al.* (2002) and Jameson *et al.* (2004) reported that tasks which utilize central executive resources (but not routine tasks such as articulatory suppression) interfere with the establishment of somatic markers. Conversely, Turnbull *et al.* (2005) failed to show any effect of a cognitively demanding secondary task on IGT performance, and concluded that intuitive decision-making (at least in the context of gambling tasks) involves processes separable from the working memory required for rational decision-making. Therefore the evidence suggests that poor decision-making may be due to either impaired cognitive processes (such as working memory) necessary to establish anticipatory emotional reactions, or specific disruption of emotion-based learning mechanisms. Either form of deficit may explain why executive dysfunction is associated with failure to learn from negative experience. The important point here is that decision-making can be undermined by too little or too much emotion, with such patients seeming to suffer a deficiency of 'emotional intelligence' despite preserved IQ (Bar-On *et al.* 2005).

The integration of cognition and emotion in risky decision-making underlies the emergence of new 'cognitive neuroeconomic' models (Kenning and Plassmann 2005). These are being applied to investigate normal human activity, such as risky sexual behaviour (Gutnik *et al.* 2006), and promise to aid our understanding of risk-taking in brain injury. Risky decisions are considered to recruit the so-called 'hot' executive functions subsumed by ventromedial neural circuits, as opposed to 'cool' decision-making in less risky scenarios which relies more on the dorsolateral prefrontal region. The distinction between 'hot' emotional executive processes and 'cool' cognitive executive processes is supported by functional neuroimaging data. A recent meta-analysis suggests that neural substrates for decision-making vary depending on the type of decision being made (Krain *et al.* 2006). This has clear clinical implications, as evidence of rational decision-making in one domain cannot be taken to indicate adequate judgement in another sphere. Therefore clinicians with responsibility for evaluating decision-making capability, be it in terms of assessing a risk or judging mental capacity, must be alert to variability in different domains of decision-making.

Conclusions: managing risk in executive disorder

This section could have been entitled 'to err is human' as it will by now be apparent that one cannot and should not try to eliminate risk-taking on the grounds that a person has a brain injury, has executive difficulties, and may do some things we regard as foolish. Experienced practitioners will have met many persons with brain injury who indulged in high-risk activities (legal or otherwise) before their injury. The consequence is often an exacerbation of a premorbid risk-taking disposition. Indeed, when coupled with a history of anti-social behaviour and resistance to authority, one could be forgiven for regarding risk management with some individuals as akin to re-arranging the furniture on the deck of the *Titanic*. This predicament was recognized by Ylvisaker and Feeney in highlighting the difficulty of working with 'the clinically challenging population of risk-taking adolescents and young adults who sometimes find themselves after a severe brain injury in a situation that they interpret as *binkification*—the typically counter-productive process of attempting to transform tough Dobermanns into passive and "socially appropriate" poodles' (Ylvisaker and Feeney 2000, p. 407). As stated in the introduction, risk is part of everyday living and should be embraced, but a duty of care and obligation to act in a person's best interests does not always sit easily with the promotion of autonomy and respect for an individual's right to make unwise decisions. Consequently, risk management is not for the faint-hearted, or the easily dispirited.

To return to our tightrope walker at the beginning of the chapter, effective management of risk is a delicate balancing act—one that improves with practice and should not be undertaken without a suitable safety net. The safety net in this instance is an appreciation of the variety of conceptual frameworks that can be used to inform the risk management process. We are at the stage where we can now outline the basis of a comprehensive approach to risk management for people with executive disorder. This can be organized around a series of key questions derived from multiple theoretical perspectives (see Appendix 3). Although the dominant actuarial approach has limited scope (not least because of the lack of quality data on relevant behaviour), much useful information from other perspectives can be practically employed. We have established that certain types of executive disorder predispose people to poor judgement, and this needs to be taken into account in clinical risk assessments. Too much or too little emotion associated with a decision can impair judgement. Similarly, in the absence of an objective measurement tool, the judgement of the assessor is also subject to a variety of influences (personal, professional, and cultural) which have to be acknowledged.

Cognitive models remind us that the beliefs that people hold about risks need to be investigated and can be challenged by tackling either the sources of information or the beliefs themselves. However one should remain alert to the possibility of risk displacement and the emergence of substitute behaviours in response to interventions. This likelihood can be minimized by understanding the function of risk-taking for the individual. Finally, the environment in which people work, live, and play can have an important influence in raising or reducing risk-taking as well as on the risk management process itself. The existence or otherwise of fair-minded systems for monitoring actions and reflecting on adverse events will affect both a willingness to accept risk and the ability to learn from experience. To paraphrase Lambert (2003)—errors of judgement (failure to *accurately* assess risk) are inevitable, errors of omission (failure to *adequately* assess risk) are preventable. It is hoped that familiarity with the theoretical perspectives introduced in this chapter will equip practitioners with the tools for an adequate evaluation of risk in most circumstances, and thereby the means to develop a comprehensive risk management intervention.

References

Adams, J. (1988). Risk homeostasis and the purpose of safety regulation. *Ergonomics* **31** 407–428.

Adams, J. (1995). *Risk*. Routledge, London.

Association of British Insurers (2005). *Care and compensation*. Association of British Insurers, London.

Audit Commission (2007). *Changing lanes: evolving roles in road safety*. Audit Commission, London.

Bar-On, R., Tranel, D., Denburg, N.L., and Bechara, A. (2005). Exploring the neurological substrate of emotional and social intelligence. In: *Social Neuroscience* (ed J.T Cacioppo and G.G. Berntson), pp. 223–37. Psychology Press, New York.

Bechara, A. (2004). The role of emotion in decision-making: evidence from neurological patients with orbito-frontal damage. *Brain and Cognition*, **55**, 30–40.

Bechara, A., Damasio, A.R., Damasio, H., and Anderson, S.W. (1994). Insensitivity to future consequences following damage to human prefrontal cortex. *Cognition*, **50**, 7–15.

Bechara, A., Damasio, H., Tranel, D., and Damasio, A.R. (1997). Deciding advantageously before knowing the advantageous strategy. *Science*, **275**, 1293–5.

Bechara, A., Damasio, H., Damasio, A.R., and Lee, G.P. (1999). Different contributions of the human amygdala and ventromedial prefrontal cortex to decision-making. *Journal of Neuroscience*, **19**, 5473–83.

Bechara, A., Damasio, H., and Damasio, A.R. (2000). Emotion decision making and the orbitofrontal cortex. *Cerebral Cortex* **10**, 295–307.

Bechara, A., Dolan, S., and Hindes, A. (2002). Decision-making and addiction. Part II: Myopia for the future or hypersensitivity to reward? *Neuropsychologia*, **40**, 1690–1705.

Better Regulation Commission (2006). *Risk, responsibility and regulation. Whose risk is it anyway?* Better Regulation Commission, London.

Bogner, M.S. (ed) (2004). *Misadventures in health care.* Lawrence Erlbaum, Mahwah, NJ.

British Psychological Society (1998). *Assessing and managing suicide risk.* British Psychological Society, Leicester.

Brower, M.C. and Price, B.H. (2001). Neuropsychiatry of frontal lobe dysfunction in violent and criminal behaviour: a critical review. *Journal of Neurology, Neurosurgery, and Psychiatry*, **71**, 720–6.

Cavell, G. (2004). Using failure, mode and effects analysis to reduce medication errors. *Health Care Risk Report*, **11**, 10–11.

Commission for Social Care Inspection (2006). *Making choices: taking risks.* CSCI, Newcastle upon Tyne.

Conner, M. and Norman, P. (2005). *Predicting health behaviour* (2nd edn). McGraw-Hill, Maidenhead.

Coyle, D. (2002). *Sex, drugs and economics.* Texere, New York.

Corbett, K. and Westwood, T. (2005). 'Dangerous and severe personality disorder': a psychiatric manifestation of the risk society. *Critical Public Health*, **15**, 121–33.

Craig, L.A., Browne, K.D., Stringer, I., and Beech, A. (2004). Limitations in actuarial risk assessment of sexual offenders: a methodological note. *British Journal of Forensic Practice*, **6**, 16–32.

Damasio, A.R., Tranel, D., and Damasio, H.C. (1991). Somatic markers and the guidance of behavior: theory and preliminary testing. In: *Frontal lobe function and dysfunction* (ed H.S. Levin, H.M. Eisenberg, and A.L. Benton), pp. 217–229. Oxford University Press, New York.

Davis, R.M. and Pless, B. (2001). BMJ bans 'accidents' (editorial). *British Medical Journal*, **322**, 1320–1.

Department of Health (2003). *Care homes for adults (18–65). and supplementary standards for care homes accommodating young people aged 16 and 17. National Minimum Standards Care Homes Regulations* (2nd edn). Stationery Office, London.

Department of Health (2007). *Independence choice and risk: a guide to supported decision making.* Department of Health, London.

Dimitrov, M., Phipps, M., Zahn, T.P., and Grafman, J. (1999). A thoroughly modern Gage. *Neurocase*, **5**, 345–54.

Dandurand, K. (2004). Prescription for error: can health care providers really 'Do no harm'? In: *Misadventures in health care* (ed M.S. Bogner), pp. 183–99. Lawrence Erlbaum, Mahwah, NJ.

Elliot, M.A., Armitage, C.J., and Baughan, C.J. (2007). Using the theory of planned behaviour to predict observed driving behaviour. *British Journal of Social Psychology*, **46**, 69–90.

Eslinger, P.J. and Damasio, A.R. (1985). Severe disturbance of higher cognition after bilateral frontal lobe ablation. *Neurology*, **35**, 1731–41.

Fellows, L.K. (2006). Deciding how to decide: ventromedial frontal lobe damage affects information acquisition in multi-attribute decision making. *Brain*, **129**, 944–52.

Fellows, L.K. and Farah, M.J. (2005). Different underlying impairments in decision-making following ventromedial and dorsolateral frontal lobe damage in humans. *Cerebral Cortex*, **15**, 58–63.

Furedi, F. (2002). *Culture of fear: risk taking and the morality of low expectation.* Continuum, London.

Greaves, R. and Harris, J. (2006). The role of the case manager in risk assessment. In: *Good practice in brain injury case management* (ed J. Parker), pp. 91–107. Jessica Kingsley, London.

Guldberg, H. (2000). Child protection and the precautionary principle. In: *Rethinking risk and the precautionary principle* (ed J. Morris), pp. 127–39. Butterworth Heineman, Oxford.

Gutbrod, K., Krouzel, C., Hofer, H., Muri, R., Perrig, W., and Ptak, R. (2005). Decision-making in amnesia: do advantageous decision require conscious knowledge of previous behavioural choices? *Neuropsychologica*, **44**, 1315–24.

Gutnik, L.A., Hakimzada, A.F., Yoskowitz, N.A., and Patel, V.L. (2006). The role of emotion in decision-making: a cognitive neuroeconomic approach towards understanding sexual risk behaviour. *Journal of Biomedical Information*, **39**, 720–36.

Hagel, B., Macpherson, A., Rivara, F.P., and Pless, B. (2006). Arguments against helmet legislation are flawed. *British Medical Journal*, **332**, 725–6.

Health and Safety Commission (2006). *Health and safety statistics 2005/06.* Health and Safety Executive, Sudbury, Suffolk.

Hinson, J.M., Jameson, T.L., and Whitney, P. (2002). Somatic markers, working memory and decision making. *Cognitive, Affective and Behavioral Neuroscience*, **2**, 341–53.

House of Lords (2006). *Government policy on the management of risk. Select Committee on Economic Affairs (5th Report).* House of Lords. Available online at http://www.publications.parliament.uk/ (accessed 17 November 2006).

Institute of Psychiatry (2002).

Jameson, T.L., Hinson, J.M.,and Whitney, P. (2004). Components of working memory and somatic markers in decision making. *Psychonomic Bulletin and Review*, **11**, 515–20.

Kenning, P. and Plassmann, H. (2005). Neuroeconomics: an overview from an economic perspective. *Brain Research Bulletin*, **67**, 343–54.

Krain, A.L., Wilson, A.M., Arbuckle, R., Castellanos, F.X., and Milham, M.P. (2006). Distinct neural mechanisms of risk and ambiguity: a meta analysis of decision making. *NeuroImage* **32**, 477–84.

Lambert, M.T. (2003). Suicide risk assessment and management: focus on personality disorders. *Current Opinion in Psychiatry*, **16**, 71–6.

McCulloch, J., Sykes, M., and Haut, F. (2005). Accidents don't happen anymore: junior doctors' experience of fatal accident inquiries in Scotland. *Postgraduate Medical Journal*, **81**, 185–7.

Marr, A. (2004). *My trade.* Macmillan, London.

Medley, A., Thompson, M., and French, J. (2006). Predicting the probability of falls in community dwelling persons with brain injury: a pilot study. *Brain Injury*, **20**, 1403–8.

Morgan, M.G., Fischoff, B., Bostrom, A., and Atman, C.J. (2002). *Risk communication. a mental models approach.* Cambridge University Press, New York.

Murphy, D. (2002). Risk assessment as collective clinical judgment. *Criminal Behavior and Mental Health,* **12**, 169–78.

Newell, S. (2001). Clinical risk assessment for an occupational therapy inpatient group programme. *British Journal of Occupational Therapy,* **64**, 200–2.

Nicholson, N., Soane, E., Fenton-O'Creevy, M., and Willman, P. (2005). Personality and domain-specific risk taking. *Journal of Risk Research,* **8**, 157–76.

Norko, M.A., Baranoski, M.V. (2005). The state of contemporary risk assessment research. *Canadian Journal of Psychiatry,* **50**, 18–26.

Oakley, R. (2001). *Inside track.* Bantam Press, London.

O'Connor, R.C., Armitage, C.J., and Gray, L. (2006). The role of clinical and cognitive variables in parasuicide. *British Journal of Clinical Psychology,* **45**, 465–81.

Oyebode, F. (2006). Clinical errors and medical negligence. *Advances in Psychiatric Treatment,* **12**, 221–7.

Park, N., Conrod, B., Hussain, Z., Murphy, K.J., Rewilak, D., and Black, S.E. (2003). A treatment program for individuals with deficits in evaluative processing and consequent impaired social and risk judgment. *Neurocase,* **9**, 51–62.

Pidgeon, N., Henwood, K., and Maguire, B. (1999). Public health communication and the social amplification of risks: present knowledge and future behaviour prospects. In: *Risk communication and public health* (ed P. Bennett and K. Calman), pp. 65–77. Oxford University Press, New York.

Pincus, J.H. (1999). Aggression, criminality and the frontal lobes. In: *The human frontal lobes* (ed B.L. Miller and J.L. Cummings), pp. 547–56. Guilford Press, New York.

Plous, S. (1993). *The psychology of judgment and decision making.* McGraw-Hill, new York.

Poortinga, W. and Pidgeon, N. (2003). *Public perceptions of risk, science and governance.* Centre for Environmental Risk, University of East Anglia.

Prins, H. (2005). Taking chances: risk assessment and management in a risk obsessed society. *Medicine, Science and Law,* **45**, 93–109.

Rakow, T., Vincent, C., Bull, K., and Harvey, N. (2005). Assessing the likelihood of an important clinical outcome: new insights from a comparison of clinical and actuarial judgment. *Medical Decision Making,* **25**, 262–82.

Reason, J. (1990). *Human error.* Cambridge University Press, New York.

Reason, J. (2000). Human error: models and management. *British Medical Journal,* **320**, 768–70.

Reason, J. (2001). Understanding adverse events: the human factor. In: *Clinical risk management* (ed C. Vincent), pp. 9–30. BMJ Books, London.

Reason, J.T., Carthey, J., and de Leval, M.R. (2001). Diagnosing 'vulnerable system syndrome': an essential prerequisite to effective risk management. *Quality and Health Care,* **10** (Suppl II), ii21–5.

Reiling, J (2006). Safe design of healthcare facilities. *Quality and Safety in Health Care,* **15** (Suppl I), i34–40.

Robinson, D.L. (2006). No clear evidence from countries that have enforced the wearing of helmets. *British Medical Journal,* **332**, 722–5.

Rolls, E.T. (1999). The functions of the orbitofrontal cortex. *Neurocase*, **5**, 301–12.

Rowe, R., Siminoff, E., and Silberg, J.L. (2007). Psychopathology, temperament and unintentional injury: cross-sectional and longitudinal relationships. *Journal of Child Psychology and Psychiatry and Allied Disciplines*, **48**, 71–9.

Royal College of Psychiatrists (1996). *Assessment and clinical management of risk of harm to other people. Royal College Of Psychiatrists Special Working Party on Clinical Assessment and Management of Risk*. RCP Council Report CR 53. Available online at: www.rcpsych.ac.uk

Royal Society (1983). *Risk assessment: a study group report*. Royal Society, London.

Royal Society (1992). *Risk: analysis, perception and management*. Royal Society, London.

Salmond, C.H., Menon, D.K., Chatfield, D.A., Pickard, J.D., and Sahakian, B.J. (2005). Deficits in decision-making in head injury survivors. *Journal of Neurotrauma*, **22**, 613–22.

Satish, U., Streufert, S., and Eslinger, P.J. (1999). Complex decision making after orbito-frontal damage: neuropsychological assessment and strategic management simulation assessment. *Neurocase*, **5**, 355–64.

Scally, G. and Donaldson, L.J. (1998). Clinical governance and the drive for quality improvement in the new NHS in England. *British Medical Journal*, **317**, 61–5.

Suzuki, A., Hirota, A., Takasawa, N., and Shigemasu, K. (2003). Application of the somatic marker hypothesis to individual differences in decision making. *Biological Psychology*, **65**, 81–8.

Thompson, M., Ellis, R., and Wildavsky, A. (1990). *Cultural theory*. Westview, Boulder, CO.

Tranel, D. (2000). Neural correlates of violent behaviour. In: *Behavior and mood disorders in focal brain injury* (ed J. Bogousslavsky and J.L. Cummings), pp. 399–418. Cambridge University Press.

Tranel, D. (2002). Emotion, decision making, and the ventromedial prefrontal cortex. In: *Principles of frontal lobe function* (ed D. Stuss and R.T. Knight), pp. 338–53. Oxford University Press, New York.

Tulloch, J. and Lupton, D. (2003). *Risk and everyday life*. Sage, London.

Turnbull, O.H., Evans, C.E.Y., Bunce, A., Carzolio, B., and O'Connor, J. (2005). Emotion-based learning and central executive resources: an investigation of intuition and the Iowa Gambling Task. *Brain and Cognition*, **57**, 244–7.

Varney, N.R. and Menefee, L. (1993). Psychosocial and executive deficits following closed head injury: implications for orbital frontal cortex. *Journal of Head Trauma Rehabilitation*, **8**, 32–44.

Walshe, K. and Sheldon, T.A. (1998). Dealing with clinical risk: implications of the rise of evidence-based health care. *Public Money and Management*, **19**, 15–20.

Walshe, K. and Shortell, S.M. (2004). When things go wrong: how health care organisations deal with major failures. *Health Affairs*, **23**, 103–11.

Walter, H., Abler, B., Ciaramidaro, A., and Erk, S. (2005). Motivating forces of human actions: neuroimaging reward and social interaction. *Brain Research Bulletin*, **67**, 368–81.

Waring, J.J. (2007). Doctors' thinking about 'the system' threat to patient safety. *Health*, **11**, 29–46.

Wilf-Miron, R., Lewnhof, I., Benyamini, Z., and Aviram, A. (2003). From aviation to medicine: applying concepts of aviation safety to risk management in ambulatory care. *Quality and Safety in Health Care*, 12, 35–9.

Williams, S. and Osborn, S. (2004). National Patient Safety Agency: an introduction. *Clinical Governance*, 9, 130–1.

Wreathall, J. and Nemeth, C. (2004). Assessing risk: the role of probabilistic risk assessment (PRA). in patient safety improvement. *Quality and Safety in Health Care*, 13, 206–12.

Ylvisaker, M. and Feeney, T. (2000). Reflections on Dobermanns, poodles, and social rehabilitation for difficult-to-serve individuals with traumatic brain injury. *Aphasiology*, 14, 407–31.

Zuckerman, M. and Kuhlman, D.M. (2000). Personality and risk-taking: common biosocial factors. *Journal of Personality*, 68, 999–1029.

Useful web-based resources

Clinical Governance Support Group A learning organization which uses its broad expertise and relationships with other organizations to promote safe patient-centred care. Website: www.cgsupport.nhs.uk. Further information on clinical governance, including policy documents is available at: www.dh.gov.uk/Policyandguidance/Healthandsocialcaretopics/Clinicalgovernance.

Clinical Risk A journal of the Royal Society of Medicine read by clinical and legal professionals, with a particular emphasis on clinical negligence. Website: www.rsmpress.co.uk.

Department for Constitutional Affairs The website www.dca.gov.uk contains details of the Compensation Act 2006, which includes provisions relating to the law of negligence and breach of statutory duty, as well as details of the Mental Capacity Act 2005. The work of the DCA has now been subsumed by the Ministry of Justice: www.justice.gov.uk.

Health and Safety Commission Government body responsible for health and safety regulation in the UK. The Health and Safety Executive is the body responsible, together with local authorities, for enforcing regulation. The website www.hse.gov.uk includes a summary of the web forum on risk aversion in society, as well as downloadable resources concerning risk management.

National Institute of Health and Clinical Excellence Provides guidance and guidelines on a multitude of health-related topics, including management of a range of mental and behavioural disorders, including secondary prevention measures. Website: www.nice.org.uk.

National Patient Safety Agency (NPSA) A UK Special Health Authority created to improve the capacity of the NHS to learn from errors and wrong-doing. Website: www.npsa.nhs.uk. Details of NPSA training programmes in Root Cause Analysis can be obtained by contacting www.rca@npsa.nhs.uk.

Quality and Safety in Health Care An international journal devoted to quality and safety issues in health care settings. Publishes a wide variety of original articles and reviews. Website: www.qshc.bmj.com.

Royal Society for the Prevention of Accidents (RoSPA) A national charity promoting greater safety awareness in all aspects of daily life. RoSPA hosts conferences and produces information about safety, and offers safety advice and training on specialized risk assessments. Website: www.rospa.com.

Appendix 1. Supported decision tool (Department of Health 2007)

What is important to you in your life?

What isn't working so well?

What could make it better?

What things are difficult for you?

Describe how they affect your life?

What would make things better for you?

What is stopping you from doing what you want to do?

Do you think there are any risks?

Could things be done in a different way which might reduce the risks?

Would you do things differently?

Is the risk present wherever you live?

What do you need to do?

What do staff/organization need to change?

What could family/carers do?

Who is important to you?

What do people important to you think?

Are there any differences of opinion between you and the people you said are important to you?

What would help to resolve this?

Who might be able to help?

What could we do (practitioner) to support you?

Agreed next steps–who will do what?

How would you like your care plan to be changed to meet your outcomes?

Record of any disagreements between people involved?

Date agreed to review how you are managing

Signatures

Appendix 2. Suicide risk matrix

Client name: _____ Date of birth: _____

Complete one column for each risk assessment. Indicate the presence of a risk factor by placing a tick in the appropriate box.

Risk Factor	Date
Predisposing factors	
S Male	
A Age (<25 years)	
D Depression	
P History of suicide attempts requiring medical attention	
E Alcohol abuse	
R Psychosis	
S Limited social support	
N No spouse	
Other psychiatric/mood disorder	
History of self-harm	
Loss or bereavement at an early age	
Observable risk factors	
Suicide plan	
Verbalizations of suicide intent	
Recent experience of failure, rejection or loss.	
Anniversary of losses	
Recent change in habits	
Deterioration in affect or behaviour	
Recent non-compliance with medication	
Psychometric assessment score (if used) *BHS/BSSI*	
Completed by (sign name)	
Signature of Senior Clinician	

© Dr Andrew Worthington

Appendix 3

RISK ASSESSMENT Risk estimation		RISK ASSESSMENT Risk evaluation	Primary risk management	Risk re-assessment	Secondary risk management
Likelihood of event occurring	Consequences of outcomes (severity)	Value (importance attached to outcomes)	Actions taken to minimize risk	Possible consequences of intervention	Any further actions required
High probability (potentially a daily event)	Risk of injury or exploitation while in community alone	B attaches high importance to his freedom to leave unit	Daily feedback on his progress to encourage his engagement	He may try to leave the unit if he finds the feedback distressing, irritating or patronising	All feedback to be recorded, noting B's response, updating risk if he is upset
	Loss of therapy input	High value attached to going back home.	Bi-weekly visits home arranged with his family	If he is allowed home he may refuse to return	
This is based on past record and B's stated intentions	Risk of alienation of family members at home with unplanned visits	He attaches low importance to complying with unit procedures.	Opportunity to earn additional 'family time' by complying with therapy sessions	May view failure to earn extra 'family time' as punishment: increase the risk of absconding, and possible increased risk to staff trying to dissuade him	B and his family to be given clear guidance on what is expected, and how to respond if he refuses to return
	Resources diverted to locate and return B to rehabilitation unit	Low importance given to listening to staff that he perceives are telling him what to do	Staff will communicate with him in a respectful non-threatening manner, accepting his frustrations		Guidelines on giving feedback and level of supervision if no extra 'family time' earned.

© Dr Andrew Worthington

Appendix 4. Principles of risk assessment associated with executive dysfunction

Based on the different approaches reviewed, there are several core principles that should dictate the evaluation of risk in persons with executive disorder. These can be arranged around five important questions for any given risky behaviour X as follows.

What attributes (personal or circumstantial) does the client possess that raise the likelihood of behaviour X?

This question asks for actuarial data that might bear on the question of how likely a person is to engage in a specific action. An illustration of how this might be used in practice is the development of a suicide risk assessment tool utilizing information about predictors of suicide from the mental health literature.

What evidence exists that this individual has previously acted in this manner?

This question reminds the clinician that the best guide to future actions is past behaviour, a core tenet of clinical risk assessment. This information is also incorporated into the suicide risk assessment decision tool in Appendix 2.

What would the client hope to achieve by such an action?

The theory of risk compensation not only incorporates the notion of value or expected utility, but also provides a mechanism for understanding how risk management strategies can sometimes increase levels of risk. An example of how this might be incorporated into a risk assessment tool is provided in Appendix 3 (in a case of risk of absconding from a rehabilitation facility).

Is the client able to understand and weigh up the costs and benefits of their behaviour before acting?

It may be important to address misinformation and underlying beliefs about risk-taking and thereby support the decision-making process. Park *et al.* (2003) reported using this kind of strategy in helping a head-injured man identify risky business decisions. However, individuals with executive disorder may be able to articulate costs and benefits rationally but still take risks regardless (e.g. because of their impulsive nature). This would suggest a more environmentally based approach to risk management, addressing the antecedent conditions to risk-taking.

What aspects of the environment need to be considered as potentially increasing the risk involved in behaviour X? Can this be reduced by modifying the environment?

It is important to recognize how a risky behaviour in one setting may not be such a risk in another context. It may be possible to promote autonomy by modifying the environment rather than the behaviour (hence a client may be less likely to smoke in his/her bedroom if given an adequate indoor smoking area instead of being told to smoke outside).

What would be the consequences for A, for his/her carer/therapist and for the organization if A carried out behaviour X?

As most risks can only be reduced and not eliminated. Risk-taking still takes place and adverse outcomes may arise. Risk management may involve a degree of restriction that needs to be balanced against the possible consequences should an undesirable behaviour occur. In general, interventions to reduce harm may be more restrictive than those that minimize other losses because the consequences are considered more serious if harm should occur.

18

The family and executive disorders

Michael Oddy and Camilla Herbert

Brain Injury Rehabilitation Trust, Horsham, West Sussex

Introduction

One of the most frequently reported and consistent findings in brain injury research concerns the impact of behavioural or personality changes associated with brain injury on the family (Rosenbaum and Najenson 1976; Perlesz *et al.* 1999; Oddy and Herbert 2003). Many studies have found such changes to be the ones that the family finds most difficult to live with and accept (e.g. Rosenbaum and Najenson 1976; Oddy *et al.* 1985; Brooks 1991; Florian and Katz 1991; Kreutzer *et al.* 1994). Family members often use phrases such as 'living with a stranger' or 'he's not the same person'. Frequently these changes are associated with damage to anterior cortical areas and with executive disorder. In this chapter we will explore the nature of these difficulties and how families can learn to live with them.

It is a commonly reported experience of families that others, both extended family and many of the health professionals they come across, do not appreciate and understand the nature and significance of many of the changes, particularly personality changes, that take place after brain injury (Gervasio and Kreutzer 1997; Knight *et al.* 1998). Personality changes following brain injury can occur in varying degrees and kinds. Often such changes may be subtle and not obvious even to close friends or family if they do not actually live with the person with the brain injury. Nevertheless, to those in the same household even subtle changes can make the person seem like a stranger, an impostor inhabiting the body of the person they knew. Understanding the nature and potential impact of these difficulties on the family is an important aspect of what rehabilitation professionals can offer families. Not only can brain injury professionals form an immediate bond with families by their familiarity with such symptoms, but they can also help the family to understand and deal with these difficulties through their theoretical understanding of the origins and operation of these changes.

It is important to emphasize the family's unique role in brain injury rehabilitation that is different from and complementary to that played by rehabilitation professionals. The family's knowledge and understanding of the person is crucial, and their relationship with the person allows them to play a different part in the rehabilitation process. The family can have an important role in motivating the individual to take part in rehabilitation, especially at early stages when the brain-injured person is unlikely to have a full awareness of their difficulties and sees little need for rehabilitation. Furthermore, their involvement is necessary because they are likely to be involved with the person with the brain injury long after the rehabilitation team has completed its work.

In the following sections we consider those changes commonly associated with executive disorders and frontal lobe injuries and their impact on both the individual and close family members.

In Chapter 1 of this book Stuss outlined four aspects of frontal lobe function which, he argues, can be differentiated. This fourfold classification will be used to consider the variety of personality and behavioural changes that the family may experience when one of their members has a brain injury.

Regulating energization

Stuss's first category is that of regulating energization. In behavioural terms this is defined as the process of initiating and sustaining behaviours over time.

Initiating behaviour

This may mean that someone who has played a leading role in the family now lacks the ability to initiate the most basic activities. They may sit around the house, requiring considerable effort on the part of others to engage them in any activity, and may appear apathetic and lacking in motivation. It will also mean that other family members (often the spouse) have to take over many of the roles that brain-injured individual previously performed. When this occurs in someone with a profound brain injury it may be understood as part of the overall and extensive change in the person concerned. In cases where there is a greater level of preserved functions, reduced initiation can appear as an incomprehensible change and may be labelled as laziness or selfishness. At its extreme, the individual may become extremely passive and this can be immensely frustrating for members of the family. It is similar to the concept of 'negative symptoms' in psychiatry, which has often been found to be associated with greater family distress (Creer and Wing 1975; Kuipers and Bebbington 1990). The family can be helped considerably by having the nature of this difficulty explained and attributed to the brain injury. A simple explanation of the nature of this deficit and suggestions as to how to prompt and help the person to initiate can enable families to cope better.

The subjective experience of the individual also needs to be considered, as they may well have clear ideas and plans that they wish to implement but be frustrated by their lack of ability to initiate or instigate these plans. This increase in frustration and irritability will in turn have an impact on other members of the family.

Sustaining behaviour

The inability to sustain goal-directed activity and the tendency to be constantly distracted is an extremely common problem following a brain injury. This also needs to be explained to both the family and the patient. Often such problems are presented in very specific or concrete terms by the family—for example, 'He just goes off at a tangent. Sometimes I don't know what he's talking about'. If these problems can be explained and categorized for the family, and the family feels that they understand why the behaviour is occurring, it is usually much easier for them to accept and cope.

Another variant on distractibility is a tendency to become 'stimulus dependent' (Lezak 1978). The person with the brain injury becomes preoccupied by a particular idea and becomes 'stuck'. This can be immensely frustrating for other members of the family. Concepts such as perseveration (repeating a response or action when it is no longer appropriate) and utilization behaviour (being unable to resist the impulse to 'utilize' objects within their visual field and reach) represent extreme examples of this. Once again a label or explanation can be very helpful for families who may be mystified or embarrassed by such behaviour. It also provides them with an explanation that they can give to wider family or friends.

Executive cognitive functions

The second functional domain described by Stuss is that of executive cognitive functions. He describes these as those higher-level cognitive functions that provide control and direction of lower-level, more automatic functions. He further divides these into task setting and monitoring.

Task setting

Some people with initiation difficulties are able to formulate ideas and plans but are unable to trigger the action needed to achieve their goals. Others, however, lack the ability to generate ideas or intentions. Families can be helped by having this explained and being shown how to help the individual to produce ideas or make choices through the provision of lists of ideas.

Monitoring

Monitoring of plans is essential to ensure that one is not distracted and for prospective memory (see this volume, Chapter 5). Families can be frustrated by lapses of memory and the burden that falls back on to them. Strategies such as lists and alarms can relieve this frustration for both individual and family.

Disinhibition, a frequent consequence of frontal brain injury, can also be seen as a consequence of a deficit in monitoring. A deficit in this system leads to 'unedited' behaviour or speech being produced which is elicited by the prevailing environment but may be an inappropriate response to it. Disinhibition can vary from the subtle to the gross. At the subtle end it can appear as a loss of the social veneer that the person once had. Examples of this include jokes which do not quite catch the mood of their audience, overly personal revelations, or remarks that can be taken as mildly critical or offensive. At the other extreme it can result in entirely inappropriate and sometimes potentially dangerous behaviour. Examples of this can be extremely offensive or critical remarks, disrobing in public, or making overtly sexual remarks to children or strangers. Needless to say, this can be experienced by other family members as extremely embarrassing. Frequently, families remark on the fact that this embarrassment is compounded by the fact that the person with the brain injury appears 'normal' in every other way. However, families can learn to predict and pre-empt such behaviour by judiciously timed intervention.

One consequence of the behavioural manifestation of executive disorder and frontal lobe injury outlined above is the common finding of social isolation in studies of those who suffer a severe acquired brain injury (Oddy *et al* 1985). However, it is not only the individual who becomes isolated but often the whole family. Changes in social behaviour make it difficult for visitors to the home to know how to respond. They can be embarrassed or even frightened by the behaviour of the person with executive deficits. A second factor is that the reduced participation of the injured individual results in a loss of opportunities for social contact for the entire family (Winstanley *et al.* 2006). As previous social contacts drop away, a new social circle of contacts made through the brain injury often becomes increasingly important. Such contacts may be made through organizations such as Headway or through the rehabilitation services. Facilitating such social contacts is an important part of what rehabilitation services have to offer the family.

A behaviour related to disinhibition is impulsivity, which can also be seen as a failure of monitoring. Impulsivity involves an immediate action before there is time for thought. Norman and Shallice's (1986) theory of executive function describes two processes, contention scheduling and a supervisory system. Contention scheduling controls routine action of a familiar kind, where well-learned behavioural routines are rolled out according to environmental cues. The supervisory system is utilized when a novel or unexpected situation arises and there are no ready prepared behavioural routines or schemas available. Impulsivity can be seen as occurring because the supervisory system fails to kick in. In response to a stimulus or set of circumstances a behaviour may be triggered immediately which would not be the response of choice had a considered thought process intervened. Such behaviour can take the form of dangerous activities, such as crossing the road without due care and attention, using equipment without adequate attention to safety considerations, or spending money in ill-advised ways. It may also take the form of a person acting out of character, without regard to their normal values, preferences, or attitudes. Clearly, significant practical problems may result, and the family may require help and advice to develop ways of recognizing, predicting, and managing these tendencies.

Behavioural/emotional self-regulatory functions

Stuss suggests that behavioural self-regulation is required in situations where cognitive analysis, habit, or environmental cues are insufficient to determine the most adaptive response. Poor emotional regulation can have a major impact on the resulting response or behaviour.

Changes in emotional lability, ranging from increased irritability through to extreme swings of mood, can be a feature of damage to the anterior parts of the brain. The metaphor of 'walking on eggshells' is frequently used to describe the care the family must take to avoid triggering an extreme reaction, and unpredictable behaviour can be extremely difficult to live with. Setting clear boundaries about what is and is not acceptable can be surprisingly effective, as can the implementation of a predictable pattern or structure to daily life. Cognitive-behavioural therapy (CBT) approaches with the individual with the brain injury may also help to establish some control over emotional responses (see this volume, Chapter 8). However, if these interventions fail, helping families identify what the triggers are and hence finding ways of avoiding them may be the best answer.

In addition to an increase in variability of mood, those with frontal brain injuries may report a tendency to be more easily provoked into an emotional response, for example being reduced to tears when a sad film is shown on television. Often the emotional expression suggests a greater affective response than the individual experiences. In contrast, other people report a blunting of emotion. Sometimes associated with this are bouts of restless and aimless uncoordinated behaviour. Affect may be disturbed with loss of interest, emotional blunting, and a general indifference to the surrounding world. Clinically, this picture can resemble a major affective disorder with psycho-motor retardation, while the indifference bears occasional similarity to the *belle indifference* sometimes noted with hysteria or dissociative conditions. The lack of concern and emotional blunting can be extremely difficult for those closest to the individual. They often 'take it personally' and feel that they must be doing something wrong. It is essential to help them understand that this can be a feature of brain injury which renders the patient unable to experience these emotions in the way they did before. It may also be important to help the person with the brain injury to express concern about family members even if they do not feel it. If this is done in a careful and sensitive way, it can eventually lead the client to experiencing more emotion as well as meeting a need within the family setting.

Meta-cognitive processes

Stuss labels the fourth functional domain 'meta-cognitive processes'. These refer to the processes of self-reflection, and are vital in integrating cognition and emotion. They are involved in 'autonoetic consciousness' (the capacity to mentally represent and become aware of subjective experiences in the past, present, and future). This allows us to mentally travel back in subjective time to re-experience our personal past, resulting in the retrieval of episodic memories. In some patients, confabulation may occur where they recall inconsistent and even impossible versions of events.

Meta-cognition or self-reflection is also vital in various aspects of social cognition, including the ability to carry out tasks often referred to as requiring 'theory of mind'—being able to understand a situation from the point of view of another, either cognitively or emotionally. The appreciation of humour also requires self-reflection (Channon *et al.* 2007). As Stuss concludes, these clearly become translated into the common family complaints that, following brain injury, individuals show a loss of the ability to empathize, a lack of concern about others, and an inability to 'read' social situations or appreciate the emotional needs of others. Once again, these can have a devastating effect in the context of close family or intimate relationships. Gosling and Oddy (1999) found that in some cases the personality changes were such that the partners no longer desired a sexual relationship with the injured person. Where the brain-injured person expressed gratitude rather than affection, relationships declined considerably and positive feelings were often reduced. In some cases where the partner had taken on a 'carer' role, personal and sexual relationships also declined and the positive feelings became those of mutual commitment. Disinhibited behaviour sometimes changed the nature of the brain-injured person's sexual advances such that these felt coercive, which was correlated with lower sexual satisfaction for the partner. In other cases reduced libido meant that the brain-injured person was not initiating behaviour in this way. Gosling and Oddy note that in half the cases studied, the women reported that they welcomed their partner's sexual advances and would welcome the resumption of a more active sexual relationship. In general, brain injury has been found to result in a reduction of sexual interest (Oddy 2001).

The impact of these changes on children is also of huge significance. Having a father or mother who lacks the ability to empathize or to experience or express the normal feelings of parenthood and who may be concrete and unyielding in their thinking and lacking in any sense of humour or self-reflection is a major challenge. Despite the obvious difficulties that children can face following a brain injury to a parent they are frequently left out of the rehabilitation process, and even within the home their needs can be inadvertently neglected as a result of all the other pressing demands. A Family Resource Pack has recently been developed by Webster and Daisley (2005) to help brain injury professionals address the needs of children in this position.

How families cope

Families show differing capacities to cope with the type of executive difficulties described above. The majority succeed remarkably well, but others struggle and may break down. The current evidence indicates that the divorce rate appears to be about twice that for the general population (Stilwell *et al.* 1997; Wood and Yurdakul 1997; Oddy and Herbert 2002). Considerable attention has been focused on what determines whether a family copes or struggles. One factor appears to be the resilience the family brings to the situation, their history of coping with adversity, and their emotional stability. For example, one study found that a history of depression was the variable most predictive of emotional well-being in close relatives after a brain injury (Gillen *et al.* 1998). The impact of different coping styles and coping strategies has been explored, although the literature remains unclear in terms of specific recommendations. There is such variability in the situations studied and the methodology used that it is difficult to draw clear conclusions. However, there does seem to be some consensus that where a solution can be found **problem-focused coping** is often effective, but in situations where there is no solution **emotion-focused strategies**, such as altering the way a problem is viewed or tackling the emotional response directly, through relaxation exercises for example, may need to be adopted (Hanks *et al.* 2007). Certainly the evidence for the efficacy of changing one's emotional response by changing one's thinking pattern is gaining increasing support from empirical studies in CBT and similar therapeutic approaches. It is clear that those who are able to view a brain injury as a manageable family challenge, rather than as a catastrophe, are more likely to be able to cope. There is less evidence for the efficacy of specific interventions to alleviate distress in the relatives of those who have experienced executive disorder in particular, but by providing information and enhancing understanding it does seem to be possible to help family members to cope with a wide range of executive impairments. It is also important to help a family adopt an 'experimental' approach to solving their problems—identifying the exact nature of the problem and devising a possible solution, and if this solution does not work then devising another solution using feedback from the experience and trying again (Zarit *et al.* 1987).

Families and rehabilitation

Family members are key informants about the premorbid nature of the person with the brain injury which may be crucial in interpreting the changes in executive function. They will also be key informants concerning the changes following the injury and the progress the person makes. In addition to being the providers of important information, they are often of vital significance in motivating the person with the brain injury. The lack of awareness of deficits that is so commonly associated with executive disorders means that the long-standing and close relationship that relatives have with the person is vital to encourage them to collaborate with the rehabilitation and to take the advice of professionals, for example regarding driving, returning to work, etc. The family can also encourage and motivate when the client becomes distressed or frustrated by the speed of their progress.

Unfortunately, in many rehabilitation services, and particularly in residential rehabilitation, it is often the least experienced and least trained members of the team who have most contact with family members. With work and family commitments to meet, visits to the rehabilitation unit will often take place in the evenings or at weekends when in most cases the clinical team is not present. Although this can be addressed to some extent through regular telephone contact and meetings during the working week to adequately support family members and enhance the transfer of rehabilitation, it is vital that training is provided to all the staff team to allow them to understand the nature of the executive deficits involved and to be able to explain these to the family.

Family members frequently report feeling that they are very much alone and that even close family who do not live in the same household fail to understand the difficulties that they face. Well-meant comments about the progress of the person with the brain injury can be experienced as a negation of the struggle for the family member. There is a further role here for the brain injury professional. By demonstrating a knowledge and understanding of the situation the family is facing, the professional can make members of the family feel that their perceptions are validated and appreciated for the first time. Clearly a professional cannot appreciate exactly how it feels to live in this situation, but the fact that they can recognize and sometimes predict the sort of changes with which the family may have to contend gives them credibility and enables the family members to feel supported. This may be far more important than any specific intervention.

Family members often become overwhelmed by the practical responsibilities that they have to take on when a member of the family has a brain injury. This is most obviously the case for couples, where there is likely to have been some division of labour. Following brain injury the uninjured partners may find themselves, or feel themselves, responsible for everything. Roles previously played by the other partner now have to be taken on, often without support or advice. These new roles may concern financial management, child care, or maintenance of the home or car. One of the seminal papers describing frontal lobe disorders by Eslinger and Damasio (1988) demonstrates the type of financial difficulties in which someone with such deficits can easily find themselves. It is normally the family who has the task of resolving such issues.

The strength of the family's influence can be both a positive and a negative force. Where long-standing dysfunction is evident in a family, the prospects for the individual regaining optimal levels of independence can be bleak as progress may become sidetracked by pre-existing disputes or patterns of behaviour. In some cases a brain injury may provide the opportunity to raise and seek help for long-standing difficulties. This is not necessarily inappropriate, and it may well be crucial to deal with such issues if brain injury rehabilitation is to be successful. The last thing that someone with executive deficits needs is a chaotic family. However, in these circumstances it is important for the rehabilitation professionals to be able to tease out what is a result of the brain injury and what are long-standing family and individual problems. This is no easy task as the two often interact, and the resulting situation may be a combination of the two.

Where a family has strong emotional and practical resources to draw upon, the outlook is much brighter. Some families are able to absorb the principles of compensation from the rehabilitation personnel they come across, and use and extend these ideas. For example, Oddy and Cogan (2004) report the case of a young woman with severe prospective and episodic memory deficits as a result of a burst anterior communicating artery aneurysm. With the help of her parents, this young woman was able to develop an extremely independent and full lifestyle despite her profound memory deficits. In this case her parents were able to extend the strategies they learnt from staff at her rehabilitation centre and tailor them to her needs after she was discharged. This family demonstrated the potential benefit of families providing not only emotional support but also active involvement in the rehabilitation process. They had a relationship with their daughter that allowed them to work constructively (but not entirely uncritically) with her, and they had the understanding and imagination to develop successful strategies that allowed desirable goals to be achieved. They were also able to provide a judicious mix of support, encouragement, and risk-taking (cf this volume, Chapter 17).

Involving the family in the rehabilitation process is not without its risks. Care must be taken to ensure that this does not place family members in roles at odds with their fundamental role within the family. This may result in more harm than good. It is always a difficult clinical judgement to make in consultation with the family as sometimes the only solution is for a family member to take on the role of a carer as opposed to their previous family relationship, such as spouse or parent. For example, in cases of people with profound brain injuries the only viable role may be to relinquish the intimate role of spouse or partner and to take on the role of carer. In some cases, involving the family members in a behavioural programme may be appropriate, but in other cases it is not. McKinlay and Hickox (1988) involved relatives in the rehabilitation of memory impairment and poor anger control using a behavioural management programme in conjunction with assertiveness training that could be implemented at home with the family as cotherapist. The results were somewhat mixed, and McKinlay and Hickox identified a number of factors, including the emotional status of the relative involved, as relevant.

An important component of the rehabilitation of executive disorders, particularly if these are severe, is the provision of a prosthetic environment. Usually this involves the provision of structure as such patients are often unable to plan and structure their own daily lives. Structure, including repetition, makes life more predicable, gives a pattern into which we all tend to fall, and eliminates some decision-making. It helps memory, both episodic and prospective, by reducing the load and giving a framework on which activities and memories can be hung. Although such an approach is axiomatic in rehabilitation centres, it is not necessarily an approach that families will take. Helping families to see the value of imposing structure and predictability on their lives is an important aspect of supporting them to manage executive deficits.

Patients suffering from executive disorders often report that fatigue is a major problem. Once again this is often best tackled by the family as a whole. Understanding that this is not laziness and that it does not always resolve spontaneously is vital advice if the family is to cope with this symptom. This may involve helping the family and the individual to identify the triggers of their fatigue. For a variety of reasons (see this volume, Chapter 10) cardiovascular fitness is often severely depleted in those who have experienced a brain injury. If that is the case, helping the family to encourage the person with the brain injury to build up their fitness through exercise may be effective. If anxiety or depression is present, tackling these may be the best way to approach the problem of fatigue. If fatigue appears to be primarily associated with cognitive activity, helping the family to reduce the informational demands on the person with the brain injury may be effective. If fatigue is the result of lack of stimulation, helping the family to encourage stimulating, productive, and enjoyable activities may be the best approach. For others, it may be necessary to ration energy expenditure or spread activity across the day or week rather than in intensive bursts.

Long-term support

Executive disorders resulting from acquired brain injury do not normally, other than in their mildest form, recover completely over time. The type of assistance required by the family is long term. Perhaps the most appropriate form of help is long-term intermittent help. Families usually go through periods of relative calm, with occasional crises cropping up from time to time. Most families are not overly demanding and will use such a service appropriately. An example is a family where the mother had a serious brain injury from a riding accident resulting in executive deficits. At the time of injury her two children were aged 10 and 12. Over the following 20 years the mother sought direct help and advice with developing strategies to deal with her deficits, her husband attended a relatives group for a period, there were periods of couple therapy, and periods when the children were showing signs of distress. The family declined the opportunity for the children to join a group of peers with a parent with a brain injury, but later one daughter, by now in her late twenties, asked for a joint session with her mother to consider unresolved issues two decades after the original accident.

Setting up support groups for family members or encouraging them to set up their own, perhaps by providing facilities, can be an important contribution to their well-being. Usually some combination of education and emotional support is an appropriate goal for such groups. Understanding the subtleties of executive disorders can be difficult, and so the support of others dealing with the same issues can be beneficial. Topics for discussion may include how to deal with embarrassing behaviour, how to motivate those with executive disorders, and how to manage lability.

Conclusions

By their very nature, executive disorders are difficult to describe and hard to understand, yet they can make a huge difference to the way an individual behaves and their ability to function in all aspects of life. These changes are clear to those closest to the individual concerned and often perceived as changes in the very essence of the individual, but are often not apparent to others with less close contact. This places family members and close others in a lonely position as they frequently have a sense of loss and often find living with these changes extremely difficult, yet others are oblivious to their predicament. Attempts to describe these changes rarely convey to the listener a full picture of the situation. This means that professional support for families and the support of others living with the same problems is a vital part of the rehabilitation of executive disorders. Such professional support involves two types of help. The first is enabling the family to see the changes in the context of the brain injury, i.e. understanding the links between brain injury and personality or behaviour, but avoiding the danger of attributing all family difficulties to the brain injury. The second is helping the family to understand the need for strategies to overcome or limit the impact of the brain injury and enabling them to provide a 'prosthetic environment' within the home to allow the person with the brain injury to function at their optimal level.

References

Brooks, D.N. (1991). The head-injured family. *Journal of Clinical and Experimental Neuropsychology*, **13**, 155–188.

Channon,S., Rule, A., Maudgil, D., *et al*. (2007). Interpretation of mentalistic actions and sarcastic remarks: effects of frontal and posterior lesions on mentalising. *Neuropsychologia*, **45**, 1725–34.

Creer, C. and Wing, J.K. (1975). Living with a schizophrenic patient. *British Journal of Hospital Medicine*, **14**, 73–82.

Eslinger, P.J. and Damasio, A.R. (1985). Severe disturbance of higher cognition after bilateral frontal lobe ablation: patient EVR. *Neurology*, **35**, 1731–41.

Florian, V., Katz, S., and Lahav, V. (1991). Impact of traumatic brain damage on family dynamics and functioning: a review. *International Disability Studies*, **13**, 150–7.

Gervasio, A.H. and Kreutzer, J.S. (1997). Kinship and family members' psychological distress after traumatic brain injury: a large sample study. *Journal of Head Trauma Rehabilitation*, **12**, 14–26.

Gillen, R., Tennen, H., Affleck, G., and Steinpreis, R. (1998). Distress, depressive symptoms and depressive disorder among caregivers of patients with brain injury. *Journal of Head Trauma Rehabilitation*, **13**, 31–43.

Gosling, J. and Oddy, M. (1999). Rearranged marriages: marital relationships after head injury. *Brain Injury*, **13**, 785–96.

Hanks, R.A., Rapport, L.J., and Vangel, S. (2007). Caregiving appraisal after traumatic brain injury: The effects of functional status, coping style, social support and family functioning. *Neurorehabilitation*, **22**, 43–52.

Knight, R.G., Devereux, R., and Godfrey, H.P. (1998). Caring for a family member with a traumatic brain injury. *Brain Injury*, **12**, 467–81.

Kreutzer, J.S., Gervasio, A.H., and Camplair, P.S. (1994). Patient correlates of caregiver's distress and family functioning after traumatic brain injury. *Brain Injury*, **8**, 211–30.

Kuipers, L. and Bebbington, P. (1990). *Working in partnership*. Heinemann, Oxford.

Lezak, M.D. (1978). Living with the characterologically altered brain injured patient. *Journal of Clinical Psychiatry*, **39**, 592–8.

McKinlay, W.W. and Hickox, A. (1987). Family-based rehabilitation after traumatic brain injury. *Journal of Clinical and Experimental Neuropsychology*, **9**, 276.

Norman, D. and Shallice, T. (1986). Attention to action: willed and automatic control of behavior. In: *Consciousness and self-regulation*, Vol 4 (ed R. Davidson, G.E. Schwartz, and D. Shapiro). Plenum Press, New York.

Oddy, M. (2001). Sexual relationships following brain injury. *Sexual and Relationship Therapy*, **16**, 247–59.

Oddy, M. and Cogan, J. (2004). Coping with severe memory impairment. *Neuropsychological Rehabilitation*, **14**, 481–94.

Oddy, M. and Herbert, C. (2003). Intervention with families following brain injury: evidence-based practice. *Neuropsychological Rehabilitation*, **13**, 259–73.

Oddy, M., Coughlan, A., Tyerman, A., and Jenkins, D. (1985). Social adjustment after closed head injury: a further follow-up seven years after injury. *Journal of Neurology, Neurosurgery, and Psychiatry*, **48**, 564–8.

Perlesz, A., Kinsella, G., and Crowe, S. (1999). Impact of traumatic brain injury on the family: a critical review. *Rehabilitation Psychology*, **44**, 6–35.

Rosenbaum, M. and Najenson, T. (1976). Changes in life patterns and symptoms of low mood as reported by wives of severely brain-injured soldiers. *Journal of Consulting and Clinical Psychology*, **44**, 881–8.

Stilwell, J., Hawley, C., and Stilwell, P. (1997). *National Traumatic Brain Injury Study*, p. 53. University of Warwick.

Webster, G. and Daisley, A. (2005). A family resource pack for working with children affected by familial acquired brain injury. *Clinical Psychology*, **46**, 26–9.

Winstanley, J., Simpson, G., Tate, R., and Myles, B. (2006). Early indicators and contributors to psychological distress in relatives during rehabilitation following severe traumatic brain injury: findings from the brain injury outcomes study. *Journal of Head Trauma Rehabilitation*, **21**, 453–66.

Wood, R.L. and Yurdakul, L.K. (1997). Change in relationship status following traumatic brain injury. *Brain Injury*, **11**, 491–502.

Zarit, S.H., Anthony, C.R., and Boutselis, M. (1987). Intervention with caregivers of dementia patients: comparison of two approaches. *Psychology and Aging*, **2**, 225–32.

19

Training support staff to work with people with executive disorders

John D. McCrea and Rashmi Sharma

Brain Injury Rehabilitation Trust, Milton Keynes

Introduction

A number of issues that the authors have encountered over almost two decades of training support staff to work with with clients with moderate to severe executive disorders are explored in this chapter. As each issue is discussed we will provide guidelines for intervention which, in our experience, has been effective. This chapter is intended as a guide to the pitfalls in training staff as experienced by the authors. Both authors work for the Brain Injury Rehabilitation Trust in the UK. The service is interdisciplinary in nature and is psychologically led, placing emphasis on reducing the impact of executive deficits following brain injury using a neurobehavioural approach (Wood and Worthington 2001). Details of the service are also available as downloadable leaflets at www.birt.co.uk.

Training staff to work with clients with executive disorders draws on education, training, neuropsychology, and management. As yet there is a relative scarcity of research specifically on this particular topic in any of the above areas of academic endeavour, and it is hoped that this chapter will stimulate discussion of how to bridge the divides between these fields.

Clients presenting with executive deficits are often able to present as articulate and intelligent. To the untrained observer, their failure to perform in everyday functional or interpersonal situations is open to misinterpretation, or indeed inappropriate labelling. Therefore we will explore a number of issues that have arisen when helping staff to interpret and respond appropriately to the behaviours encountered when dealing with such clients. As each issue is discussed we will provide guidelines for intervention which, in our experience, have been effective.

Therefore the aims of this chapter are:

- to explore and elaborate upon training issues specific to dealing with clients with executive disorders
- to provide practical pointers, with examples as appropriate, for clinicians and health/social care managers with responsibility for staff training.

We will also include a suggested training curriculum (Appendix).

The focus of this chapter is upon training inexperienced staff who do not possess relevant qualifications, although the training package used in the Trust is not provided exclusively to this group. The following assumptions are made:

- the service offered is only as good as the weakest staff member
- the client's most frequent day-to-day contact is with this staff group
- the service offered is residential (readers working in other settings should find the guidelines relatively easy to adapt as appropriate).

In the authors' experience, training is most effective if it is outcome driven. It should be possible to answer the question: 'What change has been effected by this process?' By common convention, training outcomes are often categorized into three headings.

- Knowledge—What information do we wish our staff to have?
- Skills—What tasks should staff be able to perform?
- Attitude—What perspective should staff take when interpreting client behaviour?

For more information on this conventional framework the reader is directed to any of the extensive range of web-based information on National Vocational Qualifications and Learning Disabilities Qualifications in the UK.

Setting knowledge- and skills-based objectives may seem reasonable and intuitively obvious. Setting attitudinal objectives may require justification. The approach used by the Trust, as will be described below, is essentially relational in nature. Relational neurobehaviourism places emphasis on the relationship between staff and client. Giles and Manchester (2006) observe that this relationship can be undermined by the 'fundamental attribution error' (a tendency to attribute another's unpleasant behaviour to an internal trait, i.e. to view it as under the person's control (Ross 1977)). They also observe that the fundamental attribution error is widespread in treatment settings where difficult behaviour is encountered. Therefore in order to cultivate positive working relationships between staff and clients, it is reasonable to promote appropriate staff attitudes and attribution style.

The issues

Training should provide demonstrable improvements in all three categories of learner outcome

This provides a considerable challenge to any training plan. The key words are 'demonstrable' and 'improvement'. Creating a training system that is data driven, even if the data are qualitative or anecdotal in nature, is vital in order to demonstrate its effect on the learner and the learner's performance. It also allows one to test whether the training has produced improvement. If there has been no improvement as a result of training, then the more robust the outcome data, the more likely we are to be able to decide whether the lack of improvement is a learner issue or a problem with the training system itself (training problems are more likely to be reflected in poor performance across numerous learners).

Demonstrating acquisition of knowledge is a reasonably simple affair. The simplest method is a multiple choice questionnaire (MCQ) designed around the key points of the training that has been delivered. The authors use a simple MCQ that was trialled on just over 100 staff. This distribution group is used as a benchmark, and staff tested later who fall below an agreed percentile are identified for further support. The distribution is shown in Figure 19.1.

Questionnaires also have the benefit of being quantifiable, thus avoiding the subjectivity of essay marking. For a full discussion of the issues in MCQ design and scoring, the reader is referred to the Item Writing Guide, which can be downloaded from the National Board of Medical Examiners (www.nbme.org). On occasion we have tested staff knowledge with written essays. The information gleaned in this way is by its nature more qualitative, but written essay

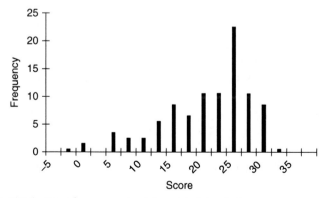

Fig. 19.1 Distribution of scores on level 1 post-training test.

assessment has the benefit of having the learner revisit the information presented in training and reliving the learning experience

Demonstrating improvement in skills is more complex. It assumes that the learner's skills have been assessed prior to training. This is impossible for new staff, as it would imply having them interact with clients and dealing with situations with no prior training. Therefore a more realistic objective for inexperienced staff would be to demonstrate the existence of skills post-training with no assumption of prior skill. Improvements in skill become a more realistic goal later in a staff member's training programme,.

Skills can be demonstrated most readily by observation against a checklist of tasks in the same way that one might prompt a client though the stages of a self-care routine. This approach is essentially the same as that used in various competence-based awards, such as the National Vocational Qualification offered in many sectors of employment in the UK. Once a task is complete, questions can be asked about why it was carried out as it was, how could it have done differently, where the learning points were, etc. Questions such as 'Why is this done this way?', 'What benefit might this approach have for the client?', or 'How does this approach promote independence?' will provide qualitative information about the learner's ability to link knowledge with skill and encourage reflective practice. Exploration of the reasoning and methodology behind the types of intervention being taught may also serve to encourage generalization of skills across a range of related situations. Exploring one's own performance of rehabilitation activities has been demonstrated to promote competency and generalization of skills across similar tasks (Arco 2002).

Demonstrating improvement in attitude is clearly the most nebulous of objectives. However, it is a valid target for training, as untrained staff can often misattribute observed behaviours in an unhelpful way. This effect is explored further below. Attitude is almost always a subjective measure based on a clinician's or manager's opinion of an individual staff member, although rating scales can obviously be applied to the information. In order to gauge change in attitude a useful strategy is to provide the new learner with a number of scenarios involving events or incidents that result from a client's executive deficits. The staff member is required to offer an explanation of the event. The responses can be rated on a number of variables such as the degree to which the staff member attributes the event to external events, client personality traits, or executive deficits. Such data can be compared with the same staff member's response style following training and with interpretation of real events observed in the workplace at any later date. The same technique (either in questionnaire or interview format) can be used on an ongoing basis during staff supervision to monitor staff attitude.

Staff expectations of training

The expectations that new staff have of the training they will receive are very variable. For example all staff, from the senior occupational therapist to the chef, were canvassed for their views on topics they would like to have included in the training programme. While some responses were quite job-specific, such as the chef asking if brain-injured people might require a special diet, *all* staff stated that they wished to learn about the brain. This was expressed in a number of ways ('the brain', 'how the brain works', 'what parts do what', etc.). It is patently obvious that knowing the location of the parietal lobe has little bearing on how one might respond to challenging behaviour (although there was a clear sense that those staff who attended the neuroanatomy course appeared, perhaps unexpectedly, to approach the newly arrived clients more confidently than those staff who had not). Clarifying expectations prior to training has proved useful, if for no other reason than that it encourages staff to seek out information actively rather than sit passively throughout. To this end a training plan with very general learner outcomes is a useful inclusion in the initial correspondence upon recruitment.

Cultivating neurobehavioural thinking

The Brain Injury Rehabilitation Trust employs a neurobehavioural approach. This is based on the premise that rehabilitation is essentially a learning process. The neurobehavioural approach incorporates constructs, theories, and procedures from cognitive, behavioural, and social psychology to promote the acquisition and spontaneous use of functional and social skills (Wood and Worthington 2001). It has been demonstrated to be particularly relevant to those whose executive deficits reduce their self-care abilities and impair their social judgement. Essentially, the approach seeks to change problematic behaviour and cultivate functional behaviours without relying on the client's ability to exercise executive control. Evidence for the efficacy of this approach with clients with executive disorders has been provided by Wood *et al.* (1999) and Worthington *et al.* (2006). Neurobehavioural thinking, or approaching situations in a neurobehavioural style, is not usually natural to newly recruited staff. Behaviourism in general is not an obvious approach. This is clearly evident from the plethora of television programmes teaching parents how to change unruly behaviour in their children, in which much time is invested in training behavioural principles. New staff are often tempted to manage situations, or 'make the problem go away', in a manner that has an immediate positive effect but longer-term negative consequences. Even when staff have knowledge and understanding, application can still fail. For example, a client at one of our units attracts staff attention by sitting outside his room opening and slamming his door, or by approaching staff more reasonably and requesting assistance. Staff are naturally instructed to respond to the latter approach only. However, one of the authors observed a trained staff member approach the client when engaged in the former behaviour and say: 'You won't get my attention by doing that. What do you want?'

The issue of linking knowledge to skill will be dealt with below.

Cultivation of of a neurobehavioural style of thinking is seen as a vital part of staff training as the model is used by the Trust not only to address specific behavioural disabilities, but also to provide a behavioural backdrop to promote the use of the various exercises and strategies developed and implemented by other clinical interventions, such as functional strategies designed by an occupational therapist. Staff training in methods of behavioural change clearly needs to address the interpersonal relationship between clients and staff, much of which is mediated by language. 'Relational behaviourism' emphasizes the relationship between staff and clients as a treatment variable. It also involves a wider range of psychological techniques such as motivational interviewing and redirection. It places less emphasis on extinction and other so-called 'time-out' procedures. A detailed description of the use of relational neurobehaviourism in a residential setting, and a comparison of operant and relational behaviourism, is given by Giles and Manchester (2006)

In terms of cultivating neurobehavioural thinking, the most effective method we have found is to introduce it in clearly defined stages as follows.

- Theory—the basic principles of reinforcement and extinction.

- Worked examples—scenarios describing appropriate staff intervention during episodes of inappropriate behaviour. These examples are explored in detail and frequent references are made to the theory already presented.

- Exercises 1—scenarios that staff are required to explore as a group. They are first required to use the theory to explain how the client in each scenario may have learnt a particular inappropriate behaviour, and then they are required to use the theory to plan an appropriate intervention. The exercises are graded in complexity. Upon completion of each exercise the trainer facilitates discussion and redirects any errors made.

- Exercises (2)—returning to less complex scenarios, the group is divided into two groups which proceed as above. Upon completion of each post-exercise discussion, the two groups are again divided. This procedure is repeated until the remaining exercises are done individually with one-to-one support and feedback.

There are two principles in operation, repetition and subdivision. Repetition leads to practice in a new style of problem-solving (rather like those worked examples we all had to endure in Maths class). Subdivision means that initially in the early exercises each member of staff can rely on the others for support, but gradually, as the group is subdivided, the trainer can identify particular individuals who need additional guidance.

In order to cultivate a neurobehavioural approach, training offered to Trust staff is substantial and repetitive. Having completed the statutory induction into social care, staff initially complete a two-day course covering the theory and methods used in the trust. Feedback from staff following training indicates that there is an optimum time for introducing theory, which is about 3 months after commencement of employment—too early and staff experience difficulty relating to the concepts; too late and we risk the development of less helpful habits and attitudes. Approximately 6 months later staff are sent on a four-day course building on the earlier theoretical work, and applying this in the design of behavioural interventions and data collection and analysis. The range of behavioural and functional skills addressed in these exercises is highly varied to help cultivate generalization of the approaches used. This second block of training is repeated on a biannual basis to help maintain gains. The training system is represented graphically in Figure 19.2.

Introducing behavioural concepts gradually

As mentioned above, the exercises used are graded in complexity. Similarly, the concepts being taught are gradually introduced. This is achieved during the post-exercise discussion when the trainer can demonstrate concepts gradually. The format we currently use is as follows:

(a) concentrating on functional behaviour and making positive reinforcement contingent upon it;

(b) creating systems whereby the above can be made practicable in a real-life residential setting;

(c) introducing the concept of extinction into the exercises;

(d) raising awareness of the risks of positive reinforcement occurring during extinction;

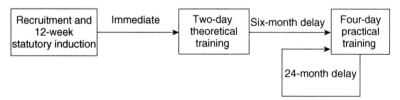

Fig. 19.2 Flowchart of main training blocks offered to Trust staff.

(e) moving away from extinction-based intervention towards a more relational approach (Giles and Manchester 2006), emphasizing redirection
and motivational techniques and relying less on extinction.

At this point, there is a reasonable probability that new staff are conversant
with a relational neurobehavioural approach and are able to think in such
terms but,as stated above, this may not necessarily translate into day-to-day
behaviour. To achieve this it is useful to create, as far as possible, a self-sustaining
behavioural culture.

Creating a behavioural culture

Training, if it is to be effective, cannot end when the projector is switched off.
To this end it is vital, as far as possible, to create a behavioural culture on the
unit. Much of the information given to staff is counter-intuitive, for example
there is a tendency for inadequately trained staff to misattribute behaviours to
factors like personality disorder, laziness, and mental illness (see discussion of
fundamental attribution errors above) Cultivating a neurobehavioural culture
is attempted, usually successfully, by training the staff behaviourally.
Essentially we not only encourage and promote a neurobehavioural style, but
we also seek to 'catch the staff out' talking in behavioural terms or acting in a
behavioural way and provide positive reinforcement in as public a way as
possible. The effect is twofold: it modifies staff behaviour and role-models
behavioural intervention to any other staff present. Obviously knowing what
acts as a reinforcer is paramount, but a safe assumption is that virtually every
employee enjoys a public 'thumbs-up' from senior staff. Secondly, during shift
handover, when recounting events from previous shifts, any behavioural
thinking that was applied to any given situation is emphasized, explored, and
as far as possible publicly recognized by clinicians and management staff. This
component of the training system is similar to that reported by Guercio *et al.*
(2002), who used public displays (noticeboard postings) of staff members'
contributions to client rehabilitation activity essentially as form of reinforcement
of staff behaviour.

Summary

Training staff to work effectively is complicated by the counter-intuitive nature
of the dysexecutive syndrome and the misattributions this can elicit from the
untrained observer. The training programme described here seeks, through
direct teaching, worked examples, and the application of behavioural techniques to the staff's own performance, to enlighten staff and encourage a more
rational interpretation of incidents and events caused by executive deficits.

The training programme aims to cultivate neurobehavioural thinking, a neuro-behavioural workplace culture, and a relational rather than purely operant style of day-to-day interaction. A vital component of the programme is the repetition of several components throughout the period of employment in order to maintain a particular style of thinking and prevent lapses of attribution and/or attitude. This is also assisted by including regular monitoring of thinking style and attitude as part of ongoing staff supervision. Staff management and supervision also includes behavioural components as a means of direct behavioural change of staff performance and as a means of role-modelling a behavioural approach.

References

Arco, L. (2002). Using self-generated feedback for generalising and maintaining staff performance in a rehabilitation program. *Behaviour Change*, **19**, 75–89.

Giles, G. and Manchester, D. (2006). Two approaches to behaviour disorder after traumatic brain injury. *Journal of Head Trauma Rehabilitation*, **21**, 168–78.

Guercio, J., Davis, P., Faw, G., *et al* (2002) Increasing functional rehabilitation in acquired brain injury treatment: effective applications of behavioural principles. *Brain Injury*, **16**, 849–60.

Ross, L. (1977). The intuitive psychologist and his shortcomings: distortions in the attribution process. In: *Advances in experimental social psychology*, Vol. 10 (ed L. Berkowitz). Academic Press, New York.

Wood, R.L., McCrea, J.D., Wood, L.M., and Merriman, R.N. (1999). Clinical and cost effectiveness of post-acute neurobehavioural rehabilitation. *Brain Injury*, **13**, 69–88.

Wood, R.L. and Worthington, A. (2001). Neurobehavioural rehabilitation: a conceptual paradigm. In: *Neurobehavioural disability and social handicap following traumatic brain injury* (ed R.L. Wood and T.M. McMillan), pp. 107–31. Psychology Press, Hove.

Worthington, A.D., Matthews, S., Melia, Y., and Oddy, M. (2006). Cost-benefits associated with social outcome from neurobehavioural rehabilitation. *Brain Injury*, **29**, 947–57.

Appendix. Sample training curriculum

Level 1

Day 1

1. Introduction to the neurobehavioural model

   History

   Structure

   Current perspectives

2. Introduction to neuroanatomy

3. Basic neurological disabilities

4. Executive disorders

   Causes

   Effects

5. Limitations on learning imposed by executive disorders

   Translating information into action

6. Using the neurobehavioural method to effect learning in the context of the executive disorders

7. The concept of behavioural disability

8. Basic behavioural analysis with detailed examples and exercises

   Behavioural ecology

   ABC analyses

   Communication value of behaviours

Day 2

1. Review of structure of neurobehavioural model

2. Examples and exercises using the neurobehavioural model to plan interventions for scenarios used for behavioural analysis on day one

3. Ethical and clinical issues in using antecedent control

4. The role of prompting/cuing in supporting behavioural learning

5. The role of motivational techniques in supporting behavioural learning

6. Using motivational techniques in day-to-day interactions with clients

7. Supporting colleagues following incidents

8. Multiple choice questionnaire

Level 2

Part 1 (days 1 and 2)

1. Revision of all material covered in basic training, including a repeat of several of the dysexecutive syndrome and intervention exercises
2. Human implications of brain injury—contentment and sense of identity
3. Types of behavioural intervention with examples

   Differential reinforcement of

   > Other behaviour

   > Incompatible behaviour

   > Low rate of response

   > Communicative behaviour

   Shaping

   Chaining

Part 2 (days 3 and 4)

1. Creating specific neurobehavioural programmes (one for each of item 3 above)

   Principles

   Group exercises with trainer and peer feedback
2. Data collection and basic analysis
3. Using and analysing graphs
4. Assessment planning exercise
5. Further exercises on programme creation
6. Motivational techniques

Optional additional modules

> Family issues and conflicts

> Taught module

> Role-play exercise

> Detailed applied behaviour analysis exercise

> History and evolution of the neurobehavioural model and the Brain Injury Rehabilitation Trust

> Using positive reinforcement effectively

> Issues of premorbid personality, treatment effects and clinical presentation

Part 4

Last word

Michael Oddy and Andrew Worthington

We have given the last word to Chloe Cook, a young woman who herself suffered a traumatic brain injury at the age of 18. In an eloquent and lively account Chloe describes the difficulties she has faced over the first few years following her injury and the inner resources she has had to draw upon. She offers sage advice to others in this position and enables this volume to finish on a positive note.

20

A personal account

Chloe Cook

I want to share with you my unexpected drama. First, I just want to give you a picture of my old self and life style.

I was a bit of a go-getter; I had a very active and what I thought was an expansive life. There I was 18 years old, just about to take the leap in to my adult life. I had been studying art at college and about to finish after a 3 year course which I largely enjoyed. In my spare time I held down two jobs, one cooking and another at a cocktail bar. In between work and play I had a very healthy social life, as most 18-year-olds do. I seemed to be always on the go—one of these people with a lot of energy who could run on little sleep. I had good multi-tasking skills and a good drive in life.

I taught myself neurolinguistic programming, which enabled me to get a clear picture of how to step into the next phase of my life. I was a month away from completing my art course, having my driving test. I had changed my diet, started a new exercise plan, and was detaching from my youthful social life. I was about to step in to three part-time jobs, working unsocial hours, working hard for 8 months in order to enable me to go travelling the world on my own for a year and a half. I would then return and go to university for four years to train to be an art therapist.

Those were my goals—to get out and play before I became a student again, to get a dose of culture.

But that old life seems like a fuzzy dream now. It is amazing how so suddenly it was like having the rug pulled from underneath my feet. Then out of the blue I managed to acquire a brain injury. I had a fall down some stairs which resulted in landing on my head.

The aftermath of that three-second fall changed my whole life. I had never broken a bone in my body, and then I fractured my skull on impact and stretched my brain stem. I had a burst blood vessel, which was putting pressure on my brain, resulting in a swelling of on the right side and me slipping in to a coma. I had to undergo open brain surgery. After the brain surgery I had seizures where I died. Luckily the medical team stabilized me, but I was in a coma with a Glasgow Coma Score of 3, with no brain activity. The doctors' diagnosis was bleak—if I did wake up, I would be a vegetable, physically and cognitively damaged.

A brain injury can have such a massive impact on your life as well as on those close to you.

I awoke a week later very confused and with a new reality to deal with. After you acquire a brain injury your memory and concentration tends to be affected. I couldn't see properly and my voice was affected. I was in a lot of pain and I couldn't feel half my body as I was paralysed down the left side, and the future looked very uncertain. I was told that I might not ever walk or use my left hand again, or see properly. Luckily enough I had the positive influence of my family to help me through and we held on to hope and created a lot of love. My family helped generate a loving gentle energy in which it was possible for me to stay calm and heal into my new reality.

The cocktail of emotions I had to go through to try to understand and deal with brain injury put life in perspective for me. This situation forced me to the present moment, the only moment that ever really existed.

I found that my brain injury sent me back to growing up emotionally. I was different and unpredictable. There were differences in the way that I processed information and my memory, and the layers of awareness in reading people had gone. My personality changed and I had a more basic understanding of things. I had constant fatigue and low tolerance to sensory stimulation so that I had become over-sensitive. On the physical side, I suffered lack of sensation and communication between brain and body, I had physical pain and nerve damage, and my sleep had been affected. My energy levels were low and so was my stamina.

So many pathways of my brain had been cut, affecting the whole wiring and activity of my mind. I had forgotten all my previous training and had to relearn how to read, write, and do everything but talk.

Every stage of the recovery has been a steep learning curve. Brain injury is so complex—every injury is unique to the individual and how their body responds. It was uncharted territory where you don't know what you don't know or where you are going. I had no map to guide me. It's hard enough for the professionals who work and advise, so what hope does the damaged individual have of self-healing? This journey has enabled me to tap into self-healing because the only truth is that healing comes from within you. Nothing outside you can heal you—it can only be a guide, a catalyst for change.

The reality of this hit me early on in my recovery—that it was down to me to do everything and that this determined the quality of the rest of my life. I would either be stuck watching the world go by, or I'd get up and try to see what I could do to move myself forward. No matter what the extent of the damage is,

I believe that it can always improve. There is always hope as long as the injured individual is alive. Progress at whatever level can be achieved.

My first task was working on my physical body. Years later I started to realize that I walked around in a confused brain fog, drifting along in a fuzzy life where nothing ever seemed fresh and clear in my mind—just confusion. I finally got the reality check that I had cognitive brain damage too. I was no longer the person that I was born. That person was dead. I have a personality transplant, like being possessed, because of my frontal lobe damage. For years I would have outbursts, but no memory or awareness of them afterwards. I had cognitive difficulties, which I have to deal with for the rest of my life.

I had social problems where I lost a lot of friends because I had lost the filter in my thoughts and so I would just say what I was thinking. Brain injury can have the effect of making you socially inappropriate because of over-stimulation. I had lost all my life skills. I would forget to eat and I had forgotten how to cook. When I tried, I would do things in the wrong order or miss stages out.

It had affected my family life so much that my parents ended up separating. Brain injury affects a whole family unit and it's a hidden disability. The damaged individual is like a vulnerable adult. Things can trigger a chemical reaction in the brain, which results in antisocial behaviour problems, never consciously done but it still destroys lives. Both parties are victims of cognitive damage.

Every stage of progress in this situation opens a doorway of new awareness and then trying to understand, remember, take control, and change. There is a big difference between understanding something and being able to deal with it.

I have seen in myself and others how brain injury can present you with a brick wall of the person's deficits and a total lack of awareness. It's almost as if brain damage can close your ears and eyes to what is right in front of you. This is because your brain is overworking to do the bare minimum.

Depression is very common, with constant dips in emotions. Throughout my recovery and coming to terms with my reality every day I would have massive emotional dips where one minute I was laughing and the next minute I was crying.

I have been positive throughout and tried to shine light on everything. I meditate every day to regulate the function of my mind, and exercise, releasing toxins. But still my highs would never last and my lows always creep up on me unexpectedly. The grieving period of acceptance can be a long and painful process for the individual, but also for the family.

You grieve the death of yourself, your life, and your reality. The heaviness, the deadness, and the lack of inspiration locks you in, as if your world is being pulled down a plug-hole. Your life feels as if it will never be easy or good again. You can't see the point of your life anymore. You have lost your identity, your friends, your family, your relationship with yourself, and your own power and independence.

Never being classed or treated as normal in society again. Not being able to provide for yourself, and becoming dependent and having to have assistance in everything. It creates a lot of confused frustration.

So mainly brain-injured people might not seem like there is much going on, but really their brain has become alien to them and they are battling to process an unprogrammed wiring of their mind. This results in a lack of response, confusion, and lack of understanding.

I found adjusting to my new situation hard. I was in shock for about a year. Everything had become a real effort of confusion with no certainties.

My lifestyle now is very different. I have spent the last three and a half years having to reprogramme my body to work and then cognitively control and improve my chaotic mind.

I find organization and general everyday things a challenge. I have now got more balance in my life and I have to work around my energy levels. My body tells me what to do. What helped me calm down and create space in my fuzzy mind, to realize and understand, build concentration and relax my body, to give me focus and a human feeling again was meditation—charging myself up with energy every day, stilling my mind so that when it does come in to action I am centred but fully alert and ready for action and learning.

I have learnt that with acceptance and staying in the present moment you can start breaking things down and take control, monitor yourself. I have to make sure what food and drinks I put in my body as everything affects my chemical reactions.

The poor concentration and memory problems have been a challenge. But anything is possible and I am learning how to deal with things bit by bit, and I remain optimistic that anything is possible. We all have endless resources within. I have just been put in a situation where I have had no choice but to tap in to these inner resources and strive for the healing of my being.

There is always hope—either you let life crush you and make it worse, or, I say, if it doesn't kill you it will make you stronger. This becomes possible when you stop resisting and learn the lesson of your drama.

Whatever damage there is can be improved, eventually, over time. You have got to live with the traits for life. You will never be the same person again but there are always ways of learning and building on what you still have—positivity, perseverance, practicality, faith, belief in change. Gratitude for what you already have in your life, even the simplest thing, like I am grateful to have the eyes to see this. You change your energy, make it feel lighter. This changes your feelings and gives you the chance to move forward.

Index

Lightning Source UK Ltd.
Milton Keynes UK
10 December 2010

164178UK00002B/2/P

80198 568056